Hairdresser to the Stars

A Hollywood Memoir
by
Ginger Sugar Blymyer

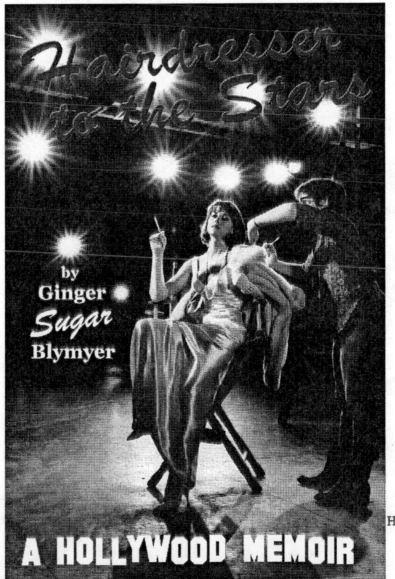

Copyright © 2000 by Ginger Sugar Blymyer

Cover Photos by Bill Ray
Cover Design by FirstWord Agency

ISBN 0-7414-0889-6

Library of Congress Number: 99-69436

Published by:

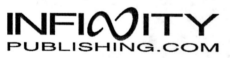

PUBLISHING.COM

519 West Lancaster Avenue
Haverford, PA 19041-1413
Info@buybooksontheweb.com
www.buybooksontheweb.com
Toll-free   (877) BUY BOOK
Local Phone   (610) 520-2500
Fax   (610) 519-0261

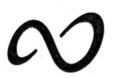

Printed in the United States of America

Printed on Recycled Paper

Hairdresser to the Stars

Table of Contents

About the Author -- 4

Introduction --- 6

Meeting Natalie Wood-- 7

Influenced By Hollywood-- 10

First Day on the Job--- 13

Makeup Department--- 17

A Career in Film-- 21

Hurrah! I'm a Hairdresser! -- 25

On My Own--- 27

How the West Was Won--- 30

The Birds --- 32

McLintock!-- 35

Wives and Lovers--- 38

Love with a Proper Stranger --- 40

Sex and the Single Girl--- 44

The Ugly Dachshund-- 49

The Great Race Continues -- 52

Inside Daisy Clover--- 61

Lord Love a Duck -- 68

This Property is Condemned -- 70

Penelope-- 79

Barefoot in the Park-- 84

Blue--- 88

The Boston Strangler-- 92

Gaily, Gaily -- 99

Bob & Carol & Ted & Alice-- 104

Dream of Kings -- 108

Grasshopper --- 111

Baby Maker--- 113

The Real Ma and Pa Kettle --- 116

Hex --- 121

Back to Hollywood-- 124

Day of the Dolphin--- 127

The Affair and Mrs. Sundance --------------------------------------- 131

The Day of the Locust--- 135

Peeper --- 138

Mandingo -- 143

Lizzie Borden -- 150

Visions-- 152

When Things Were Rotten ---- 154
Helter Skelter ---- 157
Marathon Man ---- 160
Black Sunday ---- 163
Sorcerer ---- 167
The Deep ---- 171
Santa Domingo and Bimini ---- 175
Turning Point ---- 178
The Other Side of Midnight ---- 181
Who'll Stop the Rain ---- 192
High Anxiety ---- 195
A Change of Lifestyle ---- 198
Awakening Land ---- 202
Quitting the Business ---- 211
Little Darlings ---- 215
My Last Film With Natalie ---- 218
Natalie's Death ---- 221
Meeting William Hurt ---- 225
First Meeting with Tom Cruise ---- 227
Hurrah, I'm a Grandma! ---- 230
Songwriter ---- 233
Movie Business to the Rescue ---- 237
Running Scared ---- 240
My Own Passage to India ---- 246
End of My Dream ---- 252
The Presidio ---- 257
Turner & Hooch ---- 263
Havana ---- 268
Revelations ---- 272
Rocky V ---- 274
The Jumping Off Place ---- 278
The Doctor ---- 280
Far and Away ---- 284
Stay Tuned ---- 294
Trial By Jury ---- 302
Afterward ---- 306
Expect the Unexpected ---- 310
An Ordinary Woman's Life Gone Right ---- 313
Photo Credits ---- 316
Index ---- 317

To my Beloved Spiritual Master, Adi Da Samraj, the Giver
Who in His brightness
Has broken my heart wide open so I can feel all love
Who made me understand that I cannot become happy
Because I already am happy
That is my true state
I love You with all my heart

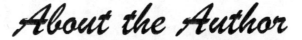

About the Author

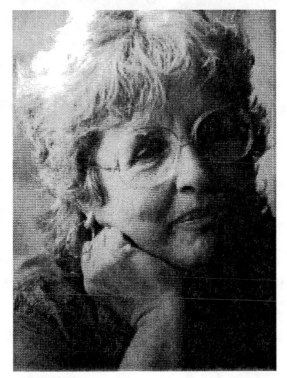

Ginger "Sugar" Blymyer began her career in Hollywood in 1954 at MGM Studios. She continued to work in Hollywood until the nineties when she retired in New Hampshire where she currently resides. Ginger has worked under many screen names, including Sugar Blymyer, Sugar Bates, and Sugar Maryce Bates.

Ginger's long career in Hollywood has afforded her many experiences with some of the most famous people in the world. Ginger's film credits include the following:

Trial by Jury	William Hurt
Stay Tuned	John Ritter, Pam Dawber
Far & Away	Tom Cruise, Nicole Kidman
The Doctor	William Hurt, Christine Lahti
Rocky V	Sylvester Stallone
Turner & Hooch	Tom Hanks
The Presidio	Sean Connery, Meg Ryan, Mark Harmon
Running Scared	Billy Crystal, Gregory Hines
Songwriter	Willie Nelson, Leslie Ann Warren, Kris Kristoferson
All the Right Moves	Tom Cruise, Lea Thompson
Little Darlings	Tatum O'Neal, Kristy McNichol
Meteor	Sean Conner, Natalie Wood, Karl Malden, Martin Landau
Who'll Stop the Rain	Tuesday Weld, Nick Nolte, Michael Moriarity
High Anxiety	Mel Brooks, Madeleine Kahn, Cloris Leachman, Harvey Korman
The Other Side of Midnight	Susan Sarandon, John Beck, Marie France Pisier
The Deep	Nick Nolte, Jacqueline Bisset
Black Sunday	Marthe Keller, Robert Shaw, Bruce Dern

Marathon Man	Laurence Olivier, Dustin Hoffman, Marthe Keller
Mandingo	Ken Norton, Susan George, Perry King
Barefoot in the Park	Jane Fonda, Robert Redford
The President's Analyst	James Colburn
Day of the Locusts	Karen Black
Lord Love a Duck	Tuesday Weld, Ruth Gordon, Roddy McDowall
Soldier in the Rain	Tuesday Weld, Steve McQueen, Jackie Gleason
The Boston Strangler	Tony Curtis
Gaily, Gaily	Melina Mercouri
Beneath the Planet of the Apes	James Franciscus, Kim Hunter
How the West Was Won	Carrol Baker, Lee J. Cobb, Henry Fonda
Mutiny on the Bounty	Marlon Brando
All Fall Down	Eva Marie Saint, Warren Beatty

Films with Natalie Wood
Love with a Proper Stranger
Sex and the Single Girl
The Great Race
Inside Daisy Clover
This Property is Condemned
Penelope
Bob & Carol & Ted & Alice
Peeper
Meteor
The Memory of Eva Ryker

Films with Elizabeth Montgomery
Mrs. Sundance
Case of Rape
Lizzie Borden
Awakening Land

Television Films
Helter Skelter
When Things Were Rotten
No Secrets
For Lovers Only

INTRODUCTION

After forty years in the movie business, I still love movies. They have taken me places I could never have gone on my own. What comes to mind at the moment are the waterfalls in *Greystroke*, the South America of *The Mission*, the Africa of *Out of Africa*, the civil war of *Gone with the Wind* the Merchant Ivory films filled with exquisite beauty, the first *Star Wars* that took me beyond the earth. I loved working on films. It was wonderful to be acquainted with the actors, actresses and the crews. My life has been full of fun and wonder, excitement and adventure - like a film in many ways. This is a memoir of my forty years in the movie business. I share my experience of what it was like to live and work in the company of fabulous entrepreneurs and studio builders. There was glamour and charm. The filmmakers were visionaries. My experience far exceeded my imagination. I was fortunate to have been there. I came in at the end of the golden age and reaped the benefits of a time that no longer exists.

In the words of Willie Nelson, "Making movies sure beats working for a living." That about sums it up.

Movies have great influence on our lives. The stars are the only royalty we have in this country. Films inspire, teach, educate and entertain us. They also help us to escape. A living art form, they are important to our lives. Art nourishes us. I am proud to have been a part of this business.

My story gives a glimpse into the wonder, talent and excitement that was present at the time I began making movies. My story begins before the television changed the industry. At that time, the industry was creative beyond belief. You only have to look at those wonderful old videos for that. After television arrived, it was never the same. In the beginning, television was also very creative. What happened? There was live television, *Playhouse 90, Naked City.* That kind of television fare no longer exists. The sponsors are necessary, but their taste is not always worthy.

I share with you a history, a view of show business at its most exciting times, just before everything changed and the times after that. It is an insider's view of Hollywood, my personal adventures behind the scenes and what it was like to be a crewmember. The opportunities I had, afforded me a fascinating life many people only dream about. It is the warm, intimate picture of people I worked with, places I traveled.

It is also my story. I began my show business career at MGM (Metro-Goldwyn-Mayer) in 1954 as a messenger. I grew up, raised a family and had fantastic adventures during my career in the movie business. Sharing that experience is a pleasure and I give you a picture of what it was like to be a hairstylist to the stars. Exciting and addictive, life behind the scenes was not always simple or easy. It is my wish that my memoirs will inspire women and men to take a chance and follow their dreams. Life works out best that way.

Chapter 1
MEETING NATALIE WOOD
Paramount Studios, Hollywood 1964

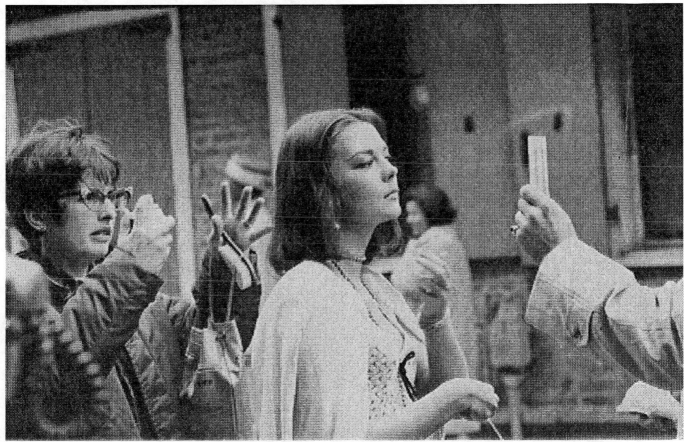

Ginger "Sugar" Blymyer and Natalie Wood, *This Property is Condemned*

"Natalie Wood's looking for a hairstylist and I suggest you to try out for the job," Nellie Manley, head hairstylist at Paramount, said excitedly as I walked into her office. My heart began to pound. My mind began to race. I was a young hairstylist with few films under my belt. I had never worked with anyone of Natalie's caliber.

All my doubts began to surface. I'd grown up watching her films and loved her ever since *Miracle on 34th Street*. Natalie had just finished filming *Splendor in the Grass* with Warren Beatty. Her next film was to be *Love with a Proper Stranger* with Steve McQueen. Was I interested? Interested! I was ecstatic.

Nervous as could be on the day of Natalie's arrival, I was ready for anything. My brushes, combs, pins and hair spray were all set out; an electric stove heating for the curling iron was on the table. Our hairdressing room wasn't fancy. It had light green walls and small dressing tables with mirrors set in rows.

I was in awe of Natalie, I couldn't imagine being good enough to get the job yet I still hoped I would be. I

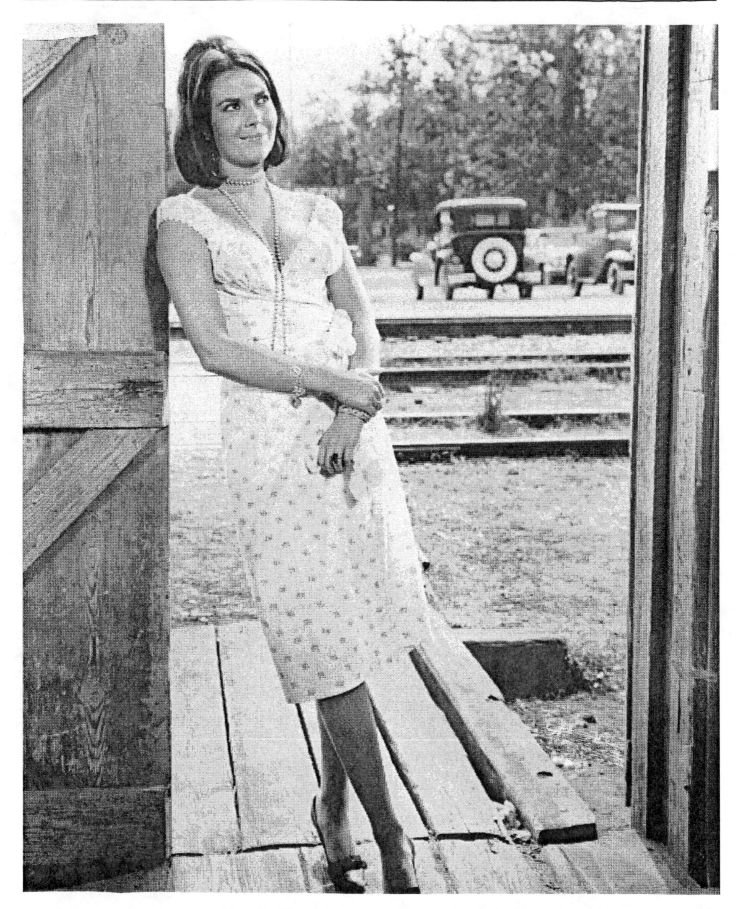

Natalie Wood, *This Property is Condemned*

sat there, desperately praying that she'd like my work. I heard some voices in the hall. It was Natalie arriving with her entourage. She walked into Nellie's office. A few moments later, Nellie called me in and introduced us. Upon meeting Natalie, I was surprised at how small and petite she actually was. Her face was as beautiful as I'd imagined. She had the biggest dark-brown eyes I'd ever seen and her mouth turned up so sweetly. I liked her right away and hoped it was mutual.

She sat at my table and described how her hair might be done to best express the character she was playing in the film. I listened carefully. I had not read the script. Although I'd been taught by the best at MGM, I was nervous, and my sweaty hands shook as I began to heat the curling iron. I began talking to myself through it silently. "Just imagine working with Natalie Wood, a really big star." I was praying, hoping I wouldn't blow this opportunity. I wondered if Natalie was used to people being so nervous around her. She probably didn't think of herself as special, but to me she was. In any case she was patient, kind, and friendly. While I was working on her hair, Natalie remarked that she was thinking of using a rinse to darken her hair. I told her I thought it was perfect as it was, and she agreed with me. When I finished, I stepped back and took a look at the results. It looked great to me.

Everyone stood up and she thanked me and left. Did I get the job? Nobody knew yet. It hadn't been offered to anyone else so far. If someone from our studio were going to do Natalie's hair, it would have to be me. Driving home that night, my imagination ran wild. What if the job was mine? My reputation would skyrocket. I'd never before imagined someone this famous wanting me to do her hair. Being chosen by a big star like Natalie (who was reputed to be difficult, but was anything but) people would think Sugar was a great hairstylist. I reveled in the possibility.

Yep! I got the job and no, I didn't faint, but I was shaky for a while. Always in my mind was the question, "Could I come up to her standards?" Natalie's entrance into my life and her subsequent support of me over the next seventeen years was a true gift and the highlight of my career. I will always be grateful to her.

Chapter 2

INFLUENCED BY HOLLYWOOD
1934 –1954

In the thirties, Los Angeles was paradise, the land of sunshine; you could swim at the beach all year long. There was no smog, no gangs, and palm trees lined the streets. Movie studios were around every corner. Hollywood was a part of our lives.

At seventeen, not being imaginative, with no drive for an exotic career, I assumed I would become a teacher. My other career choices appeared to be accounting or secretarial school. Fortunately life had other plans for me.

A Gemini, I was born on June 17, 1934 - Father's Day - to a fifty-seven-year-old man and a twenty-three-year-old woman. Being a Gemini was a wonderful birth sign and I grew up loving change, communicating, and was interested in just about everything.

My father, Maurice Zuckerman, known as M.Z., was a character, always the lover. My mother Josephine was the fourth wife of his five wives. At fourteen he'd been a sheriff in Oklahoma in 1890 and eventually migrated to California to become a potato rancher in Stockton. The title of "Potato King" was his, way back in 1925. They remained married for seven years, long enough for them to have three daughters of which I was the eldest.

In 1952, for graduation, my father bought me a Chevy Bel Aire. It was a hard top convertible, first of its kind. With transportation of my own I found new friends who helped me forget to pursue my career as a teacher. I had "too" much fun cruising the drive-ins at night instead of doing homework. Upon graduation from high school, I took a job at Hughes Aircraft, working on the assembly line soldering little goodies onto transistor boards. It was boring, but I did get a glimpse of old Howard Hughes wandering about his factory wearing rolled up faded jeans and tennis shoes without socks. I never noticed his fingernails.

After quitting the assembly line, my next job was chauffeuring for my dad who never drove his own car. This job consisted of mowing his lawn, shopping for groceries and making trips to his ranches in Utah and Oregon. My salary was $225 a month, plus meals. The job lasted nine months. It was time for me to get serious. I applied for two jobs, one at Prudential Insurance Company and the other at MGM to become a messenger.

Ah, the mind of a twenty-year-old! My reasons for applying at MGM were quite silly. My friend Patty worked as an

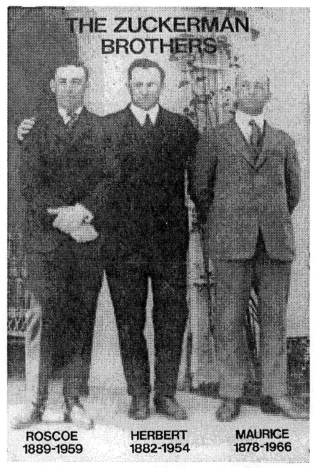

THE ZUCKERMAN BROTHERS

| ROSCOE | HERBERT | MAURICE |
| 1889-1959 | 1882-1954 | 1878-1966 |

Maurice Zuckerman, Sugar's Father

elevator operator in the Administration Building at MGM, but for a side job she played records for Lana Turner when Lana was working on a film. Patty would stand outside Lana's dressing room on the set and play her favorite records. Her life sounded exciting to me and Christmas was especially impressive. During the holidays I'd rush to visit Patty each evening, hoping for a glimpse of the baskets of presents Patty brought home each night. It was the highlight of my day. The colorful baskets of gifts inspired me to apply for a job at the studio.

I thought it would be a good idea to apply for two jobs. Both employers called me the same day for an interview. Confused, I asked my mom for advice. Wisely, she pointed out that while Prudential represented security, what did a twenty-year-old need with security? MGM sounded like it would be far more fun. "Go to MGM. Take a chance. You can always quit if you don't like it." I followed her advice.

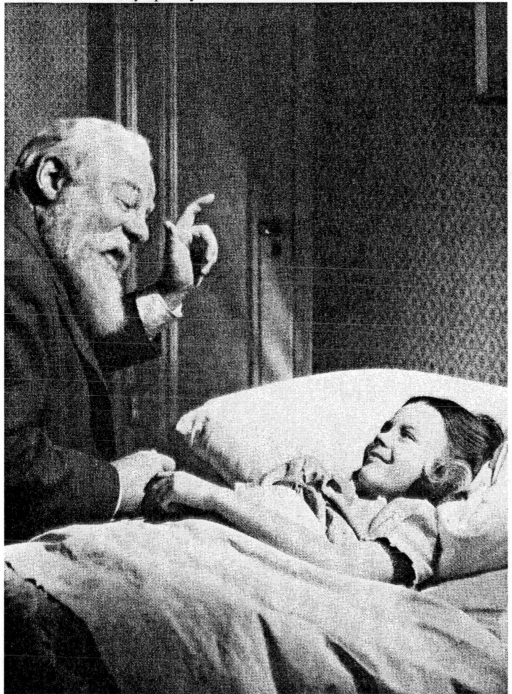

Natalie Wood and Edmund Gwenn, *Miracle on 34th Street*

My career in film actually began at fifteen when I worked as an usher at the Beverly Canon Theater in Beverly Hills. It was a small, arty theater that played foreign films. Our customers were as unique as the theater. Edmund Gwenn, who played Santa Claus in the first *Miracle on 34th Street* with Natalie Wood, came often. He was as sweet and charming as he appeared on the screen. I held back my urge to hug him. *Member of the Wedding* was my favorite film. Julie Harris was a great actress; I never tired of her performance. I must have watched that film a hundred times or more.

Because we lived so close to Hollywood, there was always the possibility we could run into a movie star. One evening, in Hollywood at the Grauman's Chinese Theater on Hollywood Boulevard, I came upon Robert Mitchum surrounded by a crowd. What an opportunity! I pushed my way in to get closer. I always carried a photo of him in my wallet. He was so powerful and handsome he made my heart beat fast. When I got close to him, I asked him to autograph the photo. He did! I was thrilled! When I showed my mother his autograph later that night she was mortified that I'd been so close to him, since he'd just been picked up for smoking the dreaded marijuana. I guess she thought the habit was catching.

I went for the interview at MGM. It was a letdown as I walked through the studio. Where was the glamour? It was drab, gray and gloomy. My interview was simple and the job was mine. Dreams do come true.

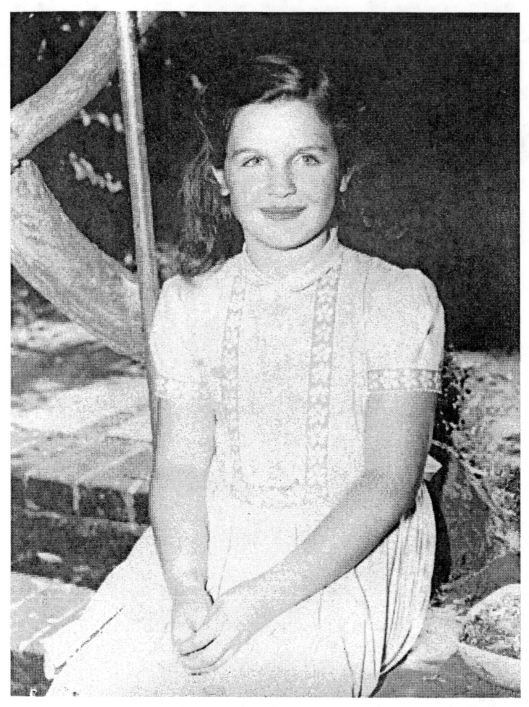

Ginger "Sugar" Blymyer, Age 10

Chapter 3

FIRST DAY ON THE JOB
MGM Studio, 1954

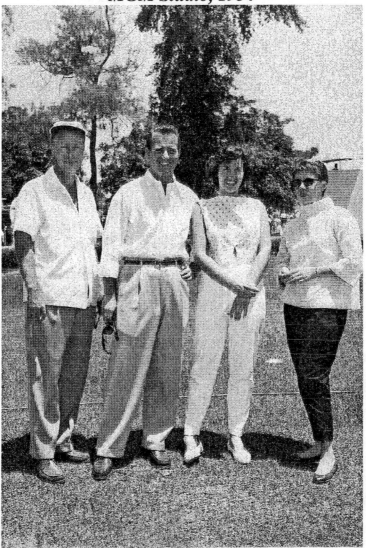

Ginger and co-workers early in her career
Left to Right: Tommy Tuttle, Stan Smith, Sugar, Shirley McShane

My stomach was full of butterflies. I wanted to look my best so I'd set my hair in pin curls the night before. It came out perfectly. Back then there were no curling irons for touching up, either your hair turned out right or you were stuck with bad hair all day. The ritual of getting dressed consisted of first putting on a merry widow bra, something like the bustiers of today. Next came the petticoats, one soft, one starched to an almost plastic consistency. On top of those went a pretty lace slip. By the time I was finished my skirt was very full giving the illusion of a small waist. I wore no makeup; only light lipstick called Pixie Pink, and rubbed my legs with baby oil to make them shine. I was ready.

MGM was located in Culver City. I parked my car as previously instructed and walked through the gate to find my time card. Having Zuckerman for a last name always made it easy to find my time card, right at the end of everyone else.

I arrived early so there was time to walk and explore on my way in. Buildings were laid out every which way in a disorderly pattern. The messenger room was right next to the drive-in gate, commandeered by Ken Hollywood. Ken was born for that job. Short and stocky, white-faced and pudgy, I was sure he'd descended from the bovine race. He was an absolute tyrant except when someone "important" came along. Then he underwent a miraculous transformation and became quite charming. But you knew it was "his" studio and you seldom entered it without being confronted by Ken.

The messenger room was full of windows. You could see everything that went on out in the street. Feeling a little nervous, I opened the screen door and looked inside. The room was large lined with bench-like couches upholstered in leather. A few girls were sitting around; others were sorting mail into the myriad of shelves and baskets located all around the room for that purpose. In the corner was a large brown desk. Our dispatcher Marlene Jost, looked up and said hello.

After introducing me to everyone, Marlene said to relax and later she explained about the five mail routes throughout the studio where we delivered and picked up mail. Messengers left every half hour to pick up mail from offices and departments around the lot - no faxes in those days. There were special messengers who awaited calls in case something had to be delivered in a hurry. In addition, the lot had its own post office.

Our crew consisted of fifteen girls and Marlene. Girls were carefully handpicked so the studio wouldn't have to worry about their behavior on the lot. My pay was $37 a week. My first check went for union dues.

"Be polite, don't show awe, be businesslike at all times when on duty," Marlene informed me. A few minutes later off I went accompanying one of the girls on her mail route. As we walked along, our arms full of envelopes, she explained where we were and who worked in each office. Although it was exciting to be inside the walls of that famous old studio, I was disappointed because of its shabby appearance. I'd expected it to look like a movie set, but it didn't really matter. I was thrilled to be there.

Following my new friend up stairs and down stairs, across bridges, in and out of buildings and offices I was getting weary. I realized I needed to build up my endurance. I also discovered that stiff petticoats and oiled legs weren't a great combination as the outdoor stairs were dirty and dusty. By the end of the day my legs and petticoats were a mess.

I'll never forget that first day's lunch. A group of us went to the commissary after finishing our route. Now this was just what I'd imagined a movie studio would feel and look like. It was bustling, full of people. Huge murals of important events at MGM covered the walls. There were hundreds of people dressed in costumes, extras in kilts working on *Brigadoon*, dancers dressed like farmers working on *Oklahoma*, extras wearing period costumes and white wigs, dancers in rehearsal outfits. Sprinkled among the extras were the "famous". I thought to myself, this is perfect; I was thrilled and tried not to stare open-mouthed.

Most items on the menu were named after a star who had considered it a favorite. I ordered the Greta Garbo sandwich. It sounded delicious - cream cheese, peanut butter, and banana on rye bread. Tasty yes, but a real sinker. No wonder Greta spent so much time swooning on the couch!

As a messenger I learned the names of the most powerful men in the studio - the producers. Dore Schary was the studio head at the time. John Houseman had the most elegant office. We were warned to stay clear of Arthur Freed as he had a thing for young girls. My favorite was Joe Pasternak with his gravelly voice. He often came into the messenger room and visited with us.

Our afternoon route took us to the third floor of the Administration Building, which was a depressing, musty place where the writers worked. The rooms were tiny with dull brown carpeting that must have been installed when the building was first built. I wondered if any of the famous writers began their careers in those dreadful little offices.

Our final run through the building included the basement. Walking through the lithograph room was always creepy. It was dark, run by a strange man with a dark sense of humor. One day as we approached, we saw a hangman's noose over his desk. We took one look, grabbed the mail, and ran out of there fast.

Production was a busy place filled with young men who were our male counterparts. There were many messengers and assistant directors on their way up, lots of cute young guys. Above the messenger room was the photo department where requests of those glossies autographed by the stars were filled. Down the hall was the censor's office. Sylvia the censor had issued a warning never to deliver mail to her office if the door was closed. I was told she often entertained a beau in her office and didn't want to be disturbed. I pictured this not-too-attractive woman panting and moaning on her couch, but I never saw any disheveled man sneak out of there to confirm my suspicions. Perhaps the censor needed to be censored.

The Film Lab had a strong chemical smell so the men would often take a break and sit on a low wall in front of the lab. Many of the girls felt awkward walking between the men who loved to make remarks and embarrass them. I soon learned to greet them first which took them off guard and they reacted in a friendly fashion.

The Props Department was incredible! There was always something unusual on the loading dock waiting to be transferred to the stages. It might be huge, gilded furniture fit for a king's palace; a stuffed bird; beds covered in golden paint; or a beaded lamp. There was a seemingly endless supply of items from every time period. I longed to spend a day going through all the back rooms of the property department.

Near our room was the scoring stage where the musicians worked. We'd see people with every sort of instrument going through the stage doors, but it was completely soundproofed so we were never able to hear any music coming from inside. The Camera Department was where all the young apprentices learned everything about cameras. Upstairs was the Editing Department. It consisted of a long walkway with little rooms opening off it. From these dark, little rooms issued squawks and squeaks from the film the editor was turning round on little wheels.

The outside route was fascinating. It included the Electrical Department where they stored all the lights including those huge lamps called brutes and the Grip Department where equipment to build set scaffolding, camera dollies (the equipment the camera sits on), gobos for lights, and wood for dolly tracks were stored. The Construction Department was filled with carpenters building sets.

Makeup Department was on the outside route, and we always hoped to see a star there. Although our routes started after most of the stars were at work, there was always a chance we'd see someone. Little did I realize I'd soon be working there.

Most fascinating was the Staff Shop where they reproduced anything in plaster. There were statues and amazing reproductions of trimmings for buildings from Greek periods. Next came the Scenic Dock where they painted the most realistic backdrops. I felt as though I could just walk right into a scene they were painting and disappear into another world.

Transportation was full of cars and limos of all vintages. We had a police and a fire department, a barbershop, a shoeshine stand, newsstand, and a hospital where Dr. Jones, a grim lady doctor, was in charge. We all tried our best to stay well so we wouldn't have to encounter Dr. Jones.

Publicity was a large and busy place filled with publicists who worked on sets with the stars. Photos were taken at the finish of a film, in the still gallery, with the stars looking their best, perfectly lit by master photographers. The walls were adorned with enormous enlargements of the stars - Elizabeth Taylor, Debbie Reynolds, Clark Gable, Mitzi Gaynor, Walter Pigeon, and more.

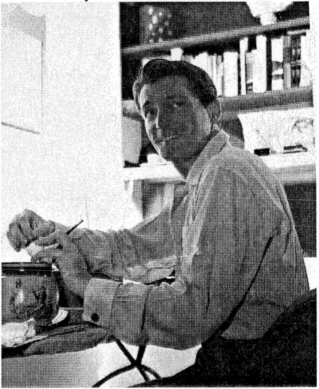

Carlos Thompson, Sugar's first Hollywood crush

Helen Rose was the reigning queen of the wardrobe department. We never saw any of her designs before they arrived on the set because the dressing rooms were located behind the office.

The talent department was located next to our room. Two attractive men, Al Trescony and Tommy Tannenbaum, who searched for new talent and trained new contract players, managed it. Roger Moore of *Bond* fame was just beginning his career. Sometimes he'd read to us in his elegant, cultured English voice. James Drury, who became *The Virginian* in the television series, was there and we were thrilled when he got a part in one of Elvis's films. Edmund Purdom was there; but soon after he starred in *The Egyptian*, we never saw him again.

Young actors often visited us and it was fun to meet them. Some went on to stardom and others got lost along the way. While under contract, they received complete training. There were teachers for voice, dance, fencing, horseback riding, and even riding sidesaddle if necessary. As a result, they were prepared for anything a film might require. The studio was like a huge family, it met all our needs and we couldn't help, but be affected by its rhythms.

A few weeks after my arrival the holidays arrived and everything ground to a halt. Our last bit of excitement on the lot was men in kilts, playing bagpipes marching into a stage for *Brigadoon*. Nothing else exciting happened until the following June. The reason for this hiatus was a tax law. In April, an inventory was taken of all films in production. Taxes were charged, even on a film in pre-production. Many people were laid off. Fortunately, the laws were eventually changed.

Messengers were invited to special events. Once we were invited to be ballroom dancers on the Peter Potter TV Show that featured dancing and music. Carlos Thompson, the romantic actor who I developed a crush on after he told me I had beautiful green eyes (my eyes are actually blue, but I had on dark glasses), appeared on this particular show. We had to dance right on stage. I was terrified. I wanted to be graceful and charming for Carlos, but I was so nervous I tripped over the cables, nearly falling on my face. So much for that romance.

Outside the drive-in gate was a grassy area with a shade tree. During my first summer we noticed a slight, plain, young man wearing glasses, stretched out under the tree reading a book, often staring into space. He was dressed in a T-shirt, khaki pants, and tennis shoes. Perhaps he was dreaming about being a star. He soon would be. We later found out that his name was James Dean and by the time we saw him on film, he was a star, no longer the plain, young man we'd seen under the tree!

Chapter 4

MAKEUP DEPARTMENT
Getting Acquainted with the Stars

The screen door to our messenger room swung open and in walked a freckle-faced young fellow with curly red hair. "This is Rusty Tamblin," my friend said as she introduced me to the young man. "He's a dancer working on *Seven Brides for Seven Brothers*. Later she told me all about him. He was an up and coming talent, under contract to the studio. A few days later Rusty asked me for a date. Impressed? Was I ever? I was going out with a real movie star. On our first date he took me to see Dave Brubeck at the Lighthouse in Long Beach. I never told him I didn't care for jazz. On our second date, we went to see a Joan Crawford movie.

Each time he arrived to pick me up the excitement level in our neighborhood elevated. Everyone peeked out from behind their curtains to get a look at him. Our relationship didn't last long, as always he dated the new messenger a couple of times and then moved on. It was great fun while it lasted and did wonders for my self-esteem.

One of the messengers, Luana - a very pretty girl - was given a screen test. The dreaded Arthur Freed had noticed her. She was carefully chaperoned, it was doubtful whether she ever ended up on the famous "casting couch" we'd all been warned about. Maybe those stories were true and maybe they weren't. I don't know. I never ended up on one.

Saturdays were quiet and often we wandered into the Talent Office where James Drury would read to us in his lovely deep voice. James became my crush and soon Carlos was left by the wayside.

Life was full of surprises these days. One day we looked up and heard the tone of Ken Hollywood's voice change and as we opened the door, Clark Gable sailed through the gate in his yellow Cadillac convertible. He waved to us and smiled to expose his lovely, big white teeth. Another day I was walking along just looking down, when I heard a low "Hello, how are you?" I looked up and there was Walter Pigeon and he was expecting a reply. "Fine" was all I could say.

Robert Russell Bennet, a well-known composer, tall, gray-haired and very dignified became my friend. One day he stopped me. "I have something for you," he said, and handed me a large envelope, in which there was a duet to sing with Santa Claus. He had written it just for me.

As messengers, one of our jobs was to take USO Tours around the studio. Proudly showing off what was now "my" studio, I'd take the tour across Overland Boulevard to the magical back lot and show them the Andy Hardy Street where Mickey Rooney lived and played with Judy Garland. We'd walk by castles, scenes from the Bible, French country sides and New York streets. The back lot became any place on earth. Actually it was only the front of buildings, but my imagination went wild and it felt real to me. One afternoon, a sarcastic young soldier on my tour complained about walking down my beloved streets. He wanted to go directly to the stage and see real "live" shooting of a film. "Why didn't you let somebody else come on this tour if all you are going to do is complain?" I admonished him. How dare he? Finally we went to the set of *Seven Brides for Seven Brothers*. At last he was satisfied. I was too, because I got to see Rusty Tamblin dancing. He flew through the air and jumped high. What a fantastic dancer he was.

Job openings inside the studio were posted on a bulletin board so anyone already working there would have first shot at it. I checked it daily. My first opportunity for advancement came when they needed extra help in the messenger office. I applied and soon I was working there occasionally helping Jean, our boss. I received a 10% raise. The next job that came up was a stock room clerk position in the Makeup Department. I had no idea what the job entailed, but it sounded interesting, so I applied. I figured I could learn whatever I needed to know. Bill Tuttle and Jack Young, the head and assistant head of makeup, interviewed me. The job entailed arriving at work at 6:00 a.m., opening the makeup stockroom and handing out supplies to makeup men and hairdressers. It also involved typing the confusing daily schedule in case Inez, the regular secretary, was ill. I was to sit at the reception desk until she came in at 10:00 a.m. Luckily, my skills were sufficient and I got the job.

Normally my day began at 6:00 a.m. when the makeup and hair people arrived. In those days, actors were allowed at least three hours for hair and makeup. It was a relaxed atmosphere. I'd come in, put the coffee on, unlock my storeroom, and set out everything they needed on the counter. I'd give the makeup people the supplies they requested and the hair stylists would come to pick up the wigs that had been locked in the storeroom overnight.

If casts of thousands were working, the Makeup Department moved beneath the rehearsal halls to an enormous room aptly named The Snake-pit. Two extravaganzas were being filmed when I began my job in Makeup. The films were *The Prodigal, a Biblical Story* and *Jupiter's Darling*, an Esther Williams swim spectacular, complete with five elephants. We made up hundreds of extras each morning. Multitudes of hair stylists and makeup men worked frantically every morning to get them all ready and on the set in time. I checked out beards and mustaches to the extras, stamping there pay vouchers so they'd be sure to return them at night (otherwise they wouldn't get paid). In the evening I'd check in all the hair and the hair people would clean and set them. When things slowed down after the morning rush, the hair and makeup people packed their cases and went to the stage for the rest of the day.

After everyone had left for the set and it was quiet, I'd bundle up hairpins and other essentials so they'd be easy to hand out during the early morning rush. If all the hairstylists weren't needed on the set, they'd stay down in the snake pit and help me sort hairpins and tell fascinating stories of the past. One of them, Edie Hubner, a round little woman with white hair, had been Jean Harlow's hairdresser.

At the time I became the stockroom clerk, MGM was in its heyday. Many people were under contract while others were there for a single film. Sydney Guilleroff was the head of the hairdressing department. In the past he had styled Greta Garbo's and Ava Gardner's hair and was now working with Elizabeth Taylor, Debbie Reynolds and Leslie Caron. When stars were working on the lot, they inevitably passed through Makeup so I got my wish to see them and feel what it was like to be in their presence.

One day a beautiful woman walked by me. Her swaying walk was familiar and very sexy. It was Marilyn Monroe and she had come to see Sydney. What a thrill! Gene Kelly was always in and out of Makeup. He worked all the time and was vibrating with energy. When I met Elizabeth Taylor in person, I was surprised at how short she was. She could put weight on easily and always had to diet. She was beautiful, friendly and generous and it didn't seem to be fair for someone to be so beautiful and still have to worry about weight like us ordinary folks.

When Elizabeth became engaged to Michael Todd, she endeared herself to me. He had given her the biggest diamond engagement ring I'd ever seen. It was a beautiful emerald cut and almost too heavy for her small hand. Michael always did things lavishly - with all his energy and nothing stood still when he was around. Elizabeth came into the Hair Department to show us her ring. She took it off offering to let each of us try the huge diamond ring on, knowing how thrilled we'd be. I think she realized we'd never own anything quite like it and she wanted to share her happiness with us. It was the diamond season. Debbie Reynolds was sporting a huge diamond from Eddie Fisher and Pier Angelli one from Vic Damone.

Never have I seen a lovelier woman than Cyd Charisse. What a fantastic dancer. She must have been born with that grace. When Leslie Caron was filming *An American in Paris,* she drove Sydney crazy trimming her hair with manicure scissors. One afternoon Lee Marvin showed up needing a shampoo. I was asked to do it. I gave him a head massage, too, which was an interesting experience. He had so many knots on his head I wish I'd been a phrenologist.

Paul Newman began to work on *Somebody Up There Likes Me*. What a gorgeous fellow, so young, so handsome, with those fabulous blue eyes. Though he was at the very beginning of his career, he was already known for his love of beer. One evening he had gone to the Pickwick Theater to see a preview. He took his six-pack and lost his checkbook. My sister, who worked at the theater, found the checkbook. She brought it to me so I could return it. When I gave it to him, Paul leaned over and gave me a big kiss of thanks in appreciation. For once in my life, I was speechless.

Marlon Brando affected me more than anyone I'd ever met. His charisma was so powerful. You couldn't measure it. He was filming *Teahouse of the August Moon* Charlie Schram applied his makeup - eyelids with straight eyelashes for a complicated Oriental look and he looked like a different person when he left Makeup each morning. At night his appliances were discarded so I collected them and gave them to a woman obsessed with Mr. Brando. One morning, sitting at the front desk, awaiting Inez's arrival, I was looking beneath the desk when I felt a touch on my hand. As I looked up, I heard Marlon Brando say, "That's a pretty ring." I nearly swooned. Something about him always made my heart beat too fast.

Rock Hudson was starring in *Something of Value,* a film about the African Mau Mau's. He was gorgeous and oh-so-nice, but I never felt attracted to him like I did to Marlon and Paul. No one knew he was gay at the time. I guess he just didn't exude the masculine aura of the other actors.

Makeup consisted of three separate departments and we all worked together. George, a mean, pinched little man who looked like Scrooge and always dressed in a gray suit, managed the accounting, in our department. He seemed angry with me, but I learned it wasn't personal. He acted angry with everyone. There was a cupboard in his office where he kept special makeup under lock and key - and he had the only key. When the makeup men needed something special they practically had to get on their knees and beg for it. Sometimes he'd warm up and I was glad to see he had a human side. He was very different when actor Louis Calhern came to visit. George would laugh and try to charm Louis. It was funny and almost embarrassing because most of the time he was so grim.

Inez, our large secretary, weighed more than 350 pounds. She had a beautiful face, white hair, and a jealous, cruel heart. If I did a favor for anyone, she was furious because she felt it was taking attention away from her. Makeup men loved to play tricks on her. For instance, at lunch time, three or four of them would each bring her back a piece of pie from the commissary. Later they would peek around the corner to see if she actually ate all the pieces. Sometimes she did.

Always erratic, occasionally Inez was nice to me, then for no reason she'd report me to Bill Tuttle for what she considered to be an infraction of her territory. Bill would call me into the office and bawl me out.

Sydney Guilleroff was wonderful to me. He'd stick up for me when Inez was mean. I really appreciated Sydney because he could be far more caustic than anyone else when he wanted to be. He passed away in June 1997 at the age of eighty-nine having written a book about his life called *Crowning Glory*. I read the book and found all sorts of surprising secrets that he'd kept to himself.

Makeup was in a long, rectangular building with a hall down the middle and makeup rooms all along it. Each makeup man had a permanent setup in the rooms with perfect lighting plus a fully stocked makeup case to take to the set when they stood by.

Johnny Truce, Gene Kelly's makeup man, had the first makeup room across from my stockroom. He also made wigs and hairpieces and did repairs if the hair lace was ripped. He also loved to gossip. We'd sit and talk while he ventilated the wigs. He'd take one hair at a time and, using a tiny needle-like hook, he'd tie it to the lace that had been fitted to a person's hairline. I tried to learn to ventilate, but gave up quickly; neither my eyes nor my patience lasted long enough.

Charlie Schram's room was next to Johnny's. He was the most talented makeup person I've ever met. His lab was a fantastic place full of plaster casts of actors' faces for sculpting appliances, scars, and aging pieces, all sorts of surprises. Charlie was strict and trained me well. For example, if I didn't put the scissors away where I found them, I wouldn't be able to use them any longer to cut the cheesecloth they used for makeup removal. He taught me to respect other people's tools.

Next in line was Lee Stanfield, a quiet, tense man. When he was laid off, I was told to clean out his room and I found gin bottles stashed everywhere. After Keester Sweeney, who had become Bill's assistant, moved on, Lee took the job of Bill's assistant. Perhaps it was too much for him because he committed suicide soon after he was laid off. I was shocked. I thought we all knew each other so well, why hadn't we noticed that he needed help?

Stan Smith in the next room was my favorite and a mentor of sorts. He and Jack Stone were the youngest men in the department and close friends. They made me laugh when one of the mean folks got after me. I developed a crush on Stan, but Stan had a crush on June Allyson. Jack, on the other hand, never seemed to have a crush on anyone. He was more interested in preparing for upcoming wars and looting whatever he could from the studio.

The hairdressing room was in the back of the department. A long counter where everyone faced the mirrors stretched from one end to the other. On the opposite side were the dryers. In those days they set hair in pin curls and then iron curled the hair to smooth it out. The coffee set up was at the end of the room and on many afternoons people dropped in for a cup. The mirrors above the counters were well lit. It was bright and very pleasant.

One day Stan goaded me, "Are you going to be a stockroom clerk for the rest of your life? Why don't you go to cosmetology school and become a hairstylist?" I'd never even thought about it. After he brought it up, the idea began to take hold in my mind. I began to watch the hairstylists more closely. I saw that they earned a lot of money, dressed stylishly, appeared to have fun. It was beginning to look like quite a good career move to me. Why not go for it? I had no other plans, and no reason not to.

Christmas season came and I cut English Holly from my bushes at home to decorate the department. The actors brought in fabulous gifts for us. Yes! I finally got my baskets of gifts. But by then this was no longer as important to me as getting to know all the people who came through the Makeup Department.

Christmas was usually rather dismal. To save money there were layoffs, production shut down and often our parties were small. Sometimes my favorite people would be missing. I'd fix eggnog and put it on the counter with cookies and other goodies. Under the counter was a bottle of gin and limejuice so I could fix Gimlets for Bill, our boss. He was usually stiff and reserved, but after a few Gimlets he became relaxed and jovial. It was good to see the other side of him.

Although I was no longer a messenger, I still vacationed with my friends in the messenger room. The next spring we all left for a vacation in Palm Springs. As we were driving toward Palm Springs, a news flash came on the car radio. James Dean was dead. He had been killed in a car crash. We couldn't believe it. We didn't want to believe it. I could hardly drive. I was crying so hard. That young man who had been sitting out under the tree in the parking lot a short while ago was dead. It just seemed like no time at all since he was talking with us. I was glad I'd been with my friends when I heard about his death.

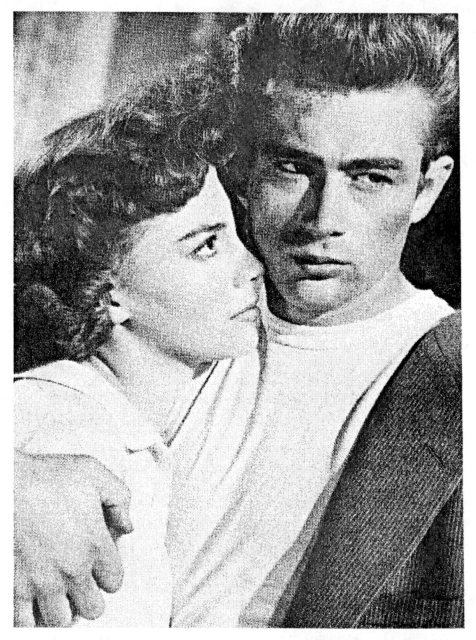

James Dean and Natalie Wood, *Rebel Without a Cause*

Chapter 5

A CAREER IN FILM
1956-1960

I seriously began to consider going to cosmetology school so I could get my license and become a studio hairdresser. Opportunity was staring me in the face, and I had no intention of letting it pass me by? Until now, I'd never had any inclination to work with hair. I had fun working with the wigs in my stockroom and watching the actors and actresses become transformed into parts they were playing. While they were testing for *Something of Value* with Rock Hudson, I braided Mau Mau hairdos and packed the hair with mud to make it look authentic. The truth was, I was getting bored in the stockroom, and a career in hairdressing was becoming more and more appealing. The pay was great. I knew it was going to be a tough haul. I'd have to take classes after work in the evenings and on weekends.

Stan, my mentor, suggested that I attend Marinello Beauty College in downtown Los Angeles. I enrolled in night classes. Little did I realize how difficult this was going to be. I'd report to MGM first thing in the morning, do my work, and when I was finished at 4:00 p.m., I'd head on down the freeway to school, a forty-five-minute drive. Most nights I was worn out. There was so much to learn. Up until that time I thought hairdressers were somewhat uneducated, but I soon found out how wrong I was. In California you had to clock in sixteen hundred hours to get a cosmetology license. That was a lot of time to spend in night school, especially when my day began at six in the morning. The good part was the people at work cheered me on and assured me they'd help me get into the union as soon as I finished.

In addition to physiology, anatomy, and pathology (disease), we were taught about chemicals and electricity. I practiced facials, manicures, cutting hair, perming, washing and setting hair. We learned how to get along with our customers and please them. We learned about sanitation.

The school charged for our work after we put in two hundred hours, but in the beginning we had to practice on willing guinea pigs. Little old ladies on fixed incomes would come to school and get their hair done for free by us, the new students, with only a fifteen-cent charge for that famous blue rinse. Once I consented to let my teacher, Mrs. Brown, give me a perm. I told her I didn't want tight curls. Big mistake! I ended up with the frizzes. I cut it all off, creating my first pixie look. Occasionally there was a bus strike, which meant no customers so we had to practice on each other. I was always a willing model because I could snooze under the dryer.

Some days I would check into school, punch my time card, then sneak out for dinner. My favorite restaurant was Clifton's Cafeteria, a restaurant complete with waterfalls, water wheels, even a photographer with a flash camera. I never wanted my picture taken because I didn't want to get caught.

Life was tough during that period. Sometimes I'd get discouraged. It was so difficult. I felt like I was working on two jobs. I'm a morning person so it was hard to learn at night. I wondered if I could keep it up long enough to finish. It was even more difficult in the summer because I went to school on Saturdays. All my friends would leave for the beach and I'd be driving in the opposite direction to that dingy, old building. But good things happened, too. I met Dorothy White Byrne and we became fast friends. She was a day student so I only saw her on Saturdays. I told her about my plan to work in the film business. A few years later she decided to become a film hairstylist too.

My friends at work kept telling me to keep up the good work. It would be worth it. The teachers told us that the students who finished night school were more respected because they had put forth so much effort. I tried to keep all that in mind, but it was still difficult.

In the meantime at MGM changes were being made. They hired a makeup apprentice, Ron Berkley. Now I was no longer the lowest person on the totem pole. I joked with Ron and told him he could take the blame for anything that went wrong, instead of me. The movie business is notorious for passing the buck. Now I had my very own flunky.

Actually we became great friends. The makeup men were so happy to have someone to teach and Ron was very clever. He was well-liked and eventually went on to become Richard Burton's makeup artist, traveling all over the world with him.

When it was quiet, we were so silly. Once Ron decided to grow a mustache, but it was a narrow one and made him look sneaky, although he was quite attractive. None of us liked the way it looked, but no way would he shave it off. One evening he wrenched his back and came to work hardly able to move. Since he couldn't fight back, we took him into Charlie's makeup room and held him still, while Charlie shaved off half his mustache leaving him with no choice, but to shave the other half himself.

Johnny Truee had the most wonderful parakeet that lived in the lab and talked more than any bird I'd ever met. First thing in the mornings I'd let him out of his cage and he'd sit on my shoulders as I opened up the stockroom. During the day he would go from person to person, ending the day parading around Inez's ample bosom. He learned to answer the phone and he'd clearly repeat "Makeup Department" along with Inez each time the phone rang. We all loved him so much. He was with us for a couple of years before tragedy struck. An actress came in for Charlie to do her makeup and her little Yorkie got hold of our sweet little bird and killed him. We were crushed.

One afternoon Louis Calhern came to the department after having been to a party where he imbibed a bit too much. Louis as usual charmed George, our accountant, but George was also worried about Louis driving home in his condition. He asked Ron if one of us would be willing to drive Mr. Calhoun's car to his home while the other followed. We did, depositing him at his elegant mansion. We were glad to oblige and when we saw his digs, a huge mansion in Beverly Hills we were thoroughly impressed.

Lovely Grace Kelly was filming *The Swan*. She was beautiful, gracious, and engaged to marry her prince. Helen Rose had designed her wedding dress and fortunately I was invited to go to the Wardrobe Department to see her try it on. The elegant dress was beautiful, covered with lace and pearls, the train filling the whole room. While this was going on, Deborah Kerr quietly came into the room and simply watched, not claiming any attention for herself, just enjoying Miss Kelly's happiness.

My social life centered around my friends at work. On Christmas Eve, Ron invited us to a party at his home in Hollywood Hills. I met a young man there, danced with him, and he asked me to go home with him to get some more liquor to take back to the party. I was wide-eyed as he opened the door to his home. A life size Santa was bobbing up and down, Christmas decorations everywhere. I'd never seen anything like it. He laughed at my astonishment and explained that his parents were florists, hence all the decorations. There was an indoor pool and he asked if I'd like a swim. He found me a suit. It was a nifty experience to have on Christmas Eve. We returned to the party with wet hair, our friends wondering what we'd been up to.

Ron and I were given tickets to the Deb Star Ball by the Makeup and Hair Department. It was a celebration of the young women from all the studios that were expected to become stars in the future. It was held at the Palladium in Hollywood. For some reason they designated Johnny Truee to be our chaperone. As if we needed one. Ron picked me up and we all met at Johnny's apartment.

I'd heard Johnny was a collector, but had no idea what I was to encounter when I went to his apartment one day. It was a museum. As soon as the door opened, I was greeted by two little Pug dogs wiggling and wagging as hard as they could. Johnny led me to his living room. Animal skins including several zebra skins were draped on the couches and on the book shelf above the couch was a complete bound set of National Geographic magazines, dating from the 1800's. There were four, three-feet-high-oriental statues carved from ivory, depicting the four seasons. In Johnny's crowded bedroom was a music box that played brass discs the size of a 76-rpm record. Fifty of these discs were piled in a corner, carefully separated by sheets of newspaper. Years later Johnny built a house to accommodate his treasures.

The holiday season was well on its way after the dance and with it came many parties. Jane Gorton, the hairstylist, offered to fix me up on a blind date with a fellow who lived with her family. The Christmas dance the studio put on each year was coming up and I had no boyfriend so I agreed. My date's name was Bill. We had something in common - a love of monkeys. I'd had a Rhesus monkey and Bill had trained a chimpanzee that traveled with him in an act where he wore a tux and played the piano. Bill was still grieving over the death of his chimp, which had become tangled in the chain of his cage while they were playing in Hawaii. For him, the loss of his chimp was like the loss of a child.

We had a wild time during the holidays. Bill was easy to talk to and my mother liked him. In those days, birth control wasn't available like it is today. I probably would have been too embarrassed to ask for it anyway. Soon I found myself expecting.

When Bill found out I was pregnant he announced he had no plans to get married, so I decided to carry on alone. There weren't many single parents around in those days, so I didn't say anything to anyone. I was happy to know I had someone growing inside of me. I'd talk to my baby and, being an optimist, I felt I'd be able to deal with whatever came up.

Three months later Bill asked me out to dinner and after a couple of drinks, shrugged his shoulders and said, "Well, I guess we might as well get married." It wasn't the romantic proposal I'd dreamed about, but it was good enough. My baby would have a father. The whole bar toasted us and bought us drinks. I felt awful the next day.

We didn't want to upset our parents, so we sneaked away to Las Vegas to get married. Our families were told we'd eloped in January, but that we had kept it a secret. Our daughter, Laurie, cooperated perfectly, arriving nine months to the day we had chosen as our anniversary. What timing.

We moved into our own apartment in Palms and I imagined a happy, married life ahead. How mistaken I was! Bill wasn't happy at all. He felt trapped. He didn't like his job as a locksmith at Douglas Aircraft and when I'd wish him a good day at work, he'd snarl at me and growl, "Don't say that, you know I won't have a nice day." He definitely was not a lot of fun, but I kept trying.

In spite of Bill's attitude, I was in heaven after Laurie arrived. She was beautiful and I loved her with all my heart and she needed me even if my husband didn't. Three months after she arrived, Bill walked out. I was heartbroken. I moved back home which made my mother happy. She loved having her first beloved grandchild with her. It took a long time to build up my self-esteem after being rejected by Bill, but an old friend, Don Gallagher, a film editor, came to my rescue. He'd had his eye on me years before, but had been married. Now he was divorced. When he heard I was free, he called and what fun we had. I began to feel good about myself again.

I was no longer working in makeup and I needed a job. My father, still hoping I'd become his secretary, offered to send me to school, but I confessed that what I really wanted to do was to finish my hairdressing course. Daddy, God bless him, agreed to finance my schooling and pay for Laurie's babysitter as well.

This time I chose a school in Santa Monica and went in the daytime. The teachers were bright and five long years after I first began cosmetology school, I graduated. Vivian Macateer, now a film hairstylist, was one of my teachers and later became a good friend. After passing the State Boards I found a job at Louis Salon de Coiffure right down the street from Fox Studios. My job taught me how much more I had to learn. Louis, who owned the little beauty shop, was an amazing character with all the charm and personality you'd expect of a Frenchman. An excellent hairstylist, he could even cut hair blindfolded. He taught me how to color hair, give perms, cut and set. Since we were so close to Fox, secretaries came to us in the evenings. Our days were long, sometimes from nine to nine. It was hard work standing on my feet all day long, but I liked it anyway. I enjoyed getting to know the customers. When I touched a person's head, they relaxed and talked to me. They felt free to confide their troubles in me. While I wasn't actually a part of their lives, I became a therapist of sorts.

Two doors down from the shop was a little bar where Louis often took his clients. From time to time a troubled woman would come in and need to talk. He'd walk her out the back door and down the alley to the bar for a drink. If we needed him, we knew where to find him. He did people more good by sitting and listening to them in that bar than many a therapist.

I realized I wouldn't be doing this kind of hairdressing forever. Nevertheless, I needed to get experience and confidence. I threw myself into the work and enjoyed myself. New Year's Eve was our busiest day ever. We worked from 6:00 a.m. to 9:00 p.m. and when I went home that night I lie down on the couch and fell asleep immediately. I never heard the year 1960 come in.

I was anxiously waiting to hear from the union. They hadn't taken anyone into the union for more than seven years, but this was about to change. Television was coming into its own and with it a great need for hair-stylists. This was 1959 and movie studios were having a difficult time admitting television was no longer just a stepchild. The union was short of hair-stylists and I was one of the first they called to come to work. Now it became difficult to work at the salon. I'd get a call the day before and have to tell Louie I wouldn't be coming to work. He understood what I'd planned on doing all along and was willing to go along with it even if he didn't like it. My first call was at MGM on the detective show *Peter Gunn*. Lola Albright was wearing a French twist and was extremely ticklish. Each time I'd run the comb up the back of her neck to catch the stray hairs that reflected the light, she would laugh hysterically.

Twilight Zone was filming at MGM and I worked on many of those stories. I also helped out with extras for *Brothers Grimm*. One scene had snow made from Ivory soap flakes falling in the streets to simulate a snowstorm. I thought they used something more sophisticated than that, but it worked and it was so pretty.

When there was spare time the new hair-stylists would go back to the department and practice using the curling iron. The curling irons were not the electric kind we have now, but the old-fashioned ones you heated in an electric oven, and we had to spin the iron to cool it off if it overheated. We were taught to work with the delicate hair lace wigs and hairpieces, all the things we never learned in school. We all knew we'd be taking a test once we had worked thirty days to qualify to join the union.

The hairstylists who work on films stay on the set to maintain the actor's hair in the style it began with at the beginning of the scene. If a hair fell out of place and the shot is printed, we had to remember and maintain it so it would match from frame to frame. We went in early and did our hairstyles. On the set we kept track of any changes that occurred, and kept records of what had been done so if they had to re-shoot a scene we'd knew what to do. I couldn't trust myself to remember.

A huge unknown factor was the weather. Hair could look just fine and then the weather would get foggy. Horrors! Right before my eyes, the hair would begin to change and become curly if it was set to be straight or straight if it was supposed to be curly. It was frustrating and sometimes impossible to stop the destruction.

Sometimes the extras upset me. They might have had a tough night before so after their hair was finished they would curl up in a corner and go to sleep. When they were called to the set, the extra would jump up so quickly that the wig might slip over one eye or something equally disastrous. Hairstylists got the blame if people didn't look right, but sometimes there was nothing we could do.

Finally after working on many shows that year, I had the thirty days required to qualify for membership in Makeup Artists and Hairstylist's Local # 706. Fortunate for me, because right after I had accumulated the thirty days, there was a writer's strike and no one had a job. Louis had let me go because Fox was also slow and his business had fallen off. He knew I'd leave eventually anyway.

Bill, in the meantime, had returned after a walk from Los Angeles to Mexico City. He decided he wanted to be married after all. I was happy about that and soon I was pregnant with my second daughter, Tanya. Two months before Tanya was born the union called and told me they had scheduled the hairdressing exam. I was excited and thrilled. I was also huge, my belly sticking out so far I could hardly reach beyond it.

I took my model with me to Warner Brothers Studio for the test. It was in the evening. I was assigned to a tiny room where I was given directions about what to do: create a hairstyle from a certain time period, use hairpieces, and put on a wig so that it was secure. I applied a man's hairpiece, a toupee, and a small fall (hair that went on the back of a man's hair). Then at the end of the evening an oral test was given and when we got to that part I was so exhausted I almost lost it. It was near 11:00 p.m. when we finished and the question I was asked was what do you do with a wet wig. The correct answer was to put it on a wig block so that it doesn't shrink. (We didn't use synthetic wigs in those days.) In my sleepy state I answered, "Dry it I guess." Quickly I recovered and realized the right answer and corrected myself. They took pity on me because of my condition and gave me credit for the right answer.

I passed. Hooray! I wanted to jump up and down. I was filled with joy. Attending the union meeting in November, I expected to be sworn in as a member, but there wasn't a quorum, so I had to wait until December. Tanya was born on November 27, 1960, so it was a slimmer me who was finally sworn in as a proper union member that December.

Chapter 6

HURRAH! I'M A HAIRDRESSER!
1962

What a journey! Reaching my goal was no small accomplishment for a Gemini who got sidetracked often. My union membership was secure and now I could work in the studios. It had taken six years of hard work to accomplish what now felt like a miracle. I was where I wanted to be and it had been well worth the effort. Now it was a matter of waiting for a call from the union, which kept a list of available hairdressers. When an employer needed a hairstylist, the union was called for the availability list. We didn't have answering machines in those days so I had to stick close to the phone so I wouldn't miss that all-important call.

MGM called first. They were filming a remake of *Mutiny on the Bounty* starring Marlon Brando. The head hairstylists assigned to the film were Lorraine Roberson and Donna McDonough. They were top of the line stylists because nearly all of the actors were wearing hair lace wigs that take a lot of work and care. Every night at the end of the shooting the wigs had to be cleaned and the hair lace pinned on a wig block so it would shrink back into place and fit the actor in the morning.

There was an opening for a hairdresser to do night work dressing the wigs. I was offered the job. I had to work in the snake pit that was dark and creepy enough during the day, but at night it was worse. I would be all alone down there. Once I descended into the "pit" the only person I saw was the policeman making his nightly rounds. Sometimes an art class was held there which provided a little company, but that was rare. Most of the time the radio was my only companion.

Each wig had been meticulously designed and made for the individual actor. The hair was specially picked out and mixed together as nobody's hair is just one single color. The wig maker ventilated the wigs, hooking one hair at a time to the net. It was expensive - at that time wigs cost $400. Now they run into thousands of dollars.

Every evening at the wrap of the day's work, Donna and Lorraine would come in and give me directions about how they wanted the wigs dressed. Donna was more particular than Lorraine. Sometimes I felt she was too demanding, but later when I was putting my own wigs on actors, I understood how important it was to have a curl fall exactly the same way each day. Most hairstylists preferred to style their own wigs, but with this large a group of actors it would have taken them most of the night.

Work wasn't steady. I'd go in for a period of time then production would slow and I'd be laid off. It was disappointing when that happened, but if a scene only had two people it was silly to call me in for work since I had to be paid for an eight-hour minimum. In addition I was at the bottom of the list along with a few other new girls.

After a few months, it was time for the crew of the *Bounty* to pack up and fly off to Tahiti for on-location filming. Lorraine and Donna wanted me to go with them. It would be for about three months. What a dilemma. Ever since reading about Gauguin, the painter who moved to Tahiti, I'd wanted to go to there. But what about my family, my babies? Later that day, while holding Tanya and Laurie on my lap, I told my husband about the offer. I thought my heart would break if I left them for such a long time. I wanted Bill to tell me "no" that he couldn't handle it alone, but he didn't. Instead he was kind and said, "We can manage if you really want to do this." No easy way out for me. I cried and cried. I didn't want to make the wrong decision. Fortunately it was made for me. The production didn't want to spend the money for another hairstylist so I couldn't go. What a relief!

After the *Bounty* crew left I began work on several different shows that were filming on the MGM lot. I was now one of the hairstylists who came in for daily calls. I carried a hair dressing case, really a piece of luggage that held just about everything I could possibly need: scissors, curling irons and stove, combs, brushes, hairpins, bobby pins, hairnets, hair sprays, crepe wool, liquid adhesive, spirit gum (glue for wigs), wig bands, and more. It's amazing how much stuff we needed. The case was heavy to carry but heaven help us if we were caught in an emergency without these necessities.

Ordinarily we had to be ready to work by 6:00 a.m. which meant getting up at 4:00 a.m. at the latest. We'd set up our hairdressing stations on tables, have coffee, and wait for the extras to pour in. The extras picked out their favorite hairstylist and would try to come to the same person each day. This made it possible to match the previous day's work. Most extras were professionals but there was the occasional flake that showed up with a hangover, still reeking with alcohol from the previous night's binge. I'd try to hold my breath until I finished with one of them. But most of the extras were great. Of course everyone wanted his or her wig to be comfortable because the days were long. I'd put myself in their places, unable to imagine myself wearing a wig all day long, so I was kind and took pains to use the minimum number of pins and still have the wig stay on all day.

We began the huge extravaganza, *How the West Was Won* and there were movie crews traveling all around the United States. Some were in South Dakota filming the buffalo. Others were down south. Our western segment called for lots of Indians to be wigged and made up plus these poor guys had to strip down to their skivvies so their skin could be sprayed a reddish bronze. How they hated it!

The first opportunity to go on location came when I was offered the job on the television series *Rawhide* starring Clint Eastwood and Sheb Wooley. Flying to Pasa Robles was exciting; I'd never before flown in a plane. It was a tiny commuter plane that took off and landed three times before we reached Pasa Robles. Our motel was brand new. I was shown to a nice room next to Sheb Wooley whom I found mightily attractive. No adjoining doors though, darn. The makeup man was Don Schoenfield, one of my favorites. On location, the atmosphere was more relaxed than in town on a stage. Everyone worked hard but it was as though all our cares were left behind at home. I had time and energy to work and play hard and lots of per diem to spend on myself.

Each segment of *Rawhide* had a different woman guest who would fly up for her part. It was my job to do her hair. Men didn't usually have hairstylists do their hair in those days unless they were wearing a wig or an unusual style. The hair and makeup would be done in a motel room and then we'd go to the location site, which was usually hot and dusty. One day we had a whole herd of cattle working with us.

I could hardly believe it when one day I found myself sitting beside the pool having a conversation with Burgess Meredith. Even though he had worked all over the world, he appeared happy just sitting by the pool at the motel talking with me. He was a man who lived in the moment.

While on location the company paid for my room and gave us a generous per diem for meals. We were expected to be able to eat at one of the best restaurants in town. One evening Burgess Meredith and Paul Brennigan (who played the cook) invited me to join them for dinner. This was steak country and I ordered a big, juicy, rare steak. When the bill came, we divided it among the three of us. They treated me as an equal - just one of the crew.

At night after the wrap we acted like high school kids. There were two cliques that formed. The Fun Group and "the others." Luckily I was invited to be a part of the Fun Group and we named ourselves "The Cheap Screw Club." The name came to us because each of us had to procure free things to bring to the parties we held each night. When it was my turn, I talked the bartender into giving me the stale popcorn left over from the night before. Clint Eastwood, his friend Bill Tompkins (also his stand-in), and Sheb Wooley were part of our group. We brought our own wine, beer, or whatever. We'd sit in someone's hotel room, laugh, sing, and talk.

The location was all too short for me and soon we returned to the studio.

Chapter 7
On My Own
1961

With very few exceptions, all hairstylists were women and all makeup people were men. Without exception on the lot a makeup man was department head of both groups, hair and makeup. The makeup men made more money than the hairstylists.

There were very few female crewmembers on the set and so hairdressers got lots of male attention. They enjoyed our company. The older hairdressers were usually nice to us, but sometimes jealousy got the better of them. The men tended to pay attention to the newcomers. Occasionally, the older hairdressers saw a naive young woman being the center of attraction and warned her to be careful. The advice often went unheeded and hearts got broken. Depending on whom we worked with, we were often criticized for the littlest thing so we had to watch our step.

At MGM, our department head, Mary Keats, wanted us to be dignified at work. She wanted us to look and act respectable. The stages or sets were dusty and dirty and it seemed silly to be so dressed up, but those were our orders so we obeyed or we were not called back.

I'd arrive at work wearing stockings, a girdle (no panty hose then), high-heeled shoes and a nice dress. Our days were long, and we had to stand up most of the day; the chairs provided on the set were only for the actors and the director. By the end of the day my feet were killing me and I could hardly wait to hurry home, remove my girdle, and change into something comfortable. Years later we got smart and began to carry little canvas stools to sit on.

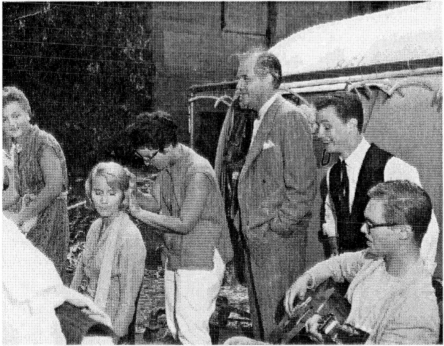

On the set of *All Fall Down*: (left to right) Angela Lansbury, Eva Marie Saint, Ginger, Karl Malden, (Not Identified), Brandon De Wilde

The summer of 1961, Mary decided I was ready to do a film of my own. This didn't mean I was going to design the hairstyles, it meant I would stand by an actress on the set all day long once the hair had been done in the main department. They finally figured out I was capable of doing hair. My first film was *All Fall Down* with Angela Lansbury, Karl Malden, Eva Marie Saint, Brandon De Wilde and a newcomer named Warren Beatty.

First thing in the morning I'd report to the hairdressing department and set things up for Sydney while he dressed Eva Marie Saint's hair. I would standby patiently and quietly and while Sydney talked and worked; I'd hand him the hairpins he needed. Being in his presence, watching his beautiful hands and his way of iron curling inspired me. He'd put Angela Lansbury's hairpiece, called a fall, on the back of her head. It fit perfectly and the rest of her hair was curled around it so it looked completely natural.

Sydney did all the talking. I tried to be quiet, which wasn't easy for me, but I succeeded most of the time. I'd been warned to let him do the talking, so I did. Sydney had always been kind to me when others weren't so I was willing to play along. It prepared me for the future when I'd be working with stars on my own.

When everyone was finished with makeup and hair, I went down to the set and was totally attentive to my actresses all day long. Making sure the hair remained just as Sydney had done it in the morning. If something needed to be changed, I'd call him to come down and make the adjustment.

John Frankenheimer, a tall, lanky, intense young man, directed the film. It was one of his first film directing jobs. Up until then he'd done fabulous, live television work on *Playhouse 90* and television shows like that. Film was different. He scared me to death; he was so wild plus he appeared to hate hairstylists. It was nothing personal. He just didn't want me or the makeup artist on the set at all; we had to sneak around to get our work done. I had hidden combs and mirrors on the set for Eva Marie so she could get a glimpse of herself and call me if she needed a repair. Maybe John, the director, didn't care about hair matching from one scene to the next, but it was important and it was my job.

Since Jack Freeman, the makeup man, and I'd been banned from the set, I would read and sometimes wander around behind the set often bumping into the cameraman, Curly Linden, who always looked annoyed when he saw me. Years later I realized he was a drinker and I must have been interrupting his nips. No wonder he was annoyed. He was a crusty character who would ask rude questions like, "Do you think you're worth the money you make? How much do you make an hour?" It wasn't any of his business, but he intimidated me and I'd reply, "Yes, I'm worth my pay." But in reality I wasn't yet sure.

Sitting around talking with the actors was the highlight of my day. Brandon de Wilde was very young and a terrific actor. I had no doubt he would be a huge success, but he died very young. It was an incredible loss. Warren Beatty was often complaining about something or other. Watching him one day, Eva Marie surmised that acting was really a feminine thing and it was difficult for men to accept all aspects of what was required. She felt that all the makeup, hair - dressing, and fussing went against what was usually done for men, so they became uncomfortable with it.

Warren Beatty was amusing, but he was also very difficult. The rest of the stars were old timers and well known. Brandon was young and such a great kid. Eva, Angela, and Karl were terrific and so professional that they often made Warren look worse. One day Warren had a scene to do with Eva Marie. The master shot had already been filmed and they were doing close-ups. Eva had finished her close-ups and was off stage doing her part for Warren's close-up. Normally Eva was sweet and relaxed. On this particular day Warren just couldn't seem to get it right. There were twenty-four takes, and in the end Eva was distressed and exhausted. When she finally finished, she came into the dressing room where I was sitting and closed the door. She was nearly hysterical from the stress of trying to help Warren get that scene right.

Warren was rather arrogant. One day on location at a gas station an onlooker for George Hamilton mistook him. Perfect! We all laughed. He'd been put in his place. Looking back now I can see Warren already knew already exactly where he was going career-wise. At one point the crew went on location to Florida for a few days. I didn't go, but heard that John, the director, had seized an opportunity to leave Warren locked in a jail cell after he had finished a scene in the cell. Warren was learning the hard way.

It felt great to have my first whole film under my belt. I didn't get any screen credit though; in those days only Sydney or department heads received credit on the screen.

At the end of shooting this film I walked up to John Frankenheimer and confessed, "You don't scare me anymore." John was surprised to hear that he had scared me at all, but then he hadn't known how insecure I was in the beginning.

How the West Was Won continued in saga style and when I finished *All Fall Down* I was assigned to go on location to Ouray, Colorado. By this time I had a terrific housekeeper, Josephina who was from Mexico, to care for my girls and Bill was working in town. We'd only be gone three weeks.

We landed in Montrose, Colorado, and were met by a chauffeured limo. We were all exhausted by the time we arrived in Ouray. It had been a long ride up into the mountains to our "home" at the Box Canyon Motel. The motel, located at the bottom of a hill, was only adequate. I shared a room with Sherry Wilson, an old friend. When we got settled, we noticed our room tilted toward the front of the motel. In fact, it tilted so much that the first night Sherry rolled out of bed. We discovered what the problem was, but there was nothing we could do. Apparently the motel had been built in the winter when the ground was frozen. In the spring when things thawed out the motel had settled at a tilt. Sherry slept with a pillow at her side so she wouldn't roll out again.

It was cold and dark the first morning and we walked up the hill looking for the café where we were going to eat breakfast. I was out of breath, because of the high altitude, and could hardly make it up the hill. We spied the brightly - lit café, already filled with wranglers and other crewmembers, and hurried toward it. After filling up on hot cereal, eggs, and coffee, off we went to get our Indian wigs ready.

Henry Hathaway, the director of this segment loved to yell and scream. We wanted to make him happy. We carefully researched material from the library. We wanted to make the Indians' hairstyles authentic. Weaving feathers and beads into the braids, we turned out some fabulous wigs and had a lot of fun creating them.

At a dress rehearsal we took our "Indians" to show Henry. We proudly paraded our Indians in front of Henry, sure that he would be as pleased as possible. We were mistaken. Henry hated what we had done. He stated flatly that he didn't care if the styles were authentic; he wanted them to look like "movie" Indians. Back to the drawing board. We gave him the standard braided look with headbands and he approved. So much for our artistic endeavors.

After we finished the wigs there was a delay in shooting and some of us were sent back to Los Angeles for a few days. I didn't want to go, but had no choice. It represented a savings to the company. One week later they had to fly us back. On the return trip something happened that made me aware of people's egos and it disappointed and hurt me a lot.

When we landed in Montrose we were met by a car, but this time it was just an ordinary station wagon. I ended up sitting in the middle of the front seat. It was getting dark and the driver handed me a message he'd been given by the production assistant. Since it was dark and I was the only one near the dash light, I read the message out loud to everyone in the car. It instructed us to report to work the next morning at 6 a.m. The makeup man, Don Cash, Sr., who was sitting in the back seat, said nothing, just listened. There was no discussion.

The message meant that by the time we got to the motel and finished our day we would have less than eight hours off before our call in the morning. This put us on what is known as a "force call" costing the company double time pay for our salaries the next day. The assistant who sent the note had assumed we would be on time. Don realized that it would be a problem and because he considered himself our boss, he should have brought up the problem, but he chose to keep his mouth shut.

The next day we all reported to work as directed. Stan Smith, my old friend and the makeup man in charge of production, came up to me, "Who do you think you are giving out calls?" I was shocked. I thought Stan and I were good friends. "All I did was read the message." "Yeah, well that's the same as giving the call." I asked him why Don hadn't cleared it up at the time and then it dawned on me - Don thought I was an upstart and wanted to get me into trouble. I was upset that Stan couldn't see what had really happened. I never trusted Don again.

Eventually we got settled in and went off to work. Our first site was in a little park where there was the local jail, the size of an outhouse. Our sheriff, dressed in a deep-blue, wrinkled shirt, baggy pants, and a very loose belt strutted about. From his belt hung his gun that dangled and swung between his legs. I hoped for his sake that it wasn't loaded.

In spite of the mix-ups at the beginning, life on that location was lots of fun. On the way home we'd buy humongous steaks and then sit outside in the evenings enjoying great meals, drinking wine, and relaxing.

On our day off we took a jeep ride through aspens and hardwoods toward Silverton. It was wonderful. We hiked up a mountain, but I had to stop half way up the hill. As I sat there all alone on a log, in the forest the rain began to fall softly and it felt mystical. It was so peaceful and quiet that I realized how badly I had needed that time alone. On location we were always with people, so busy and I was learning that quiet, peaceful moments were important.

We worked long and hard, twelve hours most days, taking advantage of every minute of daylight to film. The wranglers (cowboys who took care of the horses) were exhausted. After we finished shooting at night and were on our way home, they still had to put the horses to bed and then get them on the set early in the morning. One wrangler said he felt as if he'd just taken off his boots, thrown them across to the other side of the bed, then walked around and put them right back on without sleeping in between. I didn't envy them.

Debbie Reynolds was our saving grace. When Hathaway would scream at someone, she had a way that would calm him down. Her humor and sweetness won him over. We were extremely grateful. Hathaway reminded me of my father when he blew up. I'd always tried to avoid my father when he was mad. But Henry was our director so we had to stay there.

One day we moved to our location near the mountains. The wind blew all day long. I went into the honey wagon (combination trailer, restroom, and dressing rooms) and took a look at my face. It was dark brown, covered with dust except where my glasses had been. The day was difficult and it was exhausting work trying to keep our Indians looking good in all that wind. The next morning we got quite a shock. Looking out the window we saw three feet of unexpected snow on the ground. We packed up and flew home to Los Angeles the very next day.

Chapter 8

HOW THE WEST WAS WON
LONE PINE, 1961

Although traveling was a passion with me, I felt uncomfortable being away from my family. I often felt sad when I was not with my girls. I didn't have time to miss them while working and I was so exhausted at night, I was grateful for the quiet, but sometimes it was difficult to combine my two worlds.

Josephina, our housekeeper from Mexico, was a godsend. She looked to be in her fifties; perhaps she was younger. The years and her hard life had taken a great toll on her. Her hair was black and she wore it in two long braids. The first day we spent together, I sat at the table, dictionary in hand, trying to make conversation in Spanish and answer her questions. I'd studied French in school, but not Spanish. We worked things out, but that evening I tried to tell her, in Spanish, that I could see she was tired and had done enough for one day. In reality, I ended up telling her that she looked dirty, not tired. She laughed and laughed at my mistake. In time I learned to speak what I called kitchen Spanish.

When Josephina first came to us from Mexico, she told us about her four daughters living in Tijuana. Ernestina, the oldest, was fifteen and took care of her younger sisters while her mother was gone. One weekend we went down to meet them and see where they lived - a little wooden shack without running water. There was only a large bottle of Sparkletts water from which they drank and bathed. Electricity consisted of one light on an extension cord stretched across the yard from a neighbor's house. In spite of all the hardships the girls were clean and more content now that their mother had a job and could support them. Josephina used to go down to see them once a month. I was always nervous, praying that she would be able to get back across the border. She didn't have a green card, and it was always possible she'd get caught. She wore two dresses and carried very little so the border guards would think she was only crossing for the day.

On our drive home from Tijuana that night, I began to feel guilty. This woman was taking such good care of my kids while her children were down there all alone. At that moment we decided to help them immigrate and move in with us. The process took a year.

In anticipation of the girls' arrival we bought a huge upright freezer. When they arrived, I showed them around the house and pointed out the full freezer in the garage. We had bought two sets of bunk beds for Josephina's room. It was crowded, but that didn't matter to them, they were happy to be together. Now, despite my absences, it was easier for me, I felt my girls had plenty of family when I was gone.

A few weeks after being snowed out of Colorado we were notified the work would continue in Lone Pine, California. We packed up all our supplies and this time we went on a long bus ride to Lone Pine. Our crew filled the whole town. Motels everywhere were having a wonderful off-season business thanks to us. The makeup and hair people were put into a large motel on the edge of town. I was still rooming with Sherry, which made us both happy.

Lone Pine had a detention camp that had been set up for the Japanese/American citizens during the Second World War and it hadn't been used much since then. This camp became our makeup and wardrobe departments. It was convenient and fit our needs. We had six hairstylists working on the Indians alone. The other hairstylists and makeup worked on the stars in other places.

Each morning, two hundred Indians arrived to be wigged and made up. There were Indian wigs hanging like scalps everywhere, even from the ceiling. We'd report to work at 3:30 a.m. each morning and as soon as the cooks had something ready we'd have to eat breakfast. Union rules stated that we had to eat every six hours or there would be a meal penalty. We couldn't possibly stop to eat while we were dressing the hair, so we had to eat first. Ugh! Who wanted to eat so early? It almost turned my stomach. To make matters worse, we had to take our food back to the hair room and eat among the wigs. I'm sure we each ate at least one Indian wig by the time we finished those scenes.

Navajos transported from Arizona played our Indians. They lived in the camp and each morning lined up for breakfast, helping themselves to huge amounts of white bread along with everything else. They'd eat first and then show up at our place all showered, wearing clean, white shirts. They didn't seem to mind the wigs, but hated getting sprayed with the body makeup out in the cold. I couldn't blame them. There were always hoots and hollers and I'd wonder if it was the makeup men or the Navajos.

Around 9:00 a.m. we'd load up our stuff and get on a bus heading for location, which was way out of town. By that time we'd already been working for five and a half hours.

The first morning we arrived at the set, Hathaway was in one of his booming tempers. Stan was trying to be quiet because he had a terrible hangover. Hathaway yelled, "Who did this man's makeup?" Pointing at one actor, he screamed, "It's terrible. Get up here." Stan walked up to Henry reluctantly, looking as if he was going to his own execution. I was glad it wasn't me, and I felt sorry for him. Hathaway berated him up one side and down the other. The makeup couldn't possibly have been that bad. Hathaway's wrath was something to be avoided at all costs. Just in case, after that, I found some horse feathers used to decorate the horses' manes. I carried these in my back pocket. My plan, if I ever got yelled at, was to hand the feathers to Hathaway and say, "Oh horse feathers" and then I would walk away quickly and hitch a ride back to Los Angeles. Fortunately it never happened.

Our older hairdresser supervisor, Marie kept after us and made sure the wigs were on securely. The Indians rode horseback so fast, if one of those wigs should fall off while they were filming a huge charge on horses over a hill, Heaven Help Us. I'd stand and talk with gorgeous Gregory Peck who was working with us on this segment. His lovely voice was wonderful to hear and I loved to talk with him.

Evenings were great. Sherry met a gorgeous stunt man, Chuck Roberson, and was falling in love. Chuck stood in for John Wayne. Stunt men were always nice to us in those days simply because they liked women and always appreciated a comfortable wig. I even found my perfect dance partner one night - a huge cowboy who swung me around and I felt light as a feather. My husband Bill always made me feel clumsy when I danced, but this man made me proud of myself.

In the evenings we all gathered to eat and drink at a local bar. One evening a camera assistant took me to dinner after filling me up with "apple knockers" (vodka and apple juice) and finger sandwiches left over from our box lunches. I didn't realize how much I'd had to drink until I sat down to dinner. All of a sudden the alcohol hit me and my head began to spin; I headed for the door and cold air. My friend followed me, but when he realized I wasn't going to feel better any time soon, he took me home. Once safely back in my room I went into the bathroom where I knocked over my bottle of Vitamin C. I left the vitamins on the floor. When Sherry came in later, she found me sleeping very soundly. She was afraid I'd overdosed on vitamins. I'd overdosed all right, but not on vitamins!

Every night was a party and we all went. We weren't going to get enough sleep with those 3:30 a.m. calls anyway. Stan thought we were crazy, but actually he was just too cheap to join us. When we were told to stay out of the way at work, we'd climb on the bus and snooze. One night I actually tried going to sleep early and I felt awful the next day so I never did that again. Because we were all young, the momentum and excitement carried us through without much sleep. I was cheerful in the mornings so I was given the job of making sure the rest of our crew was up and ready to go on time. I'd knock quietly on each door and when I got an answer I'd go to the next door. Nobody was ever late.

A month after we had been back home a driver who had been on our location told my husband that he'd seen me coming out of a room, not my own, early in the morning. What a troublemaker! Luckily Bill wasn't jealous and I'd already told him about my waking up the others. That was a good example of how easily trouble could get started on location. I never understood why anyone would do that though.

The location was unique and we shared experiences that brought us all very close. One night the local Indians challenged our Navajos to a dance duel. The whole crew went into Lone Pine to watch. They built a huge bonfire and it was a fantastic sight watching the tribes drumming, dancing, singing, each trying to out-do the other.

When I first began as a stockroom clerk in the Makeup Department I wondered why there was so much hugging and kissing when Makeup and Hair got together on the big calls. It had all seemed so phony to me. As time passed, I realized how much I had grown to love my co-workers and I, too, was ready with big hugs and kisses when we rediscovered each other.

Chapter 9

The Birds
1962

The location in Lone Pine had been an exciting experience. I'd been busy at work and play. Now, back home in Los Angeles, each morning I'd get into my car and drive to work feeling sort of depressed. Life was so dull. When I reported to the Makeup Department, all I could think of was that I wanted to be on location all the time.

Meanwhile, *Mutiny on the Bounty* had returned from Tahiti after being on location for six months. Now I began working on the set, no longer banned to the snake pit at night. On gigantic Stage 30 at MGM, a huge mockup of the ship Bounty had been built. There was a tank that held tons of water. It was an impressive sight. The only way to get up on the deck of the ship was to climb a tall, steep ladder. I complained to Mary, our department head, telling her that it would be best to wear slacks on the set even though she had instructed us to dress nicely. She said, "No, it isn't lady - like." Sarcastically I asked, "Is it lady - like to walk up the ladder and have all the fellows look up our skirts?" Mary, who hadn't done much production work, stubbornly replied, "Just have the actors come down to you." What a joke! Working in the department hadn't prepared Mary for real life on the set.

In *Bounty*, Paul Baxley doubled for Marlon Brando who wore his hair long in the back in a little tail tied with a black ribbon. Paul's hair was shorter than Marlon's so I had to attach a tiny hairpiece to the back of his head. The hairdressers had brought some small French clips from Tahiti to secure the extra hair to his head. The clips held the hairpiece on the head tightly making it nearly impossible to pull loose. That was until one day when disaster fell upon me. Although I had painstakingly secured the hairpiece, it fell off. In the scene Paul was supposed to run out on the deck while the ship was burning and a sail would fall on him. He had to pull the piece of the sail off, and then jump into the sea below. It was a major stunt. Each time the ship was set ablaze, it was a complicated special effect process. The ship had been lined with pipes out of which flames shot and the ship actually looked like it was burning. It was very realistic and quite scary.

Each time they called ROLL ACTION, there were complicated problems. CUT! RESET! ONCE AGAIN! Finally the scene seemed to be working. Paul ran out on the deck, as the sail fell, he caught it, wrestled with it, and finally tore it off and leapt into the sea. But horror of horrors, Paul no longer was wearing his tail. It had come off when he pulled the sail off his head. I was mortified. I'd been responsible for ruining the scene. I felt for sure my career was finished before it started. Paul explained that he'd had a problem and had been afraid of getting burned so he had pulled off the hair in his haste. It wasn't my fault and in fact nobody was angry with me. Still I considered myself a failure. They found the little tail in the water and brought it to me. I put it on and we did many more takes. The tail never fell off again.

Peter Hurkos, the spiritualist, visited the set one-day. He walked by me and said, "I know something about you that you don't even know yet." He never did explain, but he was telling the truth - something that I didn't know yet - I was pregnant with my youngest daughter, Xochi.

Some Tahitians had come to Los Angeles with the crew. I loved them. They were like happy children, having a wonderful time. One of the men liked me and he would often go into my purse, take out my makeup, and put on lipstick and rouge amusing us and making us all laugh. They danced for us and I often wanted to join them.

The crew left for location for the second time and returned a few months later. I worked with them again this last time. That crew had been together for over a year by then and the film was still far from finished. It had turned into a lifetime job. Everyone was burned out. Marriages had broken up, affairs started and ended. It was too long a job for anyone. On the last day the producer was directing while the director, Lewis Milestone, was sitting behind the set talking to us. At the wrap the producer extended no thanks to the crew. Everyone just sighed in relief that it was finally over.

I kept on working on different projects around MGM, filling in here and there. Finally things slowed down to a halt and I was laid off. My next call came from Revue, the television arm of Universal Studios. I liked going to different studios. I especially liked the fact that they treated me with respect. No matter what I did at MGM, I was always remembered as the youngster in the stockroom. I didn't have that stigma anywhere else.

The people I had met in my travels around the studios were kind to me. I think they remembered my consideration for them when they had first begun working at MGM. That helped me a great deal with finding work and also when I had needed help.

One day I had a call on *The Virginian*. The star was James Drury, my old friend from my messenger days. He was friendly and we talked a little. He said he'd ask for me to work on the show. Of course he didn't and I knew it, but that was okay.

While working on *Frontier Circus* I met John Derek, who was truly beautiful to behold. Since it was a circus theme, wild animals were brought to the set each week. Working near them was great fun. We worked long hours, outside at night. Being pregnant, I wasn't feeling great all the time, but I was grateful for the work. Bill wasn't always able to find work and it was nearing time for the annual spring layoff.

One Thursday I was at home when the union contacted me for a Friday afternoon call at Universal. Virginia Darcy, my friend since MGM days, had given me the call. She had been Grace Kelly's hairstylist and had gone to Monaco for Grace's wedding wearing a hat covered in cherries. She did tend to stand out in a crowd.

Taking that call was the luckiest thing I could have done. People didn't like to accept a Friday call because it could mess up their unemployment for that week, but at that point I'd have taken anything. Virginia hired me and I ended up working on *The Birds* all through the spring while many others, including Bill, were out of work. Once I was hired, I wasn't likely to be laid off during the filming. It was perfect. My job on the film was quite simple. All I had to do was keep people looking messy. They had to look as if the birds had chased them. Alfred Hitchcock, the director, was an odd person, distant with the crew, but fun to work with and quite brilliant.

By that time I was getting very round due to the advanced stage of my pregnancy and I became worried, assuming I'd have to quit. I'd never seen a pregnant hairdresser on the set or, for that matter, anywhere around in the film business. We really needed the money, but my girdle was killing me. I knew I had to confess my situation to Virginia - and it was so easy! She said, "Oh, I worked when I was pregnant and you can, too." I sighed with relief as I threw away the girdle and changed into loose maternity clothes and breathed freely once again.

As soon as I told everyone I was expecting, I began to expand rapidly. Hitchcock remarked to Virginia, "I hope your assistant doesn't have her baby during a five - minute take!" When Virginia told me that, I though it was quite funny. One day when I saw Mr. Hitchcock standing alone, I walked up to him and said, "Mr. Hitchcock, I assure you I won't have this baby during your five - minute take." I must have embarrassed him because Virginia later asked me not to repeat that he'd also mentioned to her he'd like to put me on the treadmill and see what happened. I held my tongue. Actually, I really would have liked to have a photo of the portly Mr. Hitchcock and myself belly-to-belly. I doubted he'd go for it so I never mentioned it.

Rod Taylor was the star of *The Birds* along with the lovely Tippi Hendren. Both of them were exceptionally nice to work with. One of our extra girls had a crush on Rod and she would hang out in his dressing room. He was going out with Anita Eckberg at the time. Anita was a beautiful Scandinavian, Amazon-like woman. We all wondered what would happen if she ever found that girl in Rod's dressing room. The day finally came when Anita made her entrance. We were always sitting around talking while the birds were being arranged around the set. As we sat facing the dressing room, Anita entered the set. We all looked at one another and said a prayer that she wouldn't find the extra girl in Rod's dressing room. She opened the door to the dressing room and we all giggled nervously. Evidently she didn't find the girl. The extra showed up on the set the next day in one piece, no bruises or broken bones. But we did notice she didn't stick as close to Rod as before. We had great fun watching the drama and had difficulty stifling our laughter.

All my life, it seemed as though I'd been trying to diet. Now being pregnant it was worse. I was always hungry. It didn't help that we talked about food all day long. One day we had hours to sit because they had to have a hundred crows sitting atop a roof. Each crow had to be tied down by one foot. Another day they had to put hundreds of finches down a chimney and, although the set was covered in plastic, many escaped and flew up into the rafters, their chirps haunting the sound mixer from then on. Each scene took so much preparation that as a result we worked very little each day.

George, the camera operator who appeared to be a big, gruff man, brought me a lovely wicker bassinet his children had used. Everyone on the crew was excited about my baby. I was so happy working with that crew. Plus, the money got us through the spring, thanks to Virginia.

Bill had landed a job in props on *My Three Sons*, a television series with Fred MacMurray. Gene Reynolds, who became a favorite of mine, produced it. As I finished *The Birds*, the hairdressing job on that series opened up and I took it gladly. I'd never worked when I was pregnant before, but this time I felt so much better, work just seemed to agree with me. The crew was amusing, and they treated me with such care. They were always sure I had a chair, they'd pull cables out of the way so I could walk easily; they mothered me. Normally I was treated like one of the boys, but not this time.

Laurie and Tanya, now five and two years old, came in to work and met the crew. We had lunch in the commissary and Don, one of the "sons," saw me sitting at the counter with my belly hidden. He laughed and said, "Now I know how you'll look after you have the baby."

After I finished working on that show, I was sure I was finished with work until the baby was born. Then I got a desperate call from a company to do a Palmolive commercial. I told them I was very pregnant and not feeling too peppy. They said it would be okay as the hours were short. I accepted the job and quit only two weeks before my daughter Xochi arrived.

Earlier that summer we had gone to a Union dance and I learned to dance the Twist. It was easy for me. My belly went one way and I went another. While I was at the dance, Lorraine Roberson with whom I'd worked on *Mutiny on the Bounty* came over and placed her hands on my tummy, asking when the baby was due. She wanted me to help on her next film. I told her the baby was due in the middle of August and that I'd need at least six weeks after the birth before I came back to work.

Xochi arrived on August 17, 1962. What a darling baby! I was seldom able to hold her because our Josephina's daughters loved her so much. The only time I had with her was when she was nursing. My family felt complete. I had three daughters to love. And, although I worked long hours, there was always time to enjoy my girls in the evenings and on weekends.

Chapter 10

McLINTOCK!
1962

Three phone calls from Lorraine and nearly three months after Xochi was born, I accepted a job on *McLintock!* The first call came too soon after Xochi was born, the second was during the Cuban Missile Crisis and I didn't want to be away from my family if there was to be a war. The third time she called and told me the job would last a week, so I accepted. My kids were in loving hands. As it turned out, I was gone two weeks.

McLintock! was the story of a cattle baron who ran a whole town, but couldn't control his own wife, a western *Taming of the Shrew*. John Wayne and Maureen O'Hara were the stars with Andy McLagen as the director. Most of Maureen's big scenes had already been shot by the time I arrived. John Wayne was a real presence on the set and although he wasn't the director, he influenced everything that happened. Maureen was a beautiful, vivacious redhead. There were lots of tall, handsome, rugged cowboys on the set and I felt quite dainty when I stood next to them.

Our set was Old Tucson, a western movie town built out in the middle of nowhere. For years it had been used to make movies and it was also a tourist attraction with daily shows of gunfights, stunt falls, and such. The town had a saloon, a restaurant, and shops that sold saddles and other Western horse-related stuff, like old-fashioned hardware, and candies. It had a railroad station with old coaches and horses and cattle. It occurred to me this was what it was like when my father had been a sheriff in Oklahoma back in 1890. It was great to experience what the old west might have felt like to him.

There were lots of cactuses. When I first arrived, I was warned to watch out for the cactus - STAY AWAY FROM IT! Even with all the warnings, the cactus would jump out and attack me. I never learned to avoid it completely. My favorite was the huge Saguaro that stood so tall and proud. I always felt as if they were beings from the past. They brought back childhood memories of cacti dancing through the Disney film, *The Three Caballeros.*

Although there were plenty of stunt men from Hollywood, many local cowboys had been hired. The scenes with horses galloping through narrow streets, where the action was fast and dangerous frightened me. The Hollywood stunt men were worried; they knew how to look out for one another if someone fell. But the local riders were not so aware and they often thought things would look better on film if they were more reckless. It was fast and furious when they all rode together down the streets of Old Tucson in a wild rampage.

There was always a first aid person on the set in case of an accident. Union rules. It was necessary when we were shooting stunts in the country away from hospitals. The person they hired was a doozy. He was supposed to be a doctor, but that was questionable. He was a mess, always hung over, incapable of helping anyone in an emergency. The stunt men promised each other they wouldn't let him touch them if they got hurt. Instead, they'd help each other. Luckily nothing awful happened so the doctor wasn't needed for more than an occasional aspirin, and we usually had to wake him up to get it.

Chuck Roberson, John Wayne's double whom I'd met on *How the West Was Won,* was there looking very handsome as usual - actually more handsome than John Wayne himself. In the beginning, John Wayne seemed very harsh to me. For example, one day he stuffed a raw egg in Curly's (one of the stunt men) mouth and then told him to ride without breaking it. It almost made me gag. I didn't think it was a bit funny. I wasn't sure if I liked the Duke or not, but I did enjoy working on "his" film.

One day we were all weary and the sky looked as if it might rain. We wanted to go home early so we talked the Navajos into doing a rain dance. Miraculously it worked. The rain poured down and we wrapped early. Was it a coincidence? Who knows?

On my day off, two stunt men, Chuck Hayward and Jerry Gatlin, invited me to go to lunch with them. They decided to have some fun with me. I'd never eaten Jalapeno peppers before and they were aware of this. They took me to a little café where they stuffed the fresh peppers with things like tuna and olives. They were so tasty I couldn't stop eating them. We had lots of beer and lots of those peppers and other great Mexican food. On the way home they took me for ice cream. I was puzzled at this and they explained that the next day I would be saying to myself, "Come on ice cream."

I didn't get it then, but the next day I did. The result of eating all those peppers was horrific every time I went to the restroom and I finally understood why they said I'd be saying, "Come on ice cream." They laughed and laughed knowing what I was going through. I won't explain my discomfort, but soon I began to laugh with them. From then on I was more cautious.

The motel where we were staying had a huge bar with lots of round leather booths built for the movie crews. We'd rush home from work, shower off the day's dust, and then meet in the bar for a few drinks where we'd sit in a booth and play a game that was lots of fun. It involved taking a paper napkin and securing it over the top of a glass with a rubber band. A quarter was placed on the napkin. Then someone lit a cigarette and burned a hole in the napkin, carefully passing the glass and the cigarette around the table. Whoever dropped the quarter in the glass by burning the last bit of napkin, bought a round of drinks. We spent hours playing this game.

The local cowgirls loved the stunt men. Who wouldn't? And we loved to tease the guys about it. The local girls would come into the bar wearing the tightest pants we'd ever seen. One had her eye on Jerry Gatlin and he was worried. She was impossible and he couldn't avoid her. She wore the tightest pants of all. They looked as if they'd been spray painted on. We assured Jerry he had no worries - she'd never get to him, he'd always have an escape route. Obviously those pants couldn't be removed with only one hand they were so tight she'd have to use both of hers and he'd be able to get away. He relaxed a little, but still dodged her whenever possible.

Within two weeks I was back home celebrating Thanksgiving. My motherhood years were turning out a bit different than I'd pictured, but it seemed to be working and I felt happy.

I continued to work on television shows at Revue - *Bachelor Father* with John Forsythe, and a show *Going My Way* in which Gene Kelly and Barry Fitzgerald played priests. When pilot time came in the spring, I was assigned to do *The Munsters*. What a trip! It was a unique experience - a true makeup and hair show. Yvonne De Carlo wore a long, black wig with a white streak. The wig had hair lace and it took an immense amount of work to keep it in shape. Each night I had to wash the makeup out of the white streak, clean the wig, and then pin it on the block to dry for the next day.

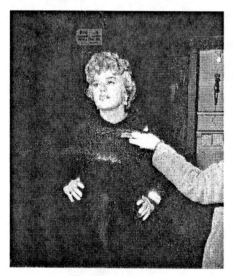

Shelly Winters

Our hours were long. We had so much work to do. There was lots of pressure and never enough time. It was funny, it was weird, and the writers hung around the set making us laugh all day and night. During those ten days of shooting we ate breakfast, lunch, and dinner at work. We were sure it was going to be a hit and it was.

There was breakaway furniture on the set and we had been warned to be careful of it because it was so easily broken. One evening around ten o'clock, I was so exhausted I forgot and sat down, not realizing it was on a breakaway chair. It cracked before I could get up and then it shattered. There I was sitting on the floor looking up at the crew who were all laughing uproariously at me. Invisibility would have been nice at that moment.

Although I had reported straight to Tucson, *McLintock!* had been produced by Paramount. That was the first time I'd ever worked for Paramount. Nellie Manley, head of the hairdressing department at Paramount, had heard good reports about me from Lorraine. Because of this, Nellie called me to work on a film. Virginia Darcy, my friend from *The Birds* was doing *Wives and Lovers*. Nellie asked me to do Shelly Winters. Shelly had a reputation for being difficult, so Virginia suggested me for the job. As she explained to Nellie, I was a happy person with a good home life who should be able to handle Shelly very well.

I was thrilled. It seemed I might just be going places. I didn't know where, but I was doing films now and I'd be able to get some good credits under my belt.

The moment I walked through the Bronson Gate at Paramount I fell in love with the lot. Finally I'd found the perfect studio. It was what I'd imagined a studio should be. The gate I walked through was the one I'd seen in so many movies and most of the buildings on the lot looked like they were from old European cities. The outside of the buildings had such character. The makeup department was housed on the third floor of a building that had the stars' dressing rooms on the ground floor. The second floor consisted of small, rather dreary rooms for the lesser actors. They brought back memories of the writers' rooms at MGM and depressed me.

Our Makeup Department was plain. All the walls were of wainscot and painted light green. The only fancy places were the two department heads' offices - Nellie Manley's and Wally Westmore's, the head of Makeup. The Hair Department was bright, though very simply decorated compared to other places I'd worked in. The mirrored workstations were small, but the atmosphere was more relaxed than MGM. It felt friendlier to me and everyone else as well. I realized I'd finally found the home I'd been searching for.

Chapter 11

WIVES AND LOVERS
1963

Paramount Studio was busy. Besides *Wives and Lovers and The Carpetbagger*, other films were being made at the studio. All the actresses and actors, working in the different films being shot on the lot, reported to Makeup in the morning. They mingled with one another. While we did our creating, Janet Leigh and Shelly Winters would chat. From time to time, Van Johnson would stick his head into the room to make some outrageous remark that always made us laugh. Other actors like George Peppard and Elizabeth Ashley would join in too. Although at first I'd had apprehensions about working with Shelly, she was great and I never suffered her famous anger or displeasure.

Janet Leigh, Tony Curtis's ex, had recently married a lawyer. He didn't understand how the movie business worked or have a clue of the toll, a long day at work, took on a person. Janet was often weary because she'd sat through one of his long business dinners when all she really wanted to do was crawl into bed and sleep. She was trying to be a good wife and she laughed about her predicament, knowing the film would eventually be finished and she'd be able to cope.

Wives and Lovers was a light-hearted script with most of the filming done on stage. If we did go on location, it was just for the day. During that film I became acquainted with the whole Paramount lot. I ate lunch in the commissary and had drinks after work at Oblath's Restaurant across the street. They were famous for their wonderful Mexican food and unforgettable cherry walnut pudding with vanilla sauce. Sometimes I'd go to Nickodells which had a great masculine feel reminding me of the Brown Derby where my father had taken me as a child. It was dark and comfortable and they served the greatest steaks and chopped Cobb salad. It usually took such a long time to get served at Nickodells, we'd have to run to get back to work on time, but it was worth it.

Wives and Lovers filmed for twelve weeks. After that I remained at Paramount working on various films being made around the lot. The studio was busy and they always needed extra hairdressers. Jerry Lewis filmed constantly. I felt uncomfortable working on his sets. He was such a control freak. He'd have all his flunkies on the set with him each day and he often belittled them, but they'd just smile and take it, knowing that if they did, he would hire them again. One day Jerry thought it would be funny to pull a grip's new alpaca sweater as far as it would go. He pulled and pulled, totally ruining it. He never stopped to realize that it had been a present from the man's daughter. Jerry offered to buy him five new ones to replace it, but that wasn't the point.

During this period, Elvis was shooting *Fun in Acapulco* in Acapulco. What a lovely man he was. We all loved him. Even then he was sweet, kind, gentle, and very handsome. Elvis loved the girls and they loved him. He was so sexy and he drove the body makeup women crazy. In this film the actresses wore bathing suits so they needed body makeup. They'd look great until Elvis got a hold of them. One day his co-star, Ursula Andress, disappeared into his dressing room. She stayed there for a while and when she was called to work on the set the body makeup lady noticed fingerprints all over her legs. They had to hold up shooting while she had her body makeup redone. Though we laughed, the body makeup woman and the assistant director, who had to wait, didn't think it was funny at all.

Elvis was much too kind and patient. I don't think he wanted to make waves. One day he prepared for a scene where he was sauntering down the cliffs of Acapulco singing a song. Since he hadn't had a chance to rehearse it yet, he was singing it for the first time. At the end of the first shot, Richard Thorpe, the director, yelled "Cut and print." Elvis looked up, shocked. He hadn't even had time to warm up and didn't like the result. Elvis asked for another shot, but the director said "It's just fine" and that settled that. It was like they hadn't even listened to him. Today a star would never let that happen. The truth was that the director wanted to bring the picture in on time so he could earn a large bonus.

A film called *For Those Who Think Young* was my next assignment. It was my first promotional film. That meant nearly all the props were given to the production for free just as long as they were shown on the screen. There were free stereos, clothes, furniture, jackets, shoes, even ice cream from Baskin and Robbins and Pepsi was everywhere. I'd never seen anything like it.

Our cast included Pamela Tiffin, Nancy Sinatra, Ellen Burstyn, and James Darren. James Darren was working in Las Vegas during the first couple of weeks. Each night after work in Hollywood he'd fly to Las Vegas to do his show, then crawl into an ambulance and be driven back to Los Angeles while he slept. Amazingly, he'd arrive rested.

The film was a beach party type frolic with college kids hoping to save their favorite club from closing. Howard Koch, Sr., one of my all time favorites, was our producer. He was a wonderful, talented and sincere man always with a ready smile for us. His son Howie, now a producer, was just a kid who helped out on the set a little.

This was a new kind of production and at times it was difficult. They were trying to save money so the budget was small. Wally Westmore insisted that Nellie work on production in the morning so she came in first thing in the morning and helped me get the many people in the cast ready. During the day I'd watch the set. After lunch it was hard because I had to do touch ups on all the cast down on the set and Nellie refused to come help me. It took me a long time to do everyone by myself. One day in particular we were shooting at the ice cream shop, the ice cream was melting and production was yelling at me, "Hurry, hurry." I called Nellie and demanded that she come down and help. She was furious and didn't talk to me for days after that, but eventually she cooled off.

Once again I became close friends with the hairdressers who were on staff at Paramount. We spent more time with each other than we did with our families. My friend from Lone Pine, Sherry Wilson, was working there as well. Being surrounded by actresses who were beautiful and slim made us aware of our deficiencies. We tried all sorts of ways to become thin and beautiful like them. Once we decided to go to a hypnotist to lose weight. We just knew this would solve everything. At first it did seem to work - that was until I had a personal appointment with the hypnotist. I sat in a darkened room all alone with him as he began to count. I was nervous. He was tracing his finger down my throat, further and further down to my chest. I sat up suddenly and ran out of the room never to return. So much for the easy way to lose weight.

One evening we were invited to a gathering about meditation on Larchmont Boulevard. It sounded interesting to us. The meeting was upstairs and I could smell incense as we walked up the stairs. We entered a large, lovely room full of flowers and cushions. A little man with a gray beard all dressed in white sat on a small stage surrounded with flowers. He smiled sweetly. The evening was enjoyable and it wasn't until years later that I realized the little man was Maharishi Mahesh Yoga, the transcendental meditation teacher.

Sherry Wilson eventually became a successful realtor in Hollywood.

Chapter 12

LOVE WITH A PROPER STRANGER
1964

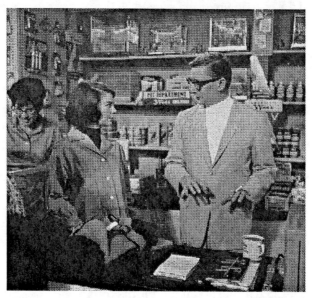

Sugar, Natalie Wood, and Robert Mulligan

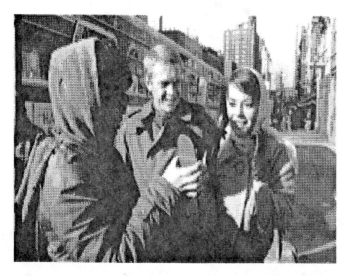

Ginger, Steve McQueen and Natalie Wood
Love with a Proper Stranger

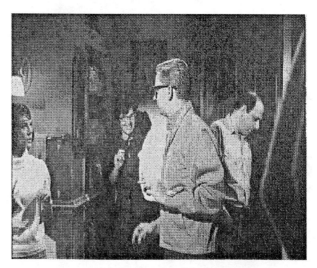

**Natalie Wood, Robert Mulligan and
Herschel Bernardi**

We began filming *Love With a Proper Stranger* on location, in New York City, the following March. This was the first time that I would work with Natalie Wood. I was excited for many reasons. First of all, I'd never been to the Big Apple. Looking out the car windows during our drive into the city, my first impression was of the fullest graveyard I'd ever seen. It was packed, no room left. Where did they put the new bodies? We stayed at the Plaza Hotel and it lived up to its reputation - luxurious and beautiful. Central Park was just across the street and there were horse drawn buggies just waiting to take us for a ride.

This was Eddie Butterworth's first time to do Natalie's makeup. He was an old friend of mine from MGM days. Natalie also had a second makeup man, her friend Bob Jiras, from New York City, who would work with us. Bob didn't always get to work with Natalie, but he was her good friend and she always

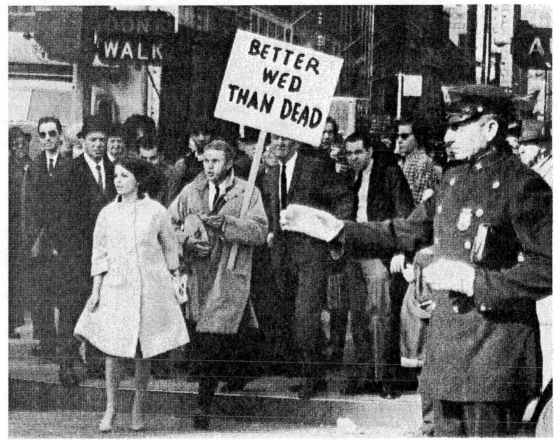

Natalie Wood and Steve McQueen in the final moments of
Love With a Proper Stranger

tried to get him on her films when she worked in the East. We called him B.J. Ann Landers (not the columnist) was Natalie's wardrobe woman and Roselle Gordon was her stand-in. Roselle didn't get to come to New York as they seldom took stand-ins on location so I didn't meet her until our return to Los Angeles.

Upon our arrival at the Plaza, the bellboy took our bags and showed Eddie and me to our rooms. He came to a door and opened it signaling for us both to go through. At first we thought they'd put us in a suite together. Eddie and I looked at each other, embarrassed. Gulp! But after we went through that one door we noticed each of us had a private door to our own room. What a relief! My room was decorated with traditional furnishings, warm and lush. The huge tub in the bathroom pleased me immensely.

Natalie had a huge suite across the street at the Sherry Netherlands where she always preferred to stay when she came to New York. Being in New York was very different from Los Angeles, which was so spread out, and nobody walked anywhere. Here I could go almost anywhere, around our hotel, on foot. I loved the freedom.

Robert Mulligan, our director, had the ability to gather the crew together and we became like a family. We trusted him and he trusted us. It was a wonderful way to work and we felt safe in that big city.

Our first day of shooting was at a park located at the foot of the United Nation's Building. We filmed little old Italian men playing Bochi Ball. That day I discovered that the "regular" coffee sold on the streets was loaded with sweet Eagle Brand canned milk. Yum, it was tasty.

Natalie taught me many tricks with her hair; after all she'd been in the business since she was five. One windy day her bangs were blowing in her face. She showed me how to hide a dark bobby pin in her bangs to hold the hair back. The bobby pins were especially made for film, painted with a flat paint that didn't reflect light. She assured me the camera would never see it. I was nervous until I saw the dailies the next evening. She was right. That trick saved me from having to panic and run in each time the wind blew.

Bob Jiras was a good friend of Natalie's and he knew her well. He clued me in on many things about her that were helpful. For example, if Natalie was getting upset she began to bite her lip, if it got worse she'd cross her legs and one leg would bounce up and down. He illustrated this as we watched her being interviewed by an obnoxious man. When B. J. saw her leg begin to bob up and down, he politely went in and interrupted the conversation, calling her to the set. He was a great buffer for her.

Natalie played the part of a girl who gets pregnant, on a one-night stand, by Steve McQueen. He doesn't even remember her so she decides to get an abortion. The abortion scene was a particularly difficult scene for our director, Bob Mulligan, as he had been raised in the Catholic faith and at one time even considered becoming a priest. Our set was located in a horrible tenement building that smelled like a giant latrine. The actress playing the abortionist was hard and cold - looking. When she pulled on her rubber gloves, they made a squeaking sound. That scene affected us all. It was terrible to see and then to realize that women had to have abortions under those conditions for so long. The horror lent itself to the scene, as Natalie became her character. She brought us all to tears. Magical things happen on the screen at times like that.

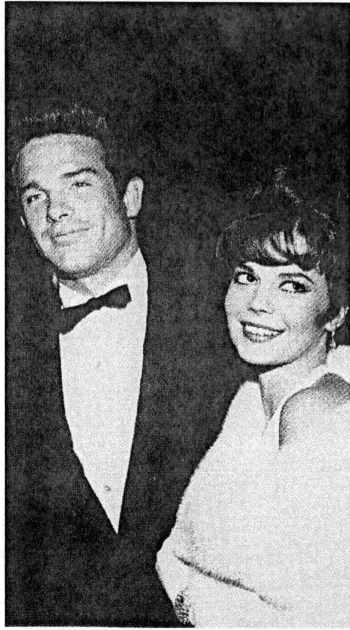

Natalie Wood and Warren Beatty

That afternoon Natalie wanted to make a phone call to Warren Beatty, who she was dating at the time. We accompanied her to an apartment where they offered to let her use their phone. The apartment was dreadful and smelled like old cabbage. Ten people must have lived in there. Later I went up on the roof of the building and looked down. All I could see was a little dark yard with a dead tree. How could anyone grow up healthy here? No wonder drugs were so popular. They brought a little happiness and distraction to the dreary lives of those who lived under these circumstances. In their shoes, I had no doubt I'd have wanted them, too.

One morning as Natalie and Steve were being made up, they began discussing what had happened the night before. They'd been at a well-known restaurant, eating dinner, when someone just pulled up a chair, joined them, and then rudely asked questions. They were eventually rescued by the headwaiter. I began to realize how lucky Eddie and I were that we could enjoy ourselves wherever we went because nobody knew us. I think even Steve was amazed at Natalie's popularity. He was great fun for her to work with and they both enjoyed it.

Warren Beatty drove Natalie crazy. He always kept her hanging. If she wanted to make plans he'd wait until the last minute to let her know if he was available. He made her life miserable. I always wondered what made him attractive to her, or any women, but I later realized it was a gift to be in a relationship with Warren because afterwards a woman would really appreciate a man who treated her nicely.

One Friday afternoon we shot outside Macy's department store. It was a madhouse. They had barricaded the street where we worked. I went into a store for something and when I returned the police wouldn't let me back through the barricade so I had to crawl under the barricade on my knees to get back to the set. My stockings were in shreds.

During the three weeks we spent in New York

the trees in Central Park began to bloom. One cool morning we set off for work wearing long underwear and all our warm clothes. Later that day the temperature rose to eighty degrees. Sweat began pouring down my body.

Those three weeks went by quickly. I became acquainted with New York and I loved it. One weekend I took a train to Connecticut, my first trip to New England, where I meet Bill's oldest brother. I fell in love with the New England countryside.

At home again in Los Angeles, we continued to shoot on the stage at Paramount. Natalie had a nice dressing room on the bottom floor of the Makeup building. One day while I was doing her hair she knocked a glass of ice tea off her dressing table, spilling it. I was relieved to see she made mistakes, too. She never tried to be perfect; it was my problem because I was still a little intimidated by her "star" status.

On occasion I'd sit and talk to Steve McQueen. He was relaxed and kind of shy and reticent in a charming way yet he was at ease talking and joking with us. I had the feeling that working with Natalie was a thrill for him. She made him comfortable and never let him feel she was more important than he was. Nevertheless, we were all aware of how important she was.

Steve was married to Neil at the time and they were considering adopting a child. He'd question me about my girls who had come from Mexico to live with us and was very interested in my experience with them.

Milt Krasner, the cameraman, became one of my all time favorites - sort of like a father. His sweetness added charm to the production.

At the end of the film we all said our goodbyes. Natalie gave me a generous gift, a gold bracelet. She always bought us jewelry and engraved it with our names. I'd never had a present like that before. It had been such fun and I felt I'd done well, but I also knew nobody had any idea what would happen in the future. I hoped I'd be able to work with her again. I didn't want to make any plans or have expectations. The business could be fickle. I did make many new friends during that production and often when I'd work at Paramount we'd find ourselves working together again.

Chapter 13

SEX AND THE SINGLE GIRL
1964

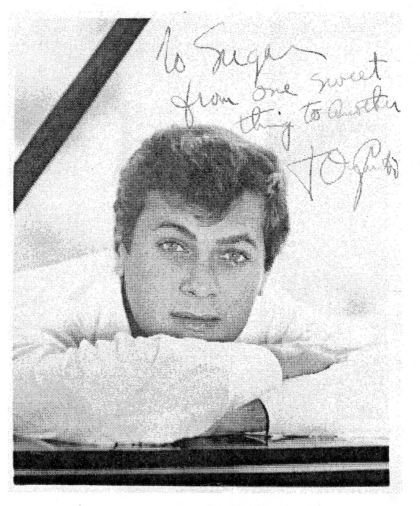

Tony Curtis

I was very happy at Paramount. I'd found my home and Nellie kept me busy. *Sex and the Single Girl*, based on the book by Helen Gurly Brown, was Natalie's next film also starring Tony Curtis, Lauren Bacall, and Henry Fonda. Sydney Guilleroff was set to design Natalie's hair even though the film would be shot at Paramount. With the exception of *Love With a Proper Stranger* Natalie had Sydney in her contract. I believe that she had something to do with the producing on *Love with a Proper Stranger* and perhaps wanted to cut expenses. Nellie assumed I would be asked to do Natalie's hair on the set again as Sydney only did the designing and left the daily work to someone else. I wasn't so sure. I'd heard rumors; many people wanted the job.

Sydney still thought of me as the stock - room clerk and although I helped him dress Natalie's new wig he never mentioned anything about me having the job on the set. It was an uncomfortable situation. One day I was so unhappy and confused that I broke down into tears. I told Nellie I needed to know what was happening. Was I going to do the picture or not? I hated playing games. A couple of days later, things came to a head and it finally was settled. I would do the film.

The night after I'd been told that I'd do the film there was a union meeting. A few of us went to a restaurant to have dinner before the meeting. Everyone was wondering who was going to do Natalie's hair. One woman was sure she already had the job. I never said anything; I kept quiet and smiled inside. This was a perfect time to keep my mouth shut and I did.

Sydney designed a perky little wig for Natalie and before the film began shooting we did hair, makeup, and wardrobe tests. I was instructed to bring the wig down from the Makeup Department to Natalie's dressing room first thing in the morning. I'd bring the wig, turn on all the lights in the dressing room, put the coffee on, and when I finished I'd go back upstairs to the Makeup Department and wait for a call from Sydney. That day we tested the wig and everyone seemed satisfied with the look. On the first day of production, as instructed, I took the wig down to the dressing room, did my duties, and as usual went back up to Makeup to wait for my call. When I went back downstairs, the wig was nowhere to be seen. Sydney was doing Natalie's own hair with the curling iron. I watched him, nervously looking around for the wig. Nobody said anything. Where on earth could it be? I was becoming more and more upset. My imagination took hold and I began to wonder how long it would take me to pay for that wig - two or three weeks' salary at least.

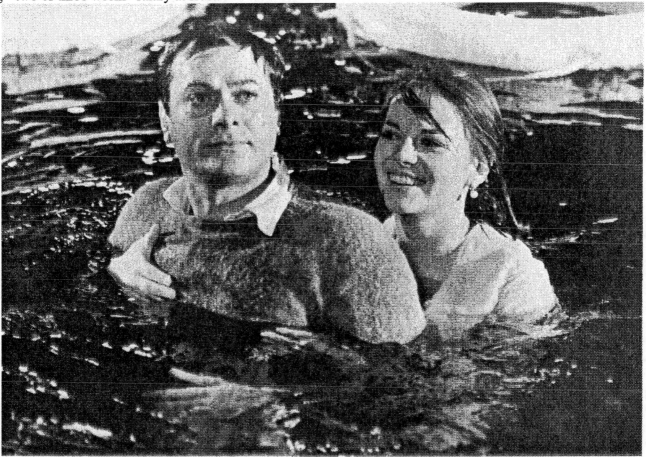

Natalie Wood and Tony Curtis, *Sex and the Single Girl*

I kept quiet while Sydney did Natalie's hair, but as soon as he finished I expressed my alarm. "Don't worry about it," he said. Easy for him to say. I was the one responsible for the wig. I tried not to worry, but just couldn't help it. B.J. was there and eventually he felt sorry for me. He explained what had happened. Natalie decided not to wear the wig so she put it in the trunk of her car and took it home. She always took her hairpieces home when a film was completed, but she took this one at the beginning. I was so relieved. Now I could now explain what happened to Nellie and it could be settled between Natalie's agent and the Hair Department. Later I asked Natalie to please put in her contract that all hairpieces went to her personally if she ordered them or used them on a film, a change that relieved me of the responsibility.

Tony Curtis was charming, boyish, handsome, and full of the devil - a great tease - embarrassing me by coming very close then saying something that made me blush. I found him funny and endearing.

Lauren Bacall was sexy with her low, charming voice. I felt sad because Natalie and Tony had fancy dressing rooms on the set while Lauren and Henry Fonda had smaller ones. I always felt that the filmmakers needed to treat the older stars with as much respect as the newer ones. But this system had been in place since movies began and nobody else appeared to be upset, at least not on the outside.

I became better friends with Natalie and her whole entourage. Now I understood how loyal she was and the same people were called back for each film. She had the largest entourage of any actress in the business. We had two makeup men, Eddie and B.J. Ann Landers was the wardrobe, Roselle was the stand-in, and Bonita Morris was body makeup. Natalie also had a secretary.

The filming began. Sydney showed up each morning and curled Natalie's hair and I'd stand by all day on the set with her. One day it rained. When it rains in Los Angeles, everything comes to a standstill, especially the freeways. It's as if people get some sort of brain damage so they don't know how to drive in the rain. There are delays that take hours. Although I set off much earlier for work this rainy day, I was still stuck in traffic, and late, but I wasn't worried. I knew Sydney would be doing Natalie's hair and I'd get to work in plenty of time to stand by on the set. Wrong! As soon as I checked into Makeup I was told to rush down to Natalie's dressing room. Sydney hadn't shown up either. Horrors! I rushed right down to her room. Her makeup was all finished and Eddie had turned on the stove for my iron so I jumped right in and began iron curling her hair. I had no time to worry or be nervous. It worked like a miracle. Her hair turned out perfectly and she was on the set in plenty of time. Sydney never returned. I wondered about that, but I never did get an explanation.

Natalie's favorite perfume was Jungle Gardenia. The scent was overpowering and we tried to avoid being around when she sprayed it. Sometimes after she'd get the dressing room warm for body makeup she'd spray and we couldn't escape. We tried not to cough, we didn't want to hurt her feelings, but I'll never forget that scent. I loved gardenias in the garden, but this was too overpowering. Whenever I smell that perfume, I am reminded of her.

Now that I was a better friend of B. J.'s, he told me how amused they had been at my nervousness when I first started working with them. He also told me the same thing had happened to a hairstylist who worked with them a few years before in New York. I laughed and wondered what it was that made some of us react like that. Natalie was so nice and easy to please. We all worked on another film in New York and I needed to hire a hairstylist so we called that person to work with us. He and I exchanged stories, laughing at ourselves.

Natalie's hair was so beautiful, full and swinging around perfectly. Between Sydney and me, we did a great job. It occurred to me that Sydney had wanted to give her a wig and she must have made the decision to use her own hair at the last minute. Over the years I learned to trust her intuition. She'd seen herself on the big screen, big as a Buick, far more often than I had.

Edith Head designed Natalie's costumes for the film. She was perfectly proportioned, but they always designed special push up bras to make her look full busted. It worked. It was great engineering. Natalie did have one imperfection, though. She had broken her left wrist and it hadn't set properly, but she refused to have it re broken. It looked a little strange and for each film a new bracelet was designed for her to cover the large bone that protruded.

Sydney gave me a clue to making things work with Natalie: He said to stick close by her and don't go off all the time with others on the set. He knew Natalie liked her own group to be nearby. She liked to work with people who were familiar; she didn't want to have to get to know new people each time she began a film. I paid heed to his advice and by the time we finished the film I felt more secure in my relationship with her. I had actually become a part of her entourage. Natalie had a wonderful way of accepting us just as we were. She didn't try to make us fill her expectations.

One time while working on a film at Fox, I was talking to a wardrobe woman who was working with Doris Day, she said, "We have a cold today." "Who has a cold?" I asked. "Oh Doris does," she replied. I wondered if that meant they all got sick too. I wouldn't want to work in a group like that.

I was very happy with Natalie. She did wonderful things and we enjoyed participating. She loved makeup and at the beginning of each film she'd ask the makeup men to shop for all sorts of new cosmetics that she'd seen or heard about. At the beginning of a film all sorts of new makeup would pour in to be tested by her. Some of it might work on the film and some might not, but the experiments were fun.

Natalie was quite a character. She had unusual tastes and her love of animals caused some trouble one evening. On the way to work she had stopped by a pet shop and bought two puppies. One was an Australian sheep dog, neither had pedigrees. She brought them to work and put them in her dressing room in the honey wagon where they wreaked havoc. Being puppies they weren't house broken and they chewed on everything including the handle of my purse. We didn't care, but the honey wagon driver was furious.

During the time we were filming *Sex and the Single Girl* at Paramount, Warner Brothers was filming *My Fair Lady* with Rex

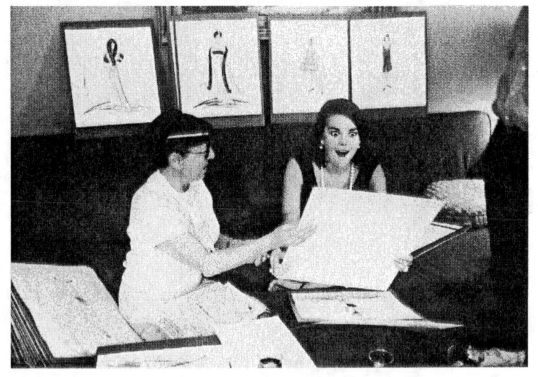

Edith Head (costume designer) shows Natalie Wood design sketches for *Sex and the Single Girl*

Harrison and Audrey Hepburn. There weren't enough hairstylists available in the industry to do all the films being made in Hollywood at the time. Normally we were not allowed to work on more than one film a day. But for this busy time all the rules changed, as they desperately needed our talent. The hair, the clothes, and especially the hats were spectacular and took hours of work to put together each morning. We all went to Warner Brothers very early in the mornings where we helped out for three hours on *My Fair Lady*. Then we reported to our own studio. The hats for *My Fair Lady* were enormous. Hair had to be built up at a certain angle so the hats would balance and be able to be pinned on to stay. It was an engineering job, but they looked wonderful once they were on. Working on two films at the same time like this was fun and it worked for everyone. What cooperation.

One morning I was outside the stage at Warners and noticed a woman standing in the sunlight. She appeared to glow. What was that about her? Then I realized it was Audrey Hepburn and she did have an inner glow, she was so lovely. I never saw her again, but I always remembered how she looked that day.

One day I was free to work all day at Warner Brothers. We were shooting in Coventry Gardens, an authentic looking marketplace from England's past. Suddenly it was announced that our President, John F. Kennedy, had been shot. I was stunned. It was impossible to believe. We all prayed, sure he would recover, but soon we were told that he had died. It was unbelievable that something like that could happen. The set was full of people, flower sellers, fruit merchants, lots of activity and we almost had a riot on the stage as a man began to shout with joy at the news. He must have been nuts. Later it was discovered that he had been hoping Kennedy would be killed. Nobody could believe it. An electrician who happened to be up in the rafters was just about to drop one of the huge lights on the makeup man, but someone ushered the man away. It was horrible.

We immediately wrapped and left work early to go home and watch the television. The whole nation was in shock. I was about the same age as Jackie Kennedy and I had children nearly the same age. I identified with her, but couldn't imagine what she must have felt. Little John John saluting at his father's grave was the most heart - breaking sight of all. We cried the whole weekend feeling robbed. For me, Kennedy had awakened a faith in the future and even in our government. All of a sudden it was gone, never to return.

The closest I came was to meeting Jackie Kennedy was while I was working at Kenneth's Salon in New York. The hairstylist had set Jackie's hairpiece for her and it came out of the drying oven with a little kink in it. I had my irons with me so I offered to take the kink out. It was nice to be able to do that for her. As I am writing this Chapter Jackie Kennedy was buried at the age of sixty-four. It reminds me of those days of sadness and disillusionment. I cried for her again today.

During that same year I worked on *Soldier in the Rain* and met Tuesday Weld for the first time. What a wild and wonderful creature. She arrived at Paramount with her long golden tresses (which were actually a fall) in tangles. Nellie took it off and washed it while I watched, positive it would disintegrate, but a few hours later it was beautiful and shining. Steve McQueen was in the film along with Jackie Gleason. We went on location to Monterrey and worked on the army base there. Our meals were wonderful. I couldn't understand why anyone in the army would complain about the food until I learned that base had the Number One mess in the country.

During this film Steve McQueen began to change. He became moody and was difficult to get along with at times. Perhaps Natalie had kept him in line, I don't know. Jackie Gleason was always a gentleman. At the end of the film Jackie gave everyone a gift. I still have mine - a little golden comedy/tragedy woman with sapphire eyes.

Working with Tuesday was fun and crazy. Always naughty, one night she put a huge piece of seaweed in the pool. It looked like an octopus and frightened the guests the next morning. Another day she drove us in her convertible down the coast to Nepenthe Restaurant for lunch, driving so fast that we all prayed we'd survive the experience. I did and had a great deal of fun working with her.

Chapter 14

THE UGLY DACHSHUND
THE GREAT RACE, 1965 (The Beginning)

Production at Paramount slowed down and I went off to work at Disney on *The Ugly Dachshund*, starring Suzanne Plechette and Dean Jones. Pat McNalley, who I knew from his MGM days, was now head of Disney Makeup. He looked much as he had then, still wearing starched white shirts and light blue faded jeans. He was gruff, but likable.

Working at Disney was a dream come true. I'd grown up on Disney and ever since I'd seen *Bambi* at age seven, I'd associated it with fantasy and fun. The studio lot was clean and beautiful. Lining the path to the commissary were topiary bushes cut to look like Mickey Mouse and Donald Duck. Perfect! The food in the commissary was healthy and offered at fair prices to the employees.

The Ugly Dachshund was a story about a Great Dane that ended up with a family of Dachshunds. It was shot totally on the studio lot. Unfortunately for the animal trainer someone poisoned some of his Great Danes right before the film began. They had been all trained and were just ready to begin working when this happened. There was no time to train new dogs, let alone find duplicates with the right temperament. I felt very sorry for the trainers.

I'd always loved Suzanne Plechette. She'd been wonderful in *The Naked City*, one of my favorite television shows. I loved her deep, sexy voice, warm humor, and her ability to laugh at herself. Dean Jones was pleasant to work with, as well. In those days he seemed to be the "chosen" one working in so many Disney movies. All the actors and actresses were easy to work with. They were appreciated and treated well, but they didn't run the show like they do now. We had no fear of getting fired or landing in trouble as long as we did our jobs well.

One afternoon after lunch I noticed a man sitting quietly at the piano in the living room. It was Walt Disney. He was thoroughly enjoying himself while watching the production. I said "Hello" and he responded, so I told him how much I enjoyed working at his studio. He smiled at me and said, "Thanks." *The Ugly Dachshund* was a short production - we were through in six weeks.

During the spring that followed that film, I had a break, which I spent at home, getting things in order, playing with the kids, and resting up for my next project. Bill was working on *Mission Impossible* as a prop man. He had long hours and was very busy, too. He was a moody man, but most of the time he was pleasant and nice to me yet something definitely was missing in our relationship. I didn't know what to do about it so I filled my life with my work. Looking back, I realize the emptiness of my relationship with my husband gave me the urge to succeed at my job. It distracted me so I didn't have to face the problems in my life. Perhaps I wasn't ready.

Over the years I've noticed that many marriages in the movie business seem to last because we never spent much time with our mates. We'd go off on our own, have our friends at work, and our egos were fed. Sometimes I seemed to forget there was life beyond the movie business. If we weren't working, our lives were empty. In those days I was a willing part of it.

Bill and I always lived beyond our means no matter how much money we made. I worked all I could and so did Bill. We lived well, but we never saved anything and therefore always needed to work.

By this time the four girls from Mexico were settled in and applying for citizenship. They were a part of our family, learning English, attending school, and enjoying their life. I felt so grateful knowing they loved my children and that they were well cared for when I was at work.

This was good because in May I learned Natalie was going to do *The Great Race* at Warner Brothers, directed by Blake Edwards. It was scheduled to start on June 17, my birthday, but there were many tests to conduct before the actual production began. This was a gigantic production, the biggest I'd ever worked on. It was Blake Edward's pet project and starred Jack Lemmon, Tony Curtis, Keenan Wynn, pre *Colombo* Peter Falk, and Natalie. But in many ways the special effects were going to be the real stars of the film.

Once again Sydney was hired to design Natalie's hairstyles. I would assist and execute the styles after they had been decided upon. Don Feld was the costume designer. He was a wonderful character, tall, slim, and wild. There was even a special designer for the hats. Susie Germaine, a good friend, was hired to do Jack Lemmon's hair and also the doubles. Jack played two parts in the film. Susie would curl his hair to make him the prince and then do a different style when he was the villain. There were five makeup men in all. Harry Ray did Jack Lemmon and Whitey Snyder did Tony Curtis. Fred Williams, Warner Brothers' makeup man was doing Natalie this time, rather than Eddie. B.J., Natalie's key makeup person, was with us once again. Ann Landers was the wardrobe, and Roselle was the stand-in again. This time Natalie had a new secretary, Mona.

Now that I was in her contract, I was only to do Natalie's hair and I would be paid even if she weren't working. I never minded helping out in the department when they needed extra help, but I didn't have to. If I did, I had to be sure I was there for Natalie when she arrived.

Sydney had ordered the most beautiful hairpieces. They were small and designed to fit different places on Natalie's head. For instance one had bangs and went on top of her head, combining with her own hair in a French twist in the back. Her hair was done in the early nineteen hundred styles. The "Gibson Girl" period is one of my favorites and I loved doing those hairstyles.

As always, Sydney was creating beautiful hairstyles, but they were impossible to work with during the actual production. He apparently believed there would always be control on the set, like in the days when he had done Greta Garbo's hair. He never considered what would happen if the hair would be blown or otherwise ruined in a scene unless it was actually supposed to happen that way. I watched and wondered how I would handle it during production.

On June 17, 1963, *The Great Race* began. Shooting started at ten o'clock, which was unusual, but Blake Edwards never liked beginning any earlier. Natalie's dressing room was filled with flowers. She was nervous. I laughed at her and asked why, when she'd been acting for so long. She explained that she was always nervous on the first day of a project, but as soon as they began to film, her nervousness disappeared.

Natalie was beautiful in her full "Gibson Girl" style dress, her hair up and full with long tendrils of hair falling in front of her ears. Her big beautiful eyes were lined, as always, with a dark pencil which the makeup men were trying to tone down so she would look more like the period. Women didn't wear makeup like that in 1910. Most stars tried to look good, but they also wanted to give the effect that they were in the correct time period for the film. Natalie didn't care about that as far as her eye makeup was concerned.

The first scene took place in a newspaper office. Natalie walked through and out onto a balcony overlooking the street

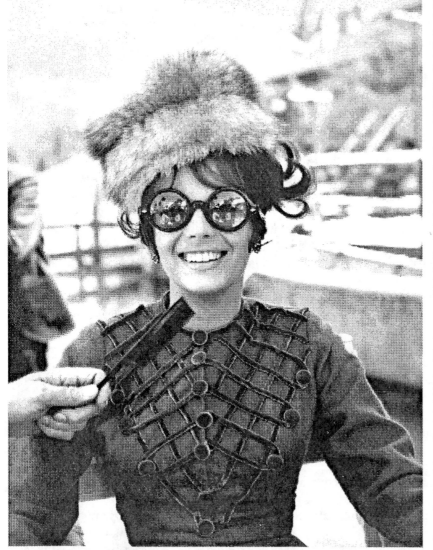

Natalie Wood. *The Great Race*

where a conversation took place. The scene was rehearsed and when everyone was satisfied the first take was called. A still photographer, a friend of Blake's, was on the set to take publicity photos. As everyone geared up to get ready for the first shot Blake said, "ROLL." At the same time goosed his photographer friend, who shouted out something obscene. He always did when he got goosed - it was a routine with them. Everyone laughed, but it distracted Natalie, who had difficulty doing her scene. She was quite annoyed.

Meanwhile, I was having my own problems. A fan was blowing, creating a breeze as Natalie stepped out on the balcony. The breeze blew the long tendrils of hair across her face. "Cut," called Blake. I went in and tried spraying the tendrils, but they still blew across her face. Neither the cameraman nor Blake liked the way it looked. I felt put in the middle. Sydney designed the hair to look one way, but it wasn't working. I was the one on the set with the problem and by this time Sydney had gone. We went back to the dressing room and I trimmed the tendrils to a length that could work with the breeze. We returned to the set and it worked just fine. I was nervous wondering what Sydney would have to say the next morning. He wasn't pleased, but I was beginning to realize how it worked with him. He had a wonderful reputation as a designer. Everyone admired him and did what he required of them. But the reality was, he got the big designing fees and the hairstylist on the set suffered with whatever was really required for a hairstyle to work on production.

The terms of Natalie's contract were amazing. She had a permanent dressing room on the lot plus another on the stage. It was lovely, but more like an apartment, and decorated especially for her. It even had a kitchen. There was a music system in each dressing room and a phone, too. Today that's the norm, but at the time it was unusual.

This was a big production for Warner Brothers, the most expensive comedy ever filmed. The heads of Makeup and Hair, Gordon Bau and Jean Burt Reilly, had their hands full staffing the film. Jean was a lovely, gentle woman. This makeup department was different from any other place I'd ever worked, much friendlier. In the center of the department was a huge room full of mirrors and makeup chairs. That's where we worked when there were crowds of people coming through the department. In the corner was a small kitchen where breakfast was cooked and served. In the morning we'd be greeted by the smell of coffee, eggs, and bacon sizzling on the grill. Old friends often sitting around and sometimes I'd see makeup people I hadn't seen in a while and meet new ones I'd only heard about, like Shot Gun Britton, John Wayne's makeup man. He was a real character, loud, funny, and dressed in red golfing trousers. When there was time to relax, we all gathered there. Through the years I met many wonderful people in that room. It rang with laughter.

The rest of the department was made up of smaller, private rooms for hair and makeup. Gordon and Jean each had their own offices, decorated to their tastes. Gordon's was very masculine, and Jean's was filled with antiques reflecting her quiet elegance.

I was excited about coming to work each day. Being on the set with Jack Lemmon and Tony Curtis was a kick. Keenan Wynn and Peter Falk were really funny. There was a pool table on the set - Peter was a wonder at pool and we always wondered how he was able to play so well with his glass eye. His mother would show up from time to time and torture him with her presence.

The Great Race was a story about a car race from New York to Paris in the early 1900s. Tony Curtis (the good guy) was always dressed in white and had a beautiful white car. Keenan Wynn was his assistant. Jack Lemmon, on the other hand, was the villain, dressed in black, always skulking around trying to destroy Tony. Jack's car was fantastic. It went up two stories high, in a scissors like effect. It belched black smoke and performed all sorts of mean tricks. Jack lived in a dreadful, old, black house where he did his experiments, assisted by Peter.

Natalie was a newspaper reporter who decided to cover the race and then entered it on her own. She tried to be independent, but was forever having troubles and being rescued by Tony.

Our schedule was set for six months of shooting, the longest film assignment I'd ever had.

Chapter 15
THE GREAT RACE CONTINUES
London, Vienna, Salzburg

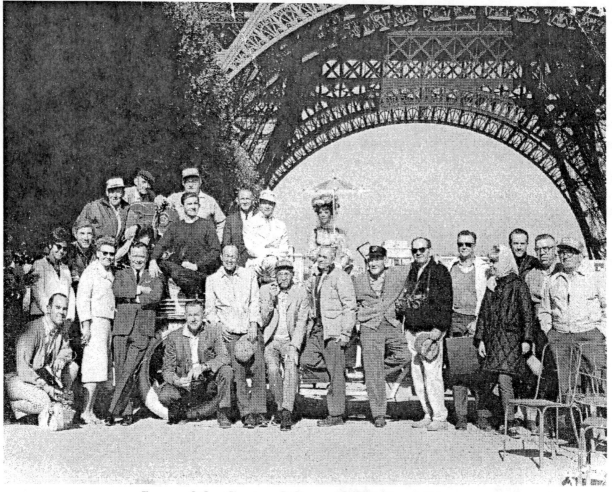

Some of the Cast and Crew of *The Great Race*

Warner's back lot was filled with crowds of people milling about the streets of New York. Gorgeous costumes, magnificent sets, thousands of people in the scene, it was the beginning of the *The Great Race*. It had taken hours to get all the people ready. First I'd worked in the main Makeup Department doing extras, and then I'd hurried to the dressing room to do Natalie's hair when she arrived a few hours later. It was exciting - everything I'd imagined working on films should be.

Despite all the activity, there wasn't a lot of pressure. The mood was rather casual most of the time because that's the way Blake ran his set. No early morning panic, no screaming or yelling to get things done.

Sydney wasn't showing up any more. He had designed a few hairdos for me and ordered all the hair goods, now he was in London working with Shirley MacLaine on *The Yellow Rolls Royce*. Natalie was concerned, as she

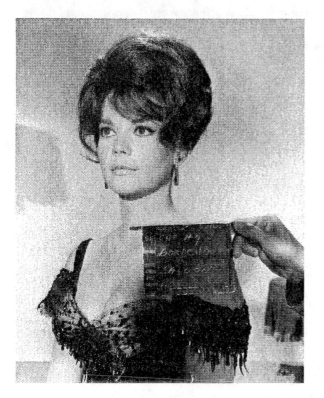

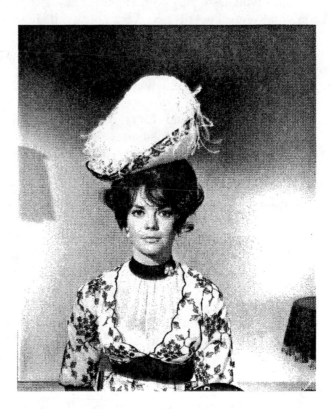

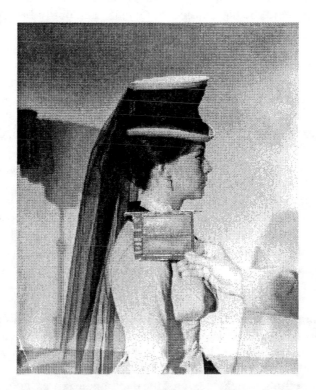

**Stills of Natalie Wood in The Great Race used by Ginger to match
hairstyles**

had demanded Sydney's services in her contract and at a high price. One day while I was doing her hair she asked, "Do you think you could design my hair, Sugar?" I hesitated for a moment, "I could. In fact, if you'd give me a try, I'd love to." I don't know how I got the nerve, but I always had a tendency to jump in when offered a great opportunity. I figured I could learn what I needed to learn. I told her I could do it. It was true.

From then on I had a wonderful time. I designed a curl that was always attractively sitting out on the right side of her hairdo no matter how her hair was done or what she was wearing. It became her trademark. Her hairpieces were the neatest one's I'd ever worked with. Sydney always demanded and got the best. Even though you are gone now, thanks Sydney.

Based in on Laurel and Hardy, it was a crazy film - a huge crew and surprisingly a leisurely pace, although one problem did occur, an assistant director's nightmare. All the stars insisted on being called from their dressing room at exactly the same time. Nobody was willing to appear on set first. This meant each star had to have their own assistant director with each assistant appearing at the dressing room door at the same moment. Watching them march to the dressing rooms at the same time made us giggle, but the production company wasn't so amused.

Special effects took hours to set up each shot and to reset after each one. While they put things back together, we'd sit around, talk and pass the time. Blake and the others had a pool table set up on the stage and it kept them busy between takes. They played for hours.

The dog trainers had a slight problem. There was a scene in which Tony Curtis sneaks into Jack Lemmon's house. He is supposed to be attacked by Jack's vicious dogs. In the script they had described the dogs as Great Danes, but when the time came to shoot the scene everyone began to realize that in no way were Great Danes mean or vicious looking. Eventually they got some footage of them barking and jumping and the editor had to use bits and pieces carefully put together to make the scene appear scary with these nice friendly dogs.

It was time to go on location in Europe. We had lots of filming to do, first in Austria - Vienna, then Salzburg - and then on to Paris. I was prepared to go, passport in hand, but I still wasn't sure they'd actually take me. Sydney was very persuasive and he kept calling from London to offer his services to Natalie for the location. He wanted to get back into the picture.

By then I had realized that Natalie was true to you as long as you were true to her. I still wondered about Sydney though. He was a master of persuasion. Natalie had told me he called, but she didn't sound interested in his offer. I had designed a great look for her and she had learned to trust me. Yet, until I boarded that plane, I wasn't sure. Fred Williams, Warner's makeup man wasn't going. We would meet Bob Jiras in New York and he'd do the European part of the film

Natalie was true to me and when the rest of the crew left to go directly to Vienna we flew to New York where I spent the evening with Natalie and her secretary, Mona. Mona was acting creepier and creepier and I wished she hadn't come, but she was Natalie's employee. She bad-mouthed Bob Jiras when he changed his plans and told us he'd meet us in Vienna instead of New York.

Natalie's plan was to go to London first, enjoy herself, get used to the time change, and stay until they needed her in Vienna. It was exciting for me as I'd never been to London.

We flew into London the next evening. I was amazed that everything was so clear. The lights at the airport spread out below us like huge butterfly wings. There was none of the expected fog.

We checked into the Dorchester Hotel. What an elegant place. My room was cozy with flowered wallpaper and, best of all, a huge bathtub with pipes on the wall to keep the bath towels warm. I ordered tea with cucumber sandwiches and a Pimm's Cup, ran a hot bath and when my food arrived I ate in the bathtub. It was a dream come true.

Natalie had the penthouse upstairs and Mona was in a room nearby. There was an eight-hour difference between Los Angeles and London time and Natalie was trying to adjust her internal clock. She was also having great fun in the evenings. Each day I'd wait in my room for Mona's call, and then I'd go up and do Natalie's hair before she went out for the evening.

The electricity was different in England, 220, not 110 and my electric stove didn't work, I had been unable to bring cans of Sterno on the plane. (Normally, I could use that to heat the irons.) So I set out to find a heat source for my irons. I'd always pictured London as foggy and cold, but it was just the opposite. I was walking around in a sleeveless dress, wearing dark glasses. So much for preconceived ideas.

I searched everywhere for something to heat the irons: the department stores, art stores, even questioning a man in the street that spoke only Welsh. Someone suggested checking out a camping store. I took a double-decker bus to where I was directed and finally found what I was looking for. It wasn't Sterno exactly, but little white pellets

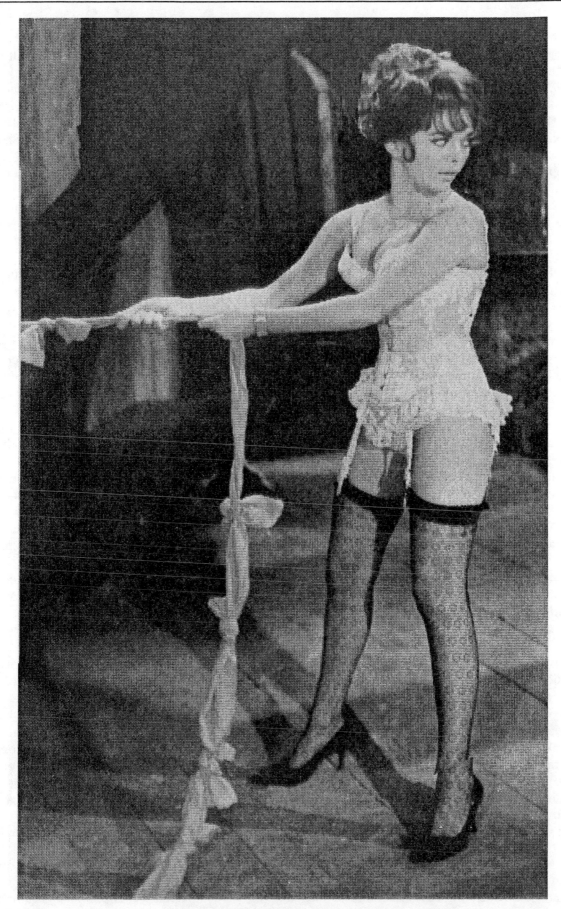

Natalie Wood in *The Great Race*

of fuel that light up with a match. The flame from the pellets gave off enough heat so my iron heated and I could curl Natalie's hair. The first evening I used the pellets, I set them in a pan on her dressing table. I lit them and it worked - that is, until the curtains blew into the flame and almost caught fire. I had to be very careful after that.

Natalie was having lots of fun, but I wasn't. Mona got weirder each day. She loved giving orders and keeping me under her thumb. Natalie slept all day and went out all night and I wanted to explore London and see the sights. Who knew when I'd ever have the chance again? Mona told me to stay in my room and not leave the hotel. I told her I'd call every hour from wherever I was and take a taxi right back if she needed me, but that wasn't good enough. She wanted complete control. She also had other weird habits. She told me she never ate anything yet one night after Natalie had finished her room service meal and rolled it into the hall, I saw Mona gulping down the left over food. It occurred to me that Mona really wanted to be Natalie Wood!

Finally after staying in my room all day waiting for Mona's call, I went to Natalie's room in tears. She asked me what was the matter and I explained how Mona kept me waiting in my room all day long each day. Natalie was utterly stunned and so sorry. She had no idea. She said from then on she'd give me a specific time to do her hair and I could do what I liked the rest of the time. I was happy, but Mona was really pissed because I went over her head.

From then on I had a great time. I walked to the Tower of London and saw the musical *Oliver* with all the beautiful little English boys. I also saw the film *Cleopatra*. Afterward I stopped in a restaurant feeling a stomachache coming on. A charming Irishman advised me to drink rum and peps. It worked. One night I went to a play where they served me a drink right at my seat during the intermission. Lovely place this great city of London.

The production company finally called us from Vienna. The next day, we went flew to that elegant, old city. Vienna's atmosphere was dark and gray and there were still bullet holes in some of the buildings left over from the Second World War. It was somber feeling, but the restaurants were great. My favorite was the basement of City Hall where we drank wine and beer and swayed together with the music. It was fun to catch up with the rest of our crew and have some company other than Mona.

My first room at the Bristol Hotel was very small. The sheets were stiffly starched and the windows were polished so clean that when I looked outside I bumped my nose on the glass. The bath was down the hall and I had to call the desk to have it drawn. It was okay, but since I loved an hour's soak I didn't feel comfortable with a shared bath. Our union contract stated that we were to have a private bath so they found me another room with my own bathtub.

Susie Germaine had already arrived and was staying at the Imperial Hotel where the rest of the crew was staying. She'd been doing Jack Lemmon's hair as well as Patty Elder's (Natalie's stunt double). Harry Ray, Jack Lemmon's makeup man; a funny little character, a real nut, was already there along with Whitey Snyder doing Tony Curtis. Bob Jiras had arrived and was working himself back into Natalie's good graces, much to Mona's displeasure. I warned B.J. about Mona's attempts to sabotage him.

The first day of production involving Natalie was to be filmed at Saint Stevens Church. I reported to work and as none of the guards knew me they wouldn't let me on the set. I tried to talk my way in, but I didn't speak Austrian so had to wait until another member of the American crew came along and explained who I was. I finally took one of the dark-blue armbands the crew wore and put it around my neck so I could go back and forth freely. Midmorning break was really nifty. I drank warm beer and ate knockwurst instead of coffee and doughnuts.

We never did work in Vienna. Natalie didn't like her costume and, rather than change it, they wrote her out of the scene. It didn't bother her. She was having a great time in the evenings with a tall, thin, amusing fellow named David Niven, Jr.

There was a huge amusement park in Vienna with the biggest Ferris wheel I'd ever seen. There was also a bumper car ride. Harry Ray had taken it and been knocked about a bit. The next night we all met in a bar at the hotel to have some drinks. Mona came with us. Harry had a few extra drinks as usual and began to describe his experience with the bumper cars. He was a skinny little guy without a bit of excess padding. He described the biggest bruise on his bum and proceeded to drop his trousers to show us. The bruise was huge, all purple and blue. We were impressed and thought it was really funny. Mona didn't think it was a bit funny. In fact, the next day she went to the producer and tried to get Harry fired for exposing himself. We never invited her anywhere again.

Mona wasn't making any friends. She drove Marty Jurow, our producer, crazy making demands in Natalie's name - things Natalie knew nothing about.

Since Natalie wasn't going to be used in Vienna, we left for Salzburg early. It was a perfect day for driving through the mountains. The flowers were bright and colorful, the lakes and rivers so clear it felt as though I was riding through a picture book. Salzburg was like summer to Vienna's wintry feeling. It felt as if *The Sound of Music* had come alive, it was so bright and cheerful.

The Salzburg Osterreichisherhof Hotel was our new home. It was right beside the river in the newer part of town. Across the river, reached by a narrow bridge, was the old town and it was ancient. Once again my room was immaculate. There were two doors that closed the room off from the hallway so it was very quiet. At least it was until I bought myself a huge harmonica that was a cross between an electronic piano and a harmonica. I loved playing it even if I didn't know how.

The countryside surrounding Salzburg was beautiful. We traveled to castles and visited the beautiful places in the country with Tony, our great driver. Our meals were sumptuous. I loved the steaks and the coffee with shlagg (whipped cream). I'd walk to the old town where the streets were so tiny and narrow that no motor vehicles could drive on them. We went to dinner at the Winkler, which overlooked the city and listened to Wayne Newton sing Aux Weidershean. I danced with Tony. I was very happy.

After a few days on our own, the rest of the film crew caught up with us. We were ready. The first day we were to work at Dumplatz Plaza. The set was all dressed and our extras were ready when it was noticed that the art director had dressed the wrong side of the Plaza. The set was all in shadow. Nobody had paid attention to the position of the sun. Another delay, but the next day the set was ready and the sun was shining where it was needed.

In the meantime, Natalie received an offer for her next film. She was reading her mail as I dressed her hair. She could hardly believe what they were offering her - $750,000. Natalie was astounded. She never imagined that she would earn that much for one film. She considered herself a rather ordinary person from an ordinary background and it was hard for her to grasp that this was happening. I found that very charming.

One night Mona asked to come to my room to talk. I couldn't turn her down. She was feeling suicidal and decided to spill her guts, which was just what I needed to hear. She told me the story of her life and how unloved she'd been. I figured I'd better listen because she was such a miserable person and although she loved controlling us, I still felt sorry for her. I wondered how it must feel to want to be Natalie without a single possibility of having something like that come true. She went on and on and it got later and later and I was exhausted. Finally she ran out of cigarettes, and as I didn't smoke, I had none to offer her. She left. I was relieved. I awoke the next morning feeling guilty. Suppose she'd gone back to her room and killed herself? I had been so selfish, not staying up longer. I showered, dressed, and went downstairs to ask if anyone had seen her. Nobody had. I was afraid to call her room, but later she appeared and was feeling just fine. She had dumped everything on me and had promptly forgotten all about it. I was exhausted and she felt great.

I awoke every morning to the lovely sound of church bells. One day, when Natalie wasn't working, we took a drive to Wolfgang Lake. We went to the Castle Costello for dinner and the waiter showed me some pictures in the men's room of dogs dressed in costumes.

We worked again at Dumplatz Plaza after many days of rain. The shot lasted exactly twenty seconds. Natalie had finished her part in Salzburg early and we departed for a weekend in Munich. She planned to do some photos with Gunther Haufman. He was Christine Kaufman's brother, who was one of Tony Curtis's wives. We had a very fast ride up the autobahn. It was beautiful, full of castles, more green trees, and lots of lakes, but as we crossed the border into Germany, the scenery changed and immediately seemed more serious, no longer like a fairy tale.

Our hotel in Munich, the Bierisherhoff, was a real change from Salzburg. It was grand, but very dark. My room had a huge tapestry hanging above the bed. Natalie's room was a bit more cheery, decorated in blonde furniture. She had a huge black mosaic tile bathtub and looked lost in it as she took a bubble bath.

Anne, the wardrobe woman ordered a flaming dish for dinner and we went out dancing afterward. They were just beginning to do the Twist dance there. The next day's lunch was at the Ratsheller of the city hall and at three o'clock we went to get Natalie ready for her photos. We worked at a beautiful park-like setting by the river with sheep grazing in the background. After finishing the shots we had dinner, and then rushed to the airport on our way to Paris.

The moment we landed in Paris a wonderful craziness enveloped me. Just imagine me, traveling first class and staying in a five star hotel in Paris! A limo picked us up at the airport and deposited us at the exquisite hotel, the Plaza Athenee. My room was perfect, as usual, opening onto a patio filled with flowers. I could look outside and see everyone and they could look in and see me. After unpacking, Ann and I took a walk through the streets of Paris, returning to the hotel with baguettes, cheese, wine, fruit, and flowers in our hands.

In the morning room service delivered a breakfast of croissants with butter and strawberry jam accompanied by strong coffee, half hot milk, my favorite. Later Ann and I went to check out the room where we would be working. I ordered a dryer and looked for different electric plugs, as the ones in Paris weren't the same as those at home. That accomplished, I dressed Natalie's hair, and then Ann and I went to lunch. We ate at the hotel - ice tea and cake - at a cost of $2.00. Later we ate dinner at a cafeteria - wine, salad, juice, cheese, bread, pork chops, potatoes, and dessert -

also $2.00. There were bargains in Paris, but not in our hotel.

The next day we went to the George Cinq Hotel because Natalie was thinking of moving there. After lunch Ann had her fortune told by a gypsy in the street. We bought more bread and wine, and felt very French.

Don Feld, our costume designer, invited us to dinner at Montmartre. He ran up the steps, his hair and scarf flying in the air and we ran after him. Crazy as ever, he filled the evening with excitement and laughter. From our table we could see the whole city with the Sacre Coeur above us. Using my high school French, I ordered French onion soup. I bought a rose from a lady in the street to take to my room.

We were ahead of our crew so we had time for sightseeing. One dreary, rainy day we went to the Impressionists' Gallery at the Louvre where I saw my favorite paintings. That night I dressed Natalie's hair for a premiere she was attending with David Niven Jr. Once again, I was amazed at her beauty.

The night my fellow makeup and hair people arrived from Salzburg, we all went out to dinner. Harry Ray entertained us by explaining how he used the bidet in his room for washing his underwear. We went to the Moulin Rouge. I never realized that breasts came in so many shapes and sizes.

A couple of days later, Ann and I were told to move to the George Cinq Hotel. Natalie liked it better there. I preferred our hotel, but after all, it was work and not a vacation - even if it felt like it at times. Moving was an ordeal, thanks to our production accountant who was a real pain. He gave us our per diem reluctantly as though it came out of his own pocket. We had to clear the changes through him and he was reluctant to okay it even though we had been told to move. I think the little guy liked to defy the lofty, and Natalie's entourage was as close as he could get.

Finally, after many days of play, we actually went to work filming under the Eiffel Tower. It was the end of the race, a gigantic scene that demanded lots of organization. During the race Natalie and Tony had fallen in love and their wedding took place as they crossed the finish line - first. Don Feld had designed a dazzling wedding gown with a veil twenty-feet long.

The first morning was spent getting the shot ready, and then the crew reported to the Eiffel Tower for lunch. This was the first time we had been reunited with our crew and they began to tease us about being on the gravy train. There were carafes of wine lined up and down our tables. Every few moments someone gave a toast to the "Gravy Train" and we all took a sip of wine. There were too many toasts, and too much wine; it was a wonderful lunch.

I didn't notice how much I'd had to drink until I went to the restroom. As I left the stall I noticed the urinals on the wall and my friend's husband was taking a leak. I'd gone into the men's room!

I'd never seen Ann drink before. She was comical, but became real panicky when she misplaced Natalie's veil for the wedding scene. We all helped each other through the afternoon. Most of the crew was in the same shape as us and the next day the wine was visibly absent from our lunch table.

That evening we went to dinner at Mouton de Pomerge, an interesting place. They served drinks in small glasses that had round bottoms, so it was immediately "bottoms up." The bread was shaped to resemble a man's privates. They presented me with a garter, the waiter happily lifting my skirt, embarrassing me as he slipped the garter up my leg. They snapped a picture and I quickly got over my embarrassment.

We worked under the Eiffel Tower a few more days, finishing the end of the race and the wedding scene where Natalie and Tony get hitched. We had a five hundred thousand-dollar confetti fight to celebrate the end of the race.

We celebrated Susie's birthday, at a little restaurant near the Beaujolais Vineyards. I used my first footstep toilet and I hated it. You don't sit; you put your feet along the sides of a hole, then you squat and hold onto handles on the side. I felt like I was going to fall in. Yuk!

Bill had joined me for a few days and we took the Bateau Mouche, which sailed up and down the river serving dinner, passing the Notre Dame Cathedral, all lit up, on the way. I bought Bill a small painting at Montmartre that night. I was having such a wonderful time that I felt I owed him something.

I had a big, surprise when I ran into Helen Gruzik, a hairstylist from home. Paris wasn't so large after all. It was nice to see a familiar face in the crowd.

Natalie loved the social scene. She had premieres and parties to attend and was having the time of her life. I dressed her hair almost every evening before she went out. Believe it or not, I was getting tired of all the wonderful food, but I couldn't turn down an invitation for an evening out. I tried cutting down on my choices, but being a curious person, it was difficult. Who knew when I'd come to Paris again? I wanted to drink in the whole experience completely.

Location neared its end and with that in sight, I began to let my feelings of being away from my children come to the surface. I wanted to go directly home from Paris to my family, but Mona wanted me to go with Natalie to New York first. She still wanted to control everything plus there was no one waiting for her at home. I was sure Natalie wouldn't need me, so I asked her if I could go straight home with the crew. She said, "Sure, go ahead. I don't need you for anything." Mona was furious with me when she found out I'd gone directly to Natalie. I had to be very careful of her; I'd seen her try to start trouble for B.J.

Our last day we finished shooting at half past ten in the morning, then Susie and I went shopping at Foquets and had an ice cream sundae at the American Drugstore. We admitted to each other that despite the excitement and fun, we were homesick.

We flew home September 24, with three months shooting still ahead of us. I'd had such a perfect time in Europe, but when I got home and saw my paycheck I was shocked. Before leaving home I was making $250 a week for forty hours. (We actually worked normal hours in those days, not the fourteen-hour ones we do now.) I'd put in many more hours than that on location, but it wasn't reflected in my paycheck. I'd spent money in Europe freely, thinking I was making lots of overtime. I got a rude awakening. I was told that overseas we had no contract so I was paid my base pay, no more. I'd earned less than I would have made if I had stayed at home. There was nothing I could do about it. I was upset. I'd spent all my salary. But I did learn to have everything in writing before I left for the next location.

Back home, I was happy to be home with my girls, enjoying their hugs and kisses and company. At the same time it was hard to settle back into normal family life after my mad dash around Europe. While I was gone I missed them so much, but I hadn't let myself dwell on it. It wasn't the norm for women to be working full time, let alone be gone from home for six weeks. I knew Josephina and her daughters gave my girls lots of love and attention and Bill was there, too. It was hard for me to acknowledge how horrible I felt, as if I was being pulled in different directions. However, I pushed the feelings away.

In the evenings, I hurried home from work, drew a bath, poured myself a glass of wine, and sank into the steaming water. The girls would gather around the tub, one sitting on the pot, and we'd talk about the day's activities. On weekends I spent as much time with them as possible. I felt so lucky to have a housekeeper. I couldn't have handled my long hours of work, the house, the meals, picking up the kids from a baby sitter, and everything else like so many mothers do today.

We went right back to work at Warners now that the biggest locations were out of the way. We shot in various locations around California - a tent scene in Pismo Beach, Lake Arrowhead for a boat race, and Lone Pine for desert work.

My favorite location was in Kentucky. It actually changed my life. Growing up in Los Angeles, I had never experienced seasons. My first taste of the crisp, cool air and the feeling of fall and excitement of the trees changing to gorgeous colors captured me. It was cold, but invigorating. I felt great. During the day we shot in the countryside where stonewalls and trees lined the roads. It actually looked like France. The trees were turning vibrant shades of red, orange, and yellow. I was hooked on the seasons.

There was a fly in the ointment. Normally, working with Natalie I had a great contract - I only had to do her hair. On this location she was only set to shoot for one day so, as per her contract, I flew back home when she did, all the time wishing I could stay in Kentucky, that beautiful place. Instead I ended up in Los Angeles for a week waiting for the crew to return.

The bar in the town of Barracho awaited us on stage at Warner Bros. Studio. Here we filmed the most extraordinary fight. Every well-known stunt person in Hollywood was in that scene. Natalie arrived at the bar dressed in a black lace dress, lovely as ever. Tony Curtis was all in white. Jack Lemmon, ever the trouble - maker in black, instigated a fight and the whole bar exploded with the fight. Chairs flew through the air, tables were overturned, the bar mirror cracked into a million pieces. People fell down staircases and off balconies. Hal Needham, now a director, had come directly from another job, using painkillers because of a prior injury, so he could do a fall off a balcony. It was a madhouse. Through it all, Tony never got a spot on his shiny, white clothes. I loved watching the cream of the stunt people in Hollywood working together.

We filmed sword fights in a castle with beautiful Chuck Hayward who grabbed Natalie, dressed in a pink corset and bloomers, and pulled her up on his horse to steal her away. Chuck was tall with dark curling hair and naughty, flirting eyes. Stunt men were really something in those days. Where have all the heroes gone? There were plenty of them in those days.

When we filmed the ocean crossing from Alaska to Russia, the stage was filled with water and icebergs with the cars sitting on the icebergs. Each day the icebergs shrank. A polar bear was brought in to sit in the back of Jack's car. The bear was truly dangerous, so they cleared most of us off the stage and filmed the bear behind glass. In the film you could tell that he was behind glass, but it was simply too dangerous to have him loose near the humans.

Natalie was always dressed in beautiful costumes even on the iceberg where she wore a gorgeous fur hood. Each time I did her hair I marveled at my good fortune. I wasn't sure where this creativity had come from, but I felt good about myself.

One day while rehearsing a romantic scene under a tree with Natalie and Tony, Blake decided they had to sing a song. He needed it instantly. This was a really big order as the scene was to be shot the next day. But no problem - we had Henry Mancini, a genius, scoring our film. He went home that night and composed "The Sweetheart Tree" for Natalie to sing. It received an Academy Award.

A Russian Village was filmed on the back lot of Colombia. In that scene, Jack, Peter and Natalie arrived in the village where all the villagers stare silently at them until Natalie, who could actually speak Russian, greets them in their language. At that point the extras were supposed to cheer with great enthusiasm. We had worked all night and it was cold and late. The extras were tired and didn't care. They didn't sound excited at all. They shot it a few more times and each time the response of the extras left a lot to be desired. Finally, Mickey McCardle, our first assistant, took the microphone from Blake and gave a passionate speech, telling the extras how we had worked all over Europe and in every instance the extras had given their all. Yet here we were in Hollywood, supposedly the place where the extras were professional and nothing was happening.

"We'll try it one more time," Mickey announced. A few minutes later Blake yelled, "ACTION," Natalie greeted the crowd and they began to cheer, but something had changed. The cheering was so loud, so wild, so wonderful, and so enthusiastic that even when Mickey yelled, "CUT" the cheering continued.

My favorite scene, at least at first, was the pie fight. As I walked through the door the stage smelled very sweet that morning. It was the frosting made from spun sugar, vanilla, and chocolate. The set was very high with stairs leading up to the second floor where a doorway opened into the building from a balcony. Cakes and pies were everywhere and a huge cake at least ten feet tall was in the center of the room.

Jack, playing the part of the tipsy prince, stepped through the door and immediately fell into the middle of the huge cake. Natalie came in right after him and took a pie directly in the face. It was difficult each time they repeated the scene because we didn't have any double wigs or costumes. As soon as they called "CUT," we rushed Natalie back to the dressing room. I took off her wig and she took off her costume. She took a shower and had her makeup redone while I dried and reset the wig and Ann washed and dried the corset. It was quite a production.

The pie fight lasted for three days and by that time we were sick of the sweet smell. Still it was amazing. By the end, Natalie was covered from head to toe in frosting; we couldn't see her face at all. What a ball she had slinging pies at people. As usual, Tony went through the scene without getting a spot on his outfit. If, by accident, a spot did appear, a wardrobe man rushed in and cleaned it right off. But in the last moment of the scene Tony finally got a pie in the chops.

It all came to an end around the Christmas of 1964. What an adventure we'd had. For the most part we were glad it was over because most of us in the industry were used to change and six months was a long time to work on one project. Nevertheless, it was a delightful time for me. I doubt that they will do a film like *The Great Race* again. I felt blessed to be a part of it plus it really cemented my relationship with Natalie.

Chapter 16

INSIDE DAISY CLOVER

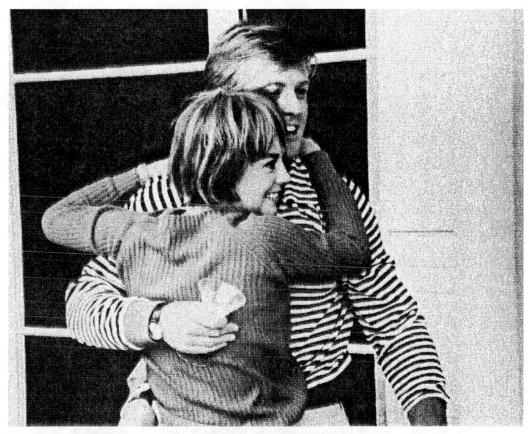

Natalie Wood and Robert Redford, *Inside Daisy Clover*

The New Year dawned and my life no longer felt much like a party. My father, who had been fifty-seven when I was born, was now eighty-six and a half and was becoming more senile by the day. Yet he insisted on remaining in his house in Santa Monica. He had been married to his fifth wife, Edith, a wonderful woman, for nearly twenty years, but finally his ways eventually drove her to drink. She left him after he broke a plate over her head (among other unpleasant incidents). I couldn't blame her, but now Daddy was alone.

I had some free time so I went to visit him. I felt very sad when I saw how far he had deteriorated both mentally and physically. Although he had plenty of money, he wouldn't pay for anyone to live with him and take care of him. There was no way he would consider a nursing home. I fed him vanilla ice cream and tried to explain in simple terms that just as a car needs fuel to run, a body needs food to survive. I asked him about his taxes and he fixed me with a blank stare. He had no idea what I was talking about. Here was man who could add a column of figures in his head. Something needed to be done as soon as possible.

I put an ad in the paper for someone to take care of him. I interviewed a couple of people, but nobody seemed right. Daddy sat there during the interviews clicking the TV to his favorite game shows to see how the interviewee's liked the show. Finally a lovely black woman showed up. I liked her. Daddy liked her too, so we hired her right then and there. Now he would be taken care of. What a relief! On Monday I visited Daddy, fed him, straightened up his house, and kissed him goodnight. I never saw him alive again. Late Tuesday night, we got a call. Daddy was dead. He had dropped a cigarette in his chair and, in his weakened condition, the smoldering fire and smoke finished him off. For some reason the woman I had hired hadn't shown up when she said she would. Maybe it was a blessing.

After the call came, we got dressed and drove to the hospital in Santa Monica. Bill didn't let me see Daddy, but he told me he was curled up like a baby and was still wearing the dark blue knit hat he always wore to keep his head warm. He had not been burned.

I had a hunch about Daddy's death. When I told him I was going to get a housekeeper for him and pay for it myself, I think he realized I no longer needed his support. He had always been there for me in times of need. He'd been weary and I believe he was waiting for a signal that I'd be okay without him. I'd always been his favorite. Perhaps my hiring the housekeeper was his signal, so he felt that he could leave.

Afterwards I realized I'd been very lucky to have him around as long as I did. After all, he was more the age of a grandfather than a father when I was born. I hadn't yet begun my spiritual studies, nor did I know about reincarnation, but I felt Daddy had gone to a better place.

Daddy came from a family of German Jews, but neither he nor his mother embraced the faith. In fact, his mother Julia was a Christian Scientist. The only experience of the Jewish faith I had was going to a synagogue to attend the weddings of some friends. We decided Daddy should have a Jewish funeral even if he hadn't practiced any sort of religion. John Rodgers, head of Fox Production at the time, was married to a nurse, Pat, who worked with my sister, Prish, in the studio hospital. John, who was Jewish, helped Prish make the arrangements for Daddy's funeral.

Daddy always said he wanted to be buried in a pine box and laid to rest in San Francisco. My sisters dressed him in one of his dark blue suits. He'd loved to gamble, especially at the horse races and always carried wooden kitchen matches in his pockets. My sisters put some of the matches in his pocket and a racing form, too, writing "I love you" on the form.

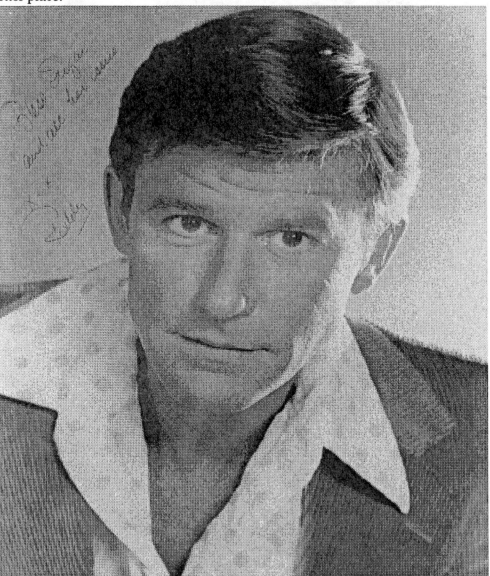

Roddy McDowall

The Temple was downtown. The Rabbi, who had obviously never met the man, described Daddy as a nice, kind person. We giggled at that. He gave a wonderful sermon describing a tree starting from a seed, growing, giving fruit, and eventually dying down in time, as it should be. I thought it described Daddy pretty well, after five wives and six children.

After the funeral was over, we ate lunch at Zucky's Deli in Santa Monica. Edith, his fifth wife, acted nervous while we were eating, as though Daddy was still going to hurry her through the meal as he had always done. We reminded her he wouldn't be doing that ever again, she could finally relax. We have a wonderful time telling "Daddy" stories, remembering what a great character he had been.

Getting Daddy from Los Angeles to San Francisco where he was to be buried posed a dilemma. Daddy always feared flying in a plane. He was so brave in many ways, but he wouldn't even get on a plane to look around. It was probably the one experience he never had while he was alive. We called the train station and they said he could travel by train, but he would have to be accompanied by someone. Nobody was able to travel with him, so as a last resort we called the airport. Yes, he could fly alone. So that's how Daddy went to his final resting place taking his first plane ride. I'll bet he turned over in his coffin during the ride.

I was preparing for *Inside Daisy Clover* so I went into Max Factor's the day after Daddy died. I'd never lost anyone so close in my life and I wasn't sure what to do. Keeping busy seemed to be the best thing. As I read the script of *Daisy* I realized that it might be a kind of catharsis for me. Daisy's mother, played by Ruth Gordon, was senile and Daisy loved her a lot. She watched after her mother, but as she became famous she was forced to put her in a home for a while. Neither of them was happy, so Daisy finally rescued her mother and took her home where, in the end, she passed away.

As I watched the most wonderful Ruth Gordon play her part, I identified her with my father and it allowed me to experience my feelings sadness and grief over the loss of Daddy.

In the film, Natalie played a young girl who was discovered by Hollywood in 1938. She lived at the beach, right on Santa Monica Pier. I was working with the Max Factor wigmakers designing a wig for Natalie - the first time I was able to design her wigs myself. I wanted her hair to look as though the sun had bleached it, but it was difficult to get the wigmakers to achieve what I envisioned. Finally, after many weeks and lots of coaxing I had the perfect finished product. It was a short pixie cut with sun streaks and I was proud of it.

Natalie met an actor who had finished his first film on Warner's lot and she decided she wanted him for our film. When Bob Mulligan, our director, and Alan Pakula, our producer met the young man, they both agreed with her and hired him. Robert Redford was introduced to us; was he ever handsome and so nice, too! We all grew to love him. He was funny, a tease, and very happy to be working with Natalie.

This was my first film with Roddy McDowall who became one of my all time favorites. I always admired him for his career choices. He was a good friend of Natalie. Christopher Plummer, playing the studio head, was sort of heavy duty, but very attractive in his own way. Katherine Bard, an executive's wife, was the real lightweight of the cast and caused the most problems. I never saw her in anything after that film.

Charlie Lang, one of the most gifted photographers of women, was our cameraman. He could do wonders for the actress and it was a joy to work with him. Natalie didn't need much help - she was only twenty-seven at the time. I always wondered if Charlie actually made the women more beautiful because of his skills or if they were actually more beautiful to begin with in those days.

Bob Clatworthy was our extraordinary art director and his assistant was Dean Tavalaris who obviously learned a lot from Bob. Dean later became most famous in his profession working with Francis Ford Coppola. I learned a lot from them. They showed me how sets were designed and built, took me through the Art Department and the display of set models, and explained how a film's budget was estimated.

Watching Andre Previn conduct the orchestra while scoring the film was a wonderful treat. Natalie had to sing in the film, but she didn't sing a complete song herself, only those parts her voice could handle well. When she got to a place where her voice couldn't carry, another singer took over. Their voices blended together in the film as though Natalie had done the whole thing. (I felt Natalie longed to be able to sing it all by herself.) My favorite song in the film was "You're Going to Hear From Me."

Conrad Hilton's home in Bel Air, a huge estate built in the thirties, was one of our sets. It was astonishing and impressed me. I sneaked upstairs to explore. The bedrooms were seductive with headboards carved with birds and snakes and silver satin bedspreads shining in the sunlight. I had the feeling those rooms could tell many a wild story. The strangest thing about the place was Conrad Hilton's own bedroom. It was a stark contrast to the seductive feel of the rest of the house. There were no frills just lots of brown leather.

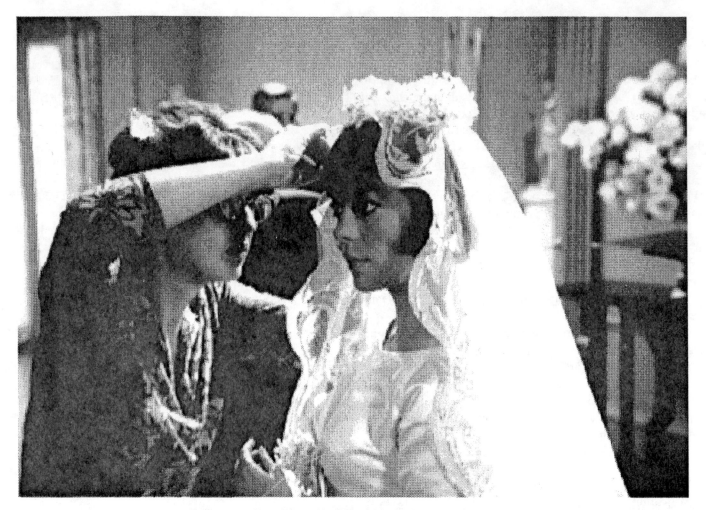

Sugar styling Natalie Wood's hair, *Inside Daisy Clover*

Our entourage was back together again. This time Natalie managed to have both her makeup men, B.J. and Eddie. In practice, Eddie did most of the makeup; B.J. was there more as a friend and to entertain Natalie. Ann Landers was handling the costumes, which were once again designed by Edith Head. Bonita Morris was body makeup and Roselle was back as stand-in. Mona was still around, but no longer in my face; she worked at home most of the time.

There was a new man in Natalie's life. David Niven Jr. hadn't lasted long. Ladislav Blatnik, an Austrian, was different from any of the men I'd seen Natalie date. He was wild and uninhibited and she was crazy about him. It was the first time I'd seen her really lost in a romance, just having fun with him, even forgetting her friends.

I was at her house one day when "Lottie" as we called him, asked Mac, the English housekeeper and me if there was any unusual food in the kitchen. He began to look through the cupboards, opening them all and then announced everything to be "boring". Since Mac was English and no gourmet cook and Natalie was often on a diet, it was a fact that everything was indeed boring. Lottie sent Mack and me to Jurgensons, an expensive, specialty food market. We were armed with a list and he told me to buy whatever else looked good - price was no object. Mac and I loaded up basket after basket oblivious of the cost. We charged hundreds of dollars of delicacies. From that day on Mac was able to come up with some amazing concoction whenever Lottie asked for something special.

Natalie's friends were somewhat resentful of this new love of hers. She had always been there for them and suddenly she was not even returning their calls. They were accustomed to Natalie answering their beck and call. It made me happy to see her indulge herself.

There was a special feeling on the set. Our crew had all worked with Bob Mulligan on *Love With a Proper Stranger* so we were already friends. On Friday evenings, at the wrap, someone would always spring for drinks and there would be a set-up on the back of the prop truck. We all sat around and had a few drinks together, director and actors included. One evening Bob Mulligan had to be somewhere to meet his wife so we all had to take him to his room to sober him up before sending him off to meet her.

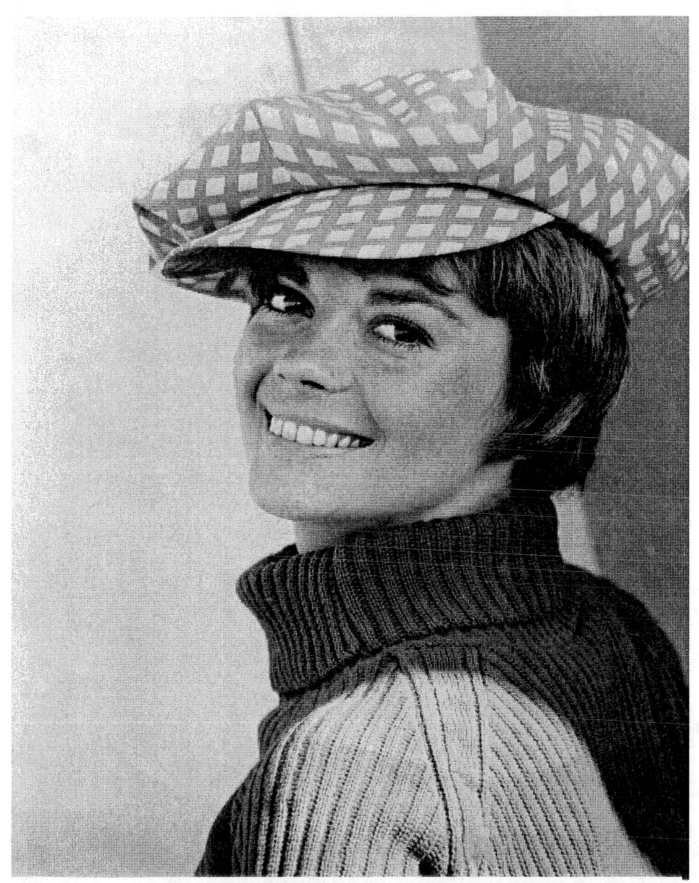

Natalie Wood, *Inside Daisy Clover*

Even though I missed Daddy, this was a fun time for me. I was in a slim phase and feeling really good about myself. On those Friday evenings, Roselle and I would go home, meet our husbands and a few other couples, and go out to an Italian restaurant and dance. I was especially enjoying myself because the style of dancing where you didn't hold on to your partner had just become popular. Bill always pointed out how I never had been able to follow very well. Now I started to feel like I was actually a very good dancer. I took off my glasses, moved to the beat of the music, and had a great time. With my glasses off, I couldn't see anybody and it seemed as though they couldn't see me either. After all those years I could dance. I knew I had it in me.

Location at the Ventura Marina was tough. We were shooting a scene on a boat when suddenly the wind came up and it got so rough that it became impossible to shoot out there. One of our crewmembers slipped and broke his leg. Finally production admitted it was impossible and quit filming for the day. In the meantime, Natalie and Bob Redford invited us to go with them for a sail on the boat. As we sailed out of the Marina, the sea calmed down and we spent the rest of the afternoon sailing up and down the coast. Not a bad day's work.

Early in the filming, Edith Head came to me and explained that she was designing a costume for Natalie that was supposed to make her look like a rag doll. She needed a yellow yarn wig to go with it and sweetly asked if I would make one. Without thinking I said "sure" never giving a thought to the fact that I'd never made a wig in my life. B.J. said I was crazy, he'd never offer to do anything like that - he was much smarter than I was.

I had no idea what to use for the base of the wig. I had to sew the yarn onto something. I bought a small pair of children's underpants and sewed the legs together to make a head shape to sew the yarn to. I assumed there would be plenty of time. Wrong! It was raining a lot so they decided to change the schedule at the last minute and the wig was needed the following Monday. By that time I discovered a small knit hat would work as a base for the wig and I had the yarn dyed the special shade of yellow requested by the cameraman. The yarn had just been delivered so I took it home and worked on the wig all weekend.

Monday morning arrived and I thought the wig looked great. It was supposed to be worn on top of the other wig Natalie was wearing. When I proudly placed the wig on Natalie's head she took one look and said, "Oh Sugar, it's too bulky, there's too much yarn. My head looks too large." My heart sank. The whole day's shooting would be held up and it was my fault. Why hadn't I listened to B.J.? How had I let Edith talk me into making the wig? Normally we would have time for fittings, but not this time.

I said a silent prayer. God must have been looking over my shoulder. As I removed the wig and hurriedly began removing yarn, strand by strand, Natalie tried on her costume. For some odd reason, it was six inches too small. They had her form in the wardrobe department so it was hard to imagine how that could have happened. Anyway, it had to go back. Next B.J. and Eddie just couldn't get the white makeup she was using to go on right. It just kept cracking. In the meantime, I kept removing yarn from the wig and by the time all the other problems were solved, her wig was perfect. I sighed with relief. My prayer had been answered.

It turned out to be a magical day. The next hurdle, once we got Natalie ready, was shooting the scene. Redford had to take the yarn wig off, but because the other wig was underneath, both wigs could come off at the same time if he wasn't careful. I began to appreciate and love Redford even more when he asked me for the best way to take the wig off. He practiced over and over and during the scene, he was so gentle carefully lifting only the yarn wig. I had no fear that the other wig would come off, too. He was just perfect.

Christopher Plummer was always a little haughty. One day he had to climb to the top of an outdoor set for a scene and he was frightened. To bolster him up, I assured him "Only the good die young" and therefore he'd have no worries. He snarled at me.

Alan Pakula, our producer, was a sweet, mild-mannered man. He was also very shy and quiet. It was his birthday and we decided to send him a belly dancer with "HAPPY BIRTHDAY" written on her belly. We hired the girl. She came first to Natalie's dressing room to disrobe so the greeting could be applied to her belly. We got Eddie's makeup case, took out all his bright colors, and painted the greeting on her belly giggling and laughing as we painted. The dancer was stunned - this was a first for her. When she was ready to go to Alan's office, we got a message he had left for the day. How disappointing. We wondered if someone had warned him about our surprise.

Thinking quickly, not wanting to waste the effort, we regrouped, erased the happy birthday greeting, redid it as "GOOD LUCK" and sent the dancer to Mike Nichols who was just beginning to film *Who's Afraid of Virginia Wolf*. Alan was quite relieved never to have received his birthday greeting.

The end of the film when Daisy decided to kill herself is one of my favorite scenes of all times. Daisy turns on the gas oven, pulls up a chair, and sticks her head in the oven. She keeps on getting interrupted and the suicide never happens. She just gives up, pours herself a cup of coffee, turns up the gas, and walks out of the house and up the beach.

The shot was the longest camera dolly shot I'd seen up to that time. The grips had to keep rebuilding the track, moving it as the tide came in. The timing had to be perfect and took hours of planning. Natalie left the house and walked up the beach as the house blew up in the background. It worked perfectly the first time. I don't know what they would have done otherwise. The house was blown to bits. There were seven cameras filming it from various angles.

    Daisy was very special to me. I felt like I was a part of the project from beginning to end plus I got a real education in moviemaking. Was it Bob Mulligan or just the time? Everyone working on the film became close friends. It was just the way I always wished working on a film would be. Looking back, I realize what a gift this was - the best total experience I ever had on a film.

Chapter 17

LORD LOVE A DUCK

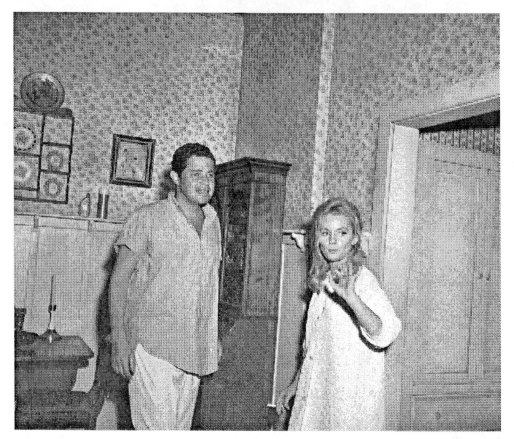

George Axelrod, director with Tuesday Weld on the set of *Lord Love a Duck*

Daisy came to an end and Natalie took some time off to rest and be with Lottie. I stayed on at Warner Brothers, working on *Hank*. It was the first television series I'd ever done. Up to this point I'd been fortunate in my career, having concentrated on film work rather than television. I felt films were more creative plus they had larger budgets and required finer work. Television schedules, on the other hand, felt rushed and the excuse of "it's only a small screen" was given all too often to justify the lack of time required to do something really well.

I thought it would be fun to try a series, but *Hank* was neither good nor clever nor did it present any challenges and soon I was bored stiff, but luck was with me. Jack Fear, the head of Columbia Studio's Production Department, called Jean. Tuesday Weld had requested me for the film she was doing and Jack wanted to trade me for another hairdresser. Jean had reminded Jack that slavery was no longer in style, but I was free to take the job. It sounded great to me.

In addition to Tuesday, *Lord Love a Duck* starred my two friends from *Daisy*, Ruth Gordon and Roddy McDowell. I didn't want Jean to think I wasn't grateful to her for giving me the *Hank* series, but I knew she'd understood that I'd much rather work on the film. I went to Goldwyn Studios for the summer. I hadn't worked on that lot before and found it small and friendly and it was, actually located in Hollywood.

Tuesday had her own large trailer right outside the stage and she often used it as a home during the week while she was working. Hayley Mills was working on the lot, too. She also had her own trailer. David Jansen of *The Fugitive* was there as well. I found him very attractive and so did the young actresses. It was amusing watching them feud over his attention. I enjoyed Tuesday's company. She tried to come across as tough, but inside she wasn't like that at all. She must have liked me, too, since she asked for me on this film.

Lord Love a Duck was a crazy satire directed by George Axelrod who had also written the script. As usual, Ruth Gordon played an outrageous older woman. She had me put her hair up in huge rollers one day and wore them through a whole scene, just loving the way she looked. She was delicious. I have no idea how old she was then, but I wished I could be as young at heart as she was and half as bright.

Tuesday had a little dog that lived with her in the trailer. I liked it well enough, but each morning when I arrived for work I had to step over a pile of dog poo that was waiting by the door. Tuesday was always still asleep. I was used to being the one who cleaned up after the animals at home, so it didn't bother me that much, but I never seemed to have enough time to clean up after both Tuesday and her dog and still get my work done. Eventually I spoke with the assistant director who agreed. Tuesday needed a nursemaid. I suggested Blanche who had worked with us on *Soldier in the Rain*, but Blanche was busy and suggested another woman who worked out well.

From then on the coffee was on and Tuesday was in the process of waking up when I arrived. That was until one morning. Tuesday must have partied late and simply fallen into bed, forgetting to take off the fall she wore in the film. Normally the wig would be hanging on the wig block waiting to be curled for the day's work. On this particular day the maid hadn't shown up either because the Watts riots were in full swing and she simply couldn't get to work. She had called the assistant and said she'd get there as soon as she could. I went into Tuesday's bedroom to wake her up. It was a struggle, but finally she got up. By that time it was very late and she wouldn't let me take the fall off to redo it.

The day was a nightmare for me. All day long her hair kept slipping because it wasn't fastened tightly enough on her head. It was messy, too. To top it off, the script supervisor kept bitching at me about it. I wanted to shut her up, but didn't want to squeal on Tuesday. It was fine in the long run, nobody noticed. Over the years I've done so much worrying about such things, but when all was said and done it always worked out. Still, I never wanted to take a chance.

We went to some unusual places like Trousdale Estates in Beverly Hills to shoot this film. I couldn't believe the houses. They were so expensive, yet in such bad taste. Our location house had a sunken living room area called a "Conversation Pit" in the film. It was tacky, but entirely appropriate for the film. We snickered a lot behind the backs of the owners. I'm afraid we weren't very kind.

It was a long, hot summer. I was slim and I felt great. My favorite lunch on the set was clam dip, potato chips, and a diet soda. We'd never heard of a low-fat diet in those days. Anyway, it worked for me (must have been that diet soda). Working with Ruth, Roddy, and Tuesday in such a crazy atmosphere was remarkable. At summer's end, after finishing with Tuesday, I headed back home to Paramount. It was still my favorite place; I was happy to return.

Natalie didn't work that summer, but she still asked me to come to her house and do her hair for special occasions. I liked going to Natalie's home in Westwood. It was quite traditional and lovely. The front door opened into a hall. Natalie's office and the bedrooms were on the first floor. The main part of the house was downstairs, overlooking beautiful gardens and a pool.

The walls of Natalie's office were decorated with pictures of her from all the films she had made. It dawned on me one day that much of my work was displayed in those pictures as well. I was impressed. Standing back looking at the photographs, I got a different perspective of myself. I had never thought of myself as an artist before. I knew I was a fairly good hairstylist and I got along well with people, yet I never had considered myself as greatly talented. That day I began to give myself some credit. I began to feel that I was really capable. Soon after this realization, Natalie decided to write into her contract that I was to be paid a $2,000 designing fee for each film, beginning with the next one. This was astonishing. At the time no other hairdresser (with the exception of Sydney who was actually known as a designer) ever received that kind of designing fee. In today's terms it might be worth nearly twenty thousand dollars. This was a real feather in my cap and it also gave the other hairdressers in the union more recognition than we'd been able to garner before. My fellow hairstylists were proud of me.

However, the accountant at Paramount didn't appear to approve of this fee. He acted like it was his money. Maybe he was afraid it would start a trend. One day he saw me in the street, opened the second floor window, and yelled down at me, "Why are you requesting a designing fee now?" I yelled back, "I have bills to pay." It really wasn't any of his business and it wasn't right that he was announcing it to anyone who walked by on the lot, but he did write out the check.

Chapter 18

THIS PROPERTY IS CONDEMNED

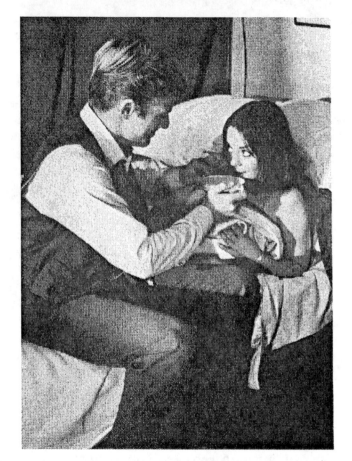

Natalie Wood and Robert Redford, *This Property is Condemned*

This Property is Condemned began shooting in the fall of 1965. Written by Tennessee Williams, the film took place in Mississippi in the 1930s. It was directed by Sydney Pollack - his second film - and produced by Ray Stark and John Houseman for Paramount and Seven Arts. Jimmy Wong Howe was the cameraman. He was an artist as well as an occasional son of a bitch, but he made the ladies look wonderful. He garnered many awards including an Oscar. We were blessed to have Robert Redford with us again plus Charles Bronson, Robert Blake, and Mary Badham, fresh from *To Kill a Mocking Bird*. Our entourage was together again, with the exception of Mona who seemed to have been lost by the wayside. Natalie had added Ralph, a masseur. It was a perfect exchange in my book. Filming began in Biloxi and it was planned to go to New Orleans and eventually finish at Paramount.

Natalie, Edith Head and I discussed Natalie's look in the film, then I ordered the wigs. The styles were fairly simple as her character was poor. After testing a variety of styles we eventually decided to go with Natalie's own hair, straight and simply parted in the middle. It worked and looked just right for the part. I assumed this basic look would make my job fairly simple, but I was fooled. The humidity of the Deep South made it difficult to keep her hair straight.

It wasn't easy to keep it looking the "same" straight all the time. I spent many hours iron curling and uncurling her hair.

As our departure date for location neared, they were unsure exactly when Natalie was going to leave for Biloxi. First, they told me I would leave on Thursday and I planned accordingly. Then, after I reported to work on Wednesday, they told me I had to leave that very afternoon. I had to be at the airport by 4:00 p.m. I panicked. Not only had I not packed, but I wouldn't be able to say goodbye to my children. It was unthinkable. I left work in tears and was totally upset by the time I got home. Still crying, I called Natalie and told her what had happened. "That's crazy," she said. "I won't even be there until tomorrow. You don't have to be there until I am. What are they thinking?" She called Production for me and told them that they would have to make other arrangements for me, as I wouldn't be leaving until the next day. Maybe they had insisted on my leaving earlier to resist Natalie's power by thwarting her through her entourage. Regardless, I got to hug my children goodbye and that's what counted.

I sat next to B.J. on the flight to New Orleans. He hated to fly and was uncomfortable especially at the take off and landing. I'd never heard him sing before, but as we landed in New Orleans, he sang, "Nearer My God to Thee," sure we would all crash and drown. What an optimist!

A limo picked us up and whisked us to Biloxi, Mississippi to the Broadwater Beach Hotel. The weather was very warm although it was October and the aftermath of Hurricane Betsy was apparent everywhere. Huge signs bent right over, trailers were overturned, and many beach side businesses were boarded up. Trees were still lying where they had been uprooted. The power of that storm was amazing.

It was late, so we stopped for dinner at the Friendship House where I had my first hush puppy. Truly delicious, Two hours later we arrived at the Broadwater Beach Hotel. What a fabulous hotel. Surrounding it were huge pine and oak trees and everywhere squirrels were running all about. Everything around the hotel was green although a little smelly because of the sulfur in the water. But we were soon used to the smell and ceased to notice it. The hotel was huge and our crew spread out everywhere. There were several pools and a large dining room where we could gather. Roselle and I had adjoining rooms. When our baggage arrived at midnight, we collapsed into bed and fell to sleep right away.

Our first day's shooting was on a train that ran across the Bay of Saint Louis in Gulfport, Louisiana. The day was hot and I was exhausted from all the rushing to get there. Wearily I sat on the steps of the train gazing down at the water beneath the tracks as we went back and forth, shot after shot. I thought to myself, "If I ever have a nervous breakdown, I'll come here and recover. It's so peaceful."

Mary Badham played Natalie's little sister. She walked up and down the railroad tracks wearing an old dress of Natalie's, so skinny and awkward with her hair hanging limp. She was perfect for the role of that tough little kid. As the film went on, she became more graceful and the awkwardness began to vanish. She was wonderful.

Robert Redford hated traveling by air so a few days later he arrived by train. B.J. got wind of this and we all got together to plan a surprise for Bob. We knew he was shy and had no desire to be noticed, but that didn't deter us.

We decided to create a silent band - something subtle. I had two Styrofoam coolie hats that I banged silently together like cymbals. I can't remember what the others played. We only wanted to embarrass Bob a little. And we did. He got off the train and tried unsuccessfully to lose us after he realized what we were up to. Eventually he gave up and greeted us with hugs and kisses; although I'm sure he wished we hadn't been so inventive.

Redford was low-key and liked to play himself down. I couldn't understand how a Leo, especially one who looked as good as he did, could do that. He had golden blonde hair and almost white eyelashes that needed to be darkened so they could be seen by the camera. He hated wearing mascara. Natalie came up with a great idea. "Let Sugar dye your eyelashes," she suggested, "and you won't need mascara." He was reluctant. After all, it wasn't the most masculine thing to do, but finally he agreed.

Natalie directed the whole operation. I hadn't dyed eyelashes since hairdressing school, so I was a bit nervous. We took Bob to Natalie's suite and had him lie down on the bed with his eyes closed. As I applied the tint to his lashes I worried, "What if I drop some dye on his skin? He'll be left with a dark mark on his face and I might not be able to remove it." But I succeeded and his lashes looked great, very natural. He no longer had to wear that "blasted" mascara.

The South's warm, sultry weather and the mixture of French and Voodoo heritage of New Orleans brought out my sensuous nature. I had the feeling this location was going to be a wild party.

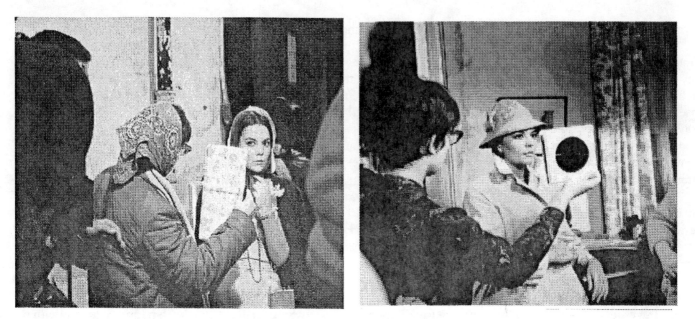

Sugar with Natalie Wood, *This Propert y is Condemned*

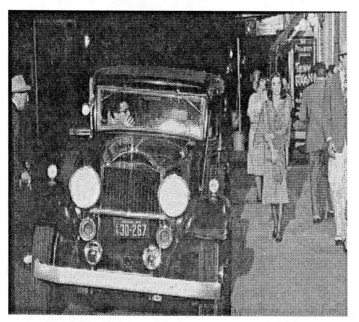

Natalie Wood on Set in New Orleans

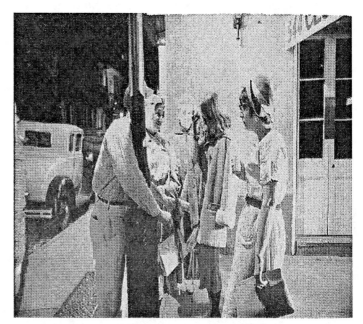

Sugar as an extra in New Orleans

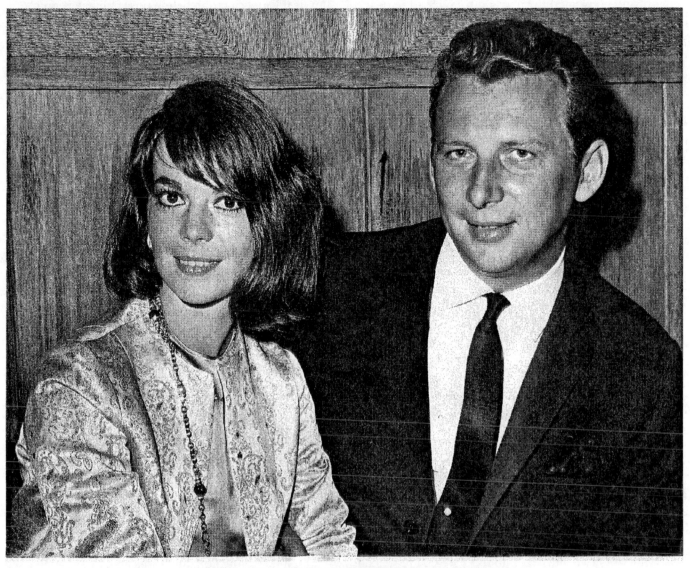

Natalie Wood with Ladislav "Lottie" Blatnik

Natalie had quite a summer and shared her adventures with us. She and Lottie had gone to Brazil, where Lottie lived during part of the year, for a vacation. The first surprise she had came during a party. Someone casually took a gun out and shot it into the ceiling. It was very scary, but not as frightening as what happened later. On a camping trip in the jungle the group decided to have a costume party. Since they hadn't planned it beforehand, the costumes had to be improvised. It was a wild scene with lots of drinking. As the party began one of Lottie's friends appeared in his "costume." As he wandered out of the jungle stark naked and covered with blood, Natalie was shocked, but everyone else burst into laughter. The man obviously had come to the party as a hamburger. To get that effect, he'd cut himself all over to make himself bloody like a piece of meat.

At this point Natalie wasn't really sure about her relationship with Lottie. I liked him, but then I only saw him occasionally when he flew down to see Natalie. I thought he was fun and witty. He hated Mona too. One day we were all talking about our experiences with Mona and Lottie made a great remark. When he saw a pretty girl, he'd often quip, "Better beneath me than beneath a truck." But when he referred to Mona, he said, "Better beneath a truck."

Now that Natalie had let Mona go, she was definitely more relaxed. We finally confessed to her all the troubles Mona had caused us, especially to B.J. and me. We admitted we hadn't told her because it didn't seem like the right thing to do since she had hired Mona and it was her business. Natalie made us promise not to ever hold our tongues if something like that should happen again.

Meanwhile, a war was going on between Sydney Pollack and Ray Stark. Sydney was the first of the new wave of directors and he wanted to have control over all parts of the film. But Ray wanted to be the boss and have control. Sydney was independent and knew what he wanted to create. He had his own ideas about camera shots - which didn't please Jimmy Wong Howe either as he was not accustomed to being told what to do. Tension built and sides were drawn with Natalie and Sydney on one side and Seven Arts on the other. In the limo on our way to work in the morning we joked, "Don't say anything important out loud." We knew "transportation" was on the "other" side and we could be taped. It was kind of silly, but had its funny moments, too.

When I called home, Laurie, my oldest daughter, sounded like an adult, even though she was only eight. Tom Collins, a neighbor and friend, was watching the house and looking after Josephina and the girls. He did the grocery shopping and anything necessary because Bill was also on location. Tom said my girls were doing well. Josephina and her girls only spoke Spanish so I really needed someone around who spoke English in case of any problems. Tom was like an uncle and he loved the kids dearly. I was able to relax knowing they were in such good hands.

Married life was feeling very flat. Bill was having his own problems and he was moody. Being around moody people always had a negative effect on me and I couldn't seem to cheer him up. While I was on location, I began to realize I was much happier away from Bill then being with him. This, of course, opened up innumerable opportunities for me to get into trouble.

Often on location, I'd been around many people during their location romances and they appeared to return home to their marriages with little problem. Sometimes I'd even eat lunch with one of the location "cuties" and then later have dinner with the wife and the same fellow. This could be rather uncomfortable, but I never looked down on anyone or judged them. It was a good thing.

My first opportunity came when a rich gentleman invited me to go flying in his new Myer's airplane. Luckily, one of the actors, a pilot who loved to fly, was sitting next to me. His ears perked up and he offered to go with us. It was fantastic flying over the Gulf of Mexico in that little plane. I was thrilled. After that the actor took me on lots of plane rides as we had so much free time.

Each time Natalie had a few days off, she left for Los Angeles and we took advantage of her absence. One night the first assistant, who was also a pilot, Roselle, Eddie Butterworth and I decided to fly to New Orleans. Things were not going too well on the set with Sydney and we weren't sure we'd get back there on location as was originally planned. One evening after work we dashed off to the Gulfport airport and hopped on a small plane for the half hour flight to New Orleans.

Upon arrival, we hailed a taxi to Bourbon Street and had our first drink at the Napoleon House in the patio of an old French home. Then we were off to the Royal Orleans Hotel for dinner - my idea of a perfect hotel - a combination of Paris and the Old South. After dinner we headed to the Absinthe House where strippers danced on the tables, and then we had coffee and beignets with powdered sugar at the Morning Call before walking the streets once more. It was a fantastic night and we were home by dawn.

After only two and a half hours of sleep, I reported to work. Despite feeling horrible, I was able to do Natalie's hair. Surprisingly, my fingers didn't even shake which earned me a black mark as everyone else was having a hard time at work. But that night I went home and passed out very early.

When we weren't working, we sat around in the restaurant and talked for hours. As usual, Charles Bronson was his obnoxious self. Once, he very slyly asked me if I did anyone's hair besides Natalie's. He had some hair he wanted doing, he said. I knew he was trying to be rude, but I happily answered, "No, I'm in Natalie's contract and take care of no one else." I know I sounded snooty, but he deserved it. He liked to get everyone's goat. One afternoon Charles Bronson and Bobbie Blake and some other actors were sitting together when the actor who had taken me flying began to talk about planes, his favorite subject. In his nasty, way Charlie remarked, "Can't you talk about anything else? All you ever talk about are planes." The actor was no match for Charlie's caustic manner so I opened my big mouth and said, "Well Charlie, you're no different." "What do you mean?" he retorted. "Well," I said, "you always say the same thing, too. Everything that comes out of your mouth is nasty so what's the difference?" He was speechless for once and stayed quiet for quite some time. Later Bobby Blake came up to me and said, "If I'm ever up against a wall, Sugar, I want you on my side." I appreciated that.

At other times Charlie told us about his childhood and how it had been growing up in the coal-mining town. It must have been tough; it still showed in his face and attitude. I had no idea what it was like to be him, but I listened and learned.

Originally our plans were to go straight to New Orleans from Biloxi, but things were really heating up between Sydney and the production company. They wanted to get him back home where they had more control over him. We hated packing up and going home, leaving behind the location atmosphere we had created. It had been such fun. At home our families were our priority. On location we could forget our responsibilities and play.

Back home, on the first day of shooting, I was stunned as I walked through the stage door at Paramount. The air on stage was so hot and humid that. I thought I was back in Biloxi. I was wearing a woolen dress. All day we glowed with sweat, just as we had down South.

We shot for a couple of weeks and suddenly our producer Ray Stark told Sydney he could only shoot only master shots - no close-ups, no over the shoulders, no singles. Normally a director shoots all these angles to give the editor as many choices as possible when he cuts the film. Natalie was outraged and went to bat for Sydney. The film looked great. Jimmy Wong Howe made Natalie look more beautiful than I'd ever seen her on film. He was a talented devil. A few days later, Ray relented and Sydney was allowed to do his work, his way and it was also decided we would go back to location to New Orleans, as originally planned, in December.

Natalie and I stayed at the Royal Orleans Hotel while the rest of the crew stayed at the nearby Monte Leon Hotel. I absolutely loved my room. It was on the top floor with little dormer windows and a window seat. The room was royal blue with touches of red and white, the coziest room I'd ever had in a hotel. The television was hidden in a cabinet. As usual, I ordered a first meal that was memorable - a dozen oysters on the half shell and hot chocolate. I was asleep by 8:30p.m.

The next day was Sunday, our day off. Roselle came over and after we collected our per diem, we walked all around the French Quarter in the rain. I loved it. We met up with some of the crew and had coffee. John, one of the crew members and I began to talk. I had known him for years, but we never had been able to just sit and talk. We ended up walking in the rain along with his son who also worked with us. After a few blocks his son left us and we continued walking. We had dinner together that night.

I didn't realize it, but this was the birth of a romance that would span two years. John was seventeen years older than I was. We were old friends. He was tall and attractive. Soon we were spending all our time off together and our feelings became more and more intense. One evening I watched as he had his picture done in pastels by an artist in the street. I felt so happy just to be with him. We listened to Dixieland bands, had a romantic dinner, and by the end of the evening I was completely in love. God, that was a romantic city. I couldn't have stopped myself from falling in love if I tried. My life at home

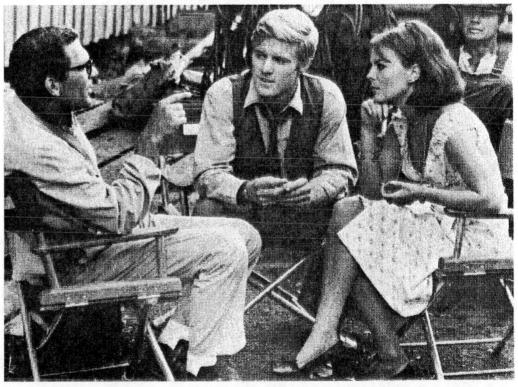

Director Sydney Pollack with Robert Redford and Natalie Wood, *This Property is Condemned*

was not fulfilling. This was just what I wanted my life to feel like. The fact that we were both married didn't seem to matter at the time.

Some of our scenes were shot in graveyards where people were buried above ground. The hurricane had blown some of the graves open and bones and teeth were scattered about the graveyard. It was weird. An eerie thing happened one morning. They were planning a funeral and someone was going to be placed in the mausoleum that afternoon. When the crypt was opened, the woman's body inside was still intact. She had red hair and was lying on a stone. But the moment they touched her she turned to dust. They just pushed her remains back so the next body could be placed where her body had been.

Natalie was very funny about her hair during the film. We hadn't cut it at all during the film. She didn't want me to and it must have grown two inches. It seems she was worried about the "double" chin she imagined she had. She was always chewing bubble gum hoping to get rid of it. She thought that if her hair were long enough her chin would be unnoticeable. She had me keep a large mirror nearby so she could see what the camera saw before every shot. Smart woman.

Howard Koch Jr., was working with us as a third assistant director. He liked hanging around with our group, but was depressed about his upcoming twentieth birthday. He felt he was getting old at twenty! We wanted to do something special for his birthday and B.J. suggested we get him a hooker. We thought that sounded like a perfect present. B.J. did the research and found out it would cost $25.00. We all contributed a dollar each and signed the card. I just happened to walk into the hotel the same time the pimp arrived and met him. He wanted to know what we were planning so I explained that we wanted a cute, young girl for Howie. I asked him if she could possibly sing "Happy Birthday" and carry a cake in to the room to him. He laughed and said he wasn't sure he could manage that. Still laughing, he confessed he'd never sold "pussy" to a woman before. Finally, after patiently listening to all my questions and requests he said, "Listen lady, just bring the money to me. I'll be in the cab outside and she'll be there for the party." Eddie actually handed him the money, but I got the credit for making the deal. It wasn't what I really wanted to be known for, but my image was rapidly changing.

The night of Howie's birthday we took him out to dinner and then went to his room, the whole crew was there. We had cans of silly soap and squirted it all over each other, playing around. There was a knock at the door. Our girl had arrived. All of the girls were curious; we'd never seen a real prostitute. Her name was Ronnie and she was young and not bad looking with only one tooth missing. In fact, she didn't look very different from anyone else, just a little hard.

The next evening Natalie was working on the street and the Production Department asked if I'd dress like an extra and stick close to her just in case there was trouble. I agreed, but I didn't realize how funny I'd look in my thirty's wardrobe. It was a cold December night, but supposed to look like summer. First of all they gave me a huge pair of long underwear to wear so I'd be warm; I had a hat and an awful dress, too. I stayed close to Natalie and it must have been helpful, but I really had to laugh at myself.

When I noticed Mike, the taxi driver who had brought us our prostitute, sitting beside the set, I walked over to him. I lifted my dress and showed him the sagging crotch of my long underwear and then asked, "Can you sell me tonight?" He laughed and laughed and later asked if he could drive me to the airport when we departed. I guess I'd made a friend.

Ronnie, our prostitute, came around now and then to visit us. She often brought a friend named Butterfly, an attractive girl - or so it seemed. But we learned more about Butterfly as she told us stories of her adventures. Men who came onto her had picked her up - they figured she was a girl, but actually she wasn't. Still, she looked feminine to me and quite pretty with her hair combed in a ducktail. Who would have known? She told us how when she'd take off in a car with a man and begin to respond to him, her manhood would begin to make its presence known. Then on realizing the truth he'd beat her up and throw her out of the taxi. So much for the street life in New Orleans. I felt sorry for these young people. They'd chosen a tough life.

I didn't feel sorry for myself though. I decorated my room for Christmas, invited John up and life was wonderful for the moment. I felt appreciated and so did he. Our only problem was we had to go home soon and as we were both married it wouldn't be a pretty picture. What was I going to do? I figured I'd decide what to do when I went home on Christmas Eve.

But it was Christmas and I didn't want to ruin the day for everyone so I didn't say anything until Christmas night when Bill and I went to Natalie's house for a party. After a few drinks, I confessed to Natalie about my affair. She was amazed, as she had thought that my life was really good. She found it was strange that something like this would happen and ruin things. I realized at that moment that I'd never shared my problems; nobody knew my marriage was so empty. Driving home from the party later that night, I confessed my infidelity to Bill. He was calm. His response was to ask, "Why didn't you tell me before?" He didn't understand that I didn't want to ruin Christmas, but I had anyway.

It was awful. Bill insisted I call John and talk with his wife. I called, feeling so small. John asked me to come over and later I sat with his wife having coffee. It was humiliating. I wanted to disappear.

By now everyone on the set knew what was happening. It was obvious John was staying with his wife and it was the end of the location romance for him, but I was heart broken. Bill and I talked and I explained how he was never affectionate. I longed for affection. He replied, "Well, don't we have three lovely girls?" "Yes," I said. It was true, but I thought there was more to a relationship than that. I said then, "You never say you love me." He replied, "I build you things, don't I?" It seemed we were always speaking different languages.

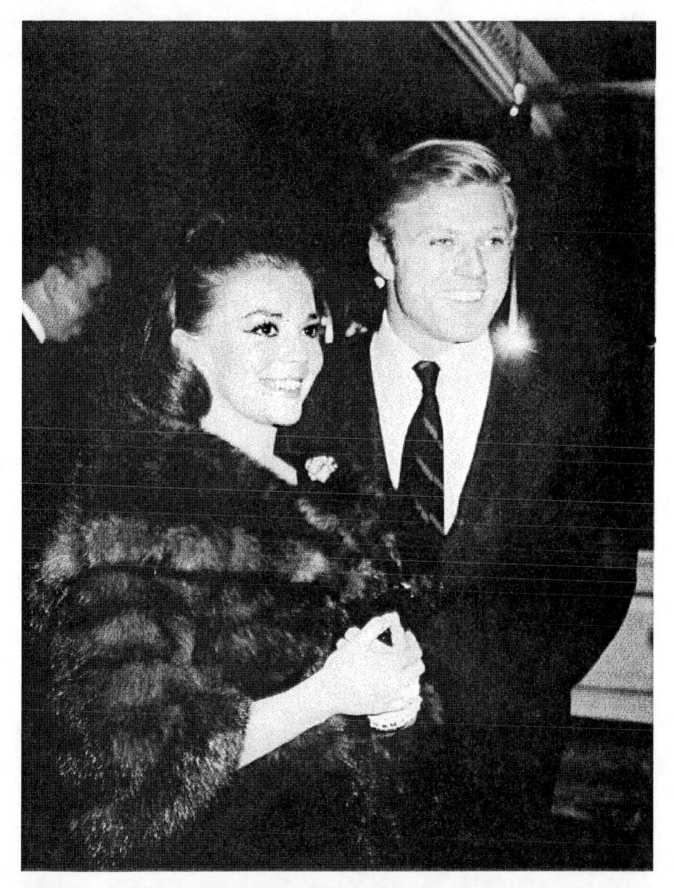

Robert Redford and Natalie Wood, press screening of *This Property is Condemned*

One day I was sitting on the set in tears when Eddie and Roselle came up to me. They were actually happy to see me crying. I thought it was strange, but they told me they felt I'd never shown my real feelings. I always acted so happy. They were glad to see I had feelings like everyone else. I thought they were just awful. I didn't want anyone to see me so unhappy. But I couldn't help it that day.

The film was finished and Bill and I decided to patch things up as best we could. John stayed with his wife. I wasn't happy with my situation and I had no clue to the future, but there didn't seem to be much of a choice at that point. It was a location romance, after all.

Chapter 19

PENELOPE

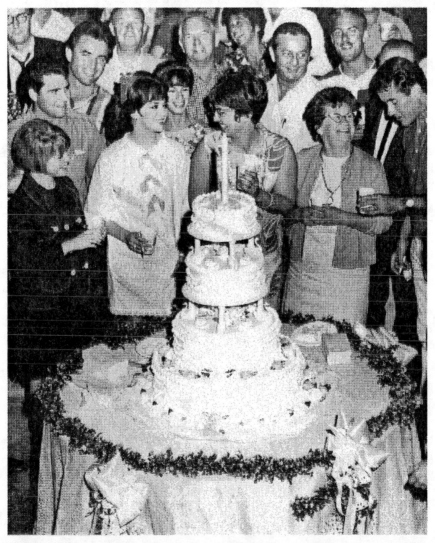

Natalie Wood celebrates Sugar's birthday with a cake used in
Penelope

After *This Property is Condemned* finished, I decided to take some time off, stay home and make some sense of my life. I was twenty-nine years old. In Astrological terms, it was my first Saturn Return - a time to evaluate life and look in new directions. And so I did. I began to study psychology and spirituality, to ask questions of myself and of life. I began to understand that my life experiences, both good and not so good, were gifts, opportunities for growth. Up until then, I hadn't understood this simple truth. I simply accepted what life handed me and dealt with it as best I could. Now I discovered what it was I liked about myself, who I was becoming. I found a new confidence.

A couple of weeks later, I began working on *The President's Analyst* starring James Colburn, Godfrey Cambridge and Severn Darden. It was a strange story in which the telephone company was eventually exposed as the villain.

Our cameraman, William Fraker was a sweet, white-haired man with a white beard. He wasn't really old, but he liked us all to think he was. I wonder why? Bill would often call me up to arrange the actress, Joan Delaney's hair, so it would look good in her close-ups. I always appreciated that from a cameraman. The best ones would call me to come and look through the lens, to see what the camera saw - you can't always tell just by looking with the naked eye.

One sunny morning, on location, James Colburn walked through a field of flowers with his arm around a curvy, naked woman. I wondered how she could be so casual while walking in front of the whole crew, without a stitch of clothing. It would have been extremely difficult for me because I didn't have a "great" looking body. It was healthy, but ordinary to look upon. Even if I'd had a spectacular body, I don't know if I could have pulled that off.

When *President's Analyst* finished, Nellie asked if I'd like to go on a publicity tour, with three sets of twins, for a film called *Gunn*. It sounded great to me. I met the twins and found that there were two real sets and one had been "created" by publicity. Our first assignment was a trip on a paddleboat junket in Long Beach Harbor. That evening I met the girls at the studio and dressed their hair. We took a bus to Long Beach. We arrived at the harbor and boarded a boat filled with publicity people. There was an abundance of good food, music and booze.

It was quite a night. Once I'd retouched the girl's hair, I was free to do whatever I wanted to do. I joined in the festivities. It was a good thing the ride back to the studio took a long time; it gave me a chance to sober up so I could drive home from the studio.

We took off on the actual publicity junket the next week. First we flew to Atlanta and stayed at the Hyatt Hotel. It was fantastic. There was a lobby, open with fountains and an elevator, which took us to the restaurant at the top of the building. The studio hadn't sent a wardrobe person on the tour. Apparently, the girls had a choice between a hairdresser and a wardrobe person and they figured their hair would be a bigger problem than their clothes. I became hair, wardrobe, makeup person and mother, all combined in one. In some ways the twins seemed rather helpless and they needed guidance from me. The only other person with us was a publicity man, who showed up in New York City and Denver. Other wise we were met by a local publicist.

The dresses the studio sent for the girls had been worn on the film. They were low cut and sexy and didn't fit worth a damn. It was fine on the set, as long as there was a wardrobe person nearby to tape them together here and there to keep the girls from being exposed completely. There was nobody doing that at the publicity parties and so the girls opted to wear some strange paper dresses the studio had sent along for them. Each day I had to cut the dress to the right length for each of them. It was very strange. One evening, we were invited to a Playboy Club. I pitied the poor bunny waitresses all dressed in the steel-like outfits. Their hips were bruised from wearing those costumes.

In New York City, we had an impressive arrival. Our plane was late, so the publicist rushed us out of the airport over to the heliport. We were loaded into a helicopter and soon were flying above Manhattan.

When summer arrived, Natalie had another film to do called *Penelope*. Our director was Arthur Hill and the cameraman was the wonderful Harry Stradling, Sr., Ian Bannen, Dick Shawn and a friend of Natalie's, Norma Crane, were also in it. The film was made at MGM. I hadn't worked there in many years. Sydney Guilleroff was still working there.

Natalie was in a dilemma. What were we to do about Sydney? He always designed the hair for films made and MGM and here I was, in her contract as the hair designer. My ego had never been a big problem, so we discussed it. We decided that Sydney could do the designing and I would get my two thousand dollar designing fee anyway. I was okay with that and Natalie relaxed. Not having to cross Sydney was a relief.

The film was silly little story about a bank president's wife that is a bank robber and a kleptomaniac. Natalie needed to have different looks. She had four wigs in different colors and they thought she could use rubber face masks as a disguise.

Bill Tuttle, head of makeup, always did the important makeup jobs if possible. He had designed a mask that fit over Natalie's face. She hated it. He took her into his special makeup room and tried doing something different. He was putting rubber on her face, then stretching it to make wrinkles and drying it with a dryer. Natalie hated that too. Finally, Eddie Butterworth came up with a better idea on his own. He was very capable. Natalie felt Bill was pompous. He seemed to want to make things look good, not caring how it felt to her. Natalie refused to put up with that sort of treatment and I didn't blame her.

Sydney ordered three wigs for Natalie. They were awful, way too much hair in them. I let him do as much designing as he wanted to, and then I took over and thinned the wigs so they didn't look quite so "wiggy." The blonde

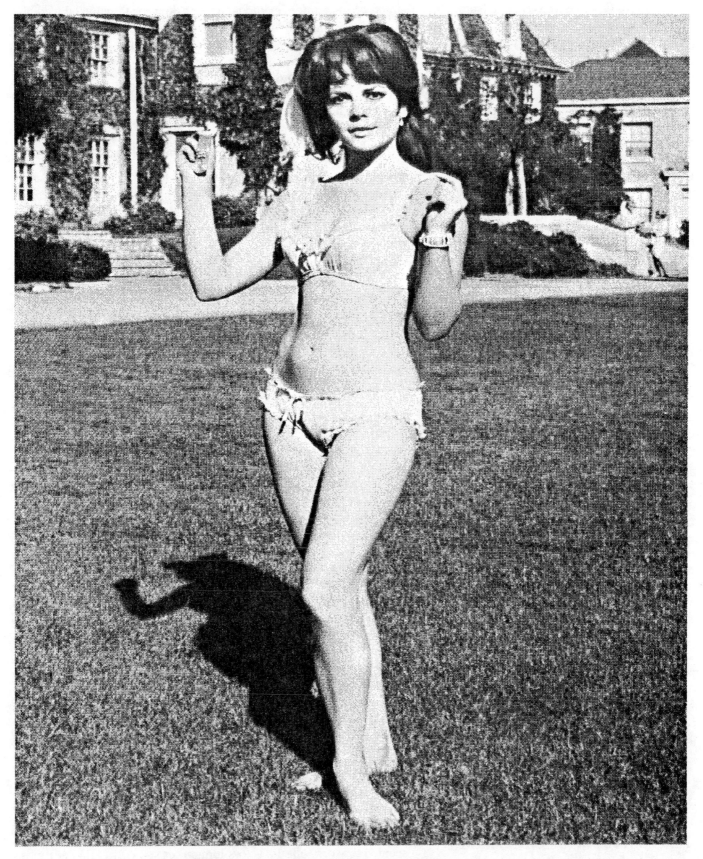

Natalie Wood in *Penelope*

wig did look great when I was finished.

One day while we were in a Natalie's dressing room, a gentleman knocked at the door. Natalie introduced him as Leon Uris, the author. As she was having her makeup done, I sat and talked with him. I'd read so many of his books and really admired his writing. I was disappointed. He was such a good writer, but so dull in person. I hoped she wasn't dating him.

Actually, at this time she was dating Arthur Lowe, Jr., a humorous man despite the fact that he always looked so sad. Natalie told me a story about him that explained his demeanor. When he was a child, he lived on an island in New York in a huge mansion. He spent his childhood surrounded with towering, dark trees and hedges. From then on, in my mind, I could always picture this little boy crouching down, trying to escape the wind blowing as he ran from place to place. Arthur still seemed to be crouching away from something. He appeared much older than he actually was.

Arthur often brought his adopted children from his former marriage to Linda Christian with him when he visited Natalie. They were the children of Tyrone Power, their father's beauty shone through them. Natalie loved children and enjoyed having them with her. I enjoyed seeing them too, remembering how handsome their father had been. He'd been my favorite after I saw him in *Captain from Castile*.

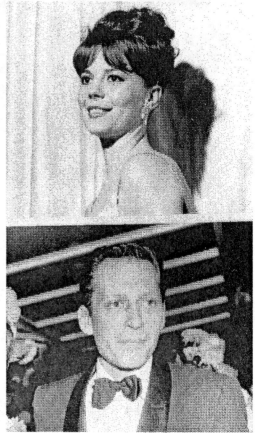

Natalie Wood and Arthur Loew, Jr.

One day, we shot in Central Park. The teamsters were supposed to be watching Natalie's trailer, but someone broke in. I had left my purse in her trailer and they stole my per diem out of it. Usually, the teamsters would have made an excuse, but an amazing thing happened. They collected the amount of money that had been stolen and presented it to me.

While we were shooting, a young girl of about twelve began hanging around the set. She was well dressed and a bit chubby. She showed up each day, always finding out where we were shooting somehow. Her name was Dianne. She attached herself to me when he realized I was friendly and also Natalie's hairstylist. After that, she became my friend and showed up at the set each day taking pictures.

We had problems with the crowds of people in the streets. New York is a difficult place to shoot. Things changed suddenly sometimes. One day, the script supervisor told me they were shooting a scene, so Natalie and I went to the hotel to put her red wig on for the scene, only to find out as we arrived on the set that it wasn't actually the scene they were shooting. I was really embarrassed and we had to rush back to the hotel to put on the blonde wig. I felt humiliated, even though it wasn't my fault. Nobody wants to hold up production.

Arthur Miller was nice and he never appeared to really direct anyone. I heard him described by one of Natalie's friends, as having very good taste. By that, they meant he hired good actors, let them do their own thing and then chose the best take possible. It seemed to work, but the actors longed for some direction at times.

The cameraman, Harry Stradling, Sr. was a true artist. He

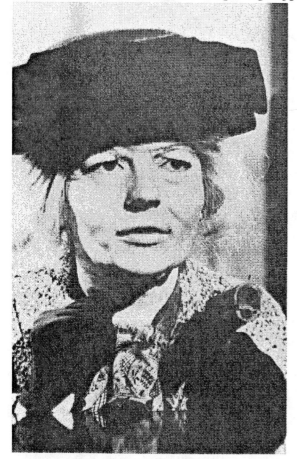

Natalie Wood disguised as an elderly woman in *Penelope*

would call me to look through the lens. It was Panavision and distorted things a little. He would show me how to place Natalie's hair so she looked the most beautiful. His close-ups of Natalie were as beautiful as the one Jimmy Wong Howe had done, yet somehow different. Whatever happened to those artists? Doesn't anyone remember how they did it?

Working at MGM brought back some difficult times I'd had when I was young, working in the stock room. It hadn't been wonderful for me to work there. It was different now. I was working in the dressing room of a star, not in the department. I felt so much better when I worked at the other studios. Perhaps it was me, but I doubted it.

This was a low period in Natalie's life. I'd never seen her like this. I sensed that all her friends were getting married, having children, but somehow she wasn't finding the man of her dreams. I found that funny because she was the woman of so many men's dreams. She appeared to have everything, but what she really wanted was a family and it didn't seem to be happening. She was seeing her "shrink" as she put it, as often as possible, trying to work it all out.

Chapter 20

BAREFOOT IN THE PARK

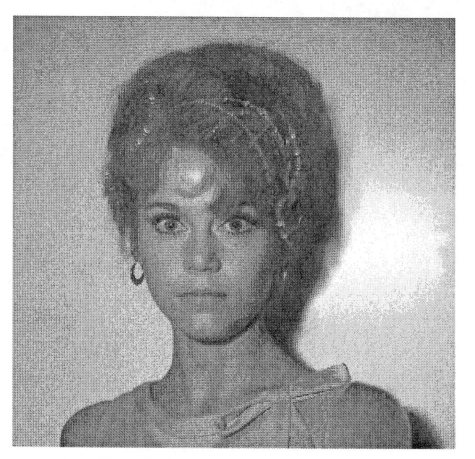

Jane Fonda, *Barefoot in the Park*

During that year I made an effort to patch up my marriage, ignoring the most helpful route, which would have been to visit a counselor. Instead Bill and I foolishly bought a larger home in Agoura, in an area called Lake Lindero. It was about as close to country as one could get in our area. It was a large home, including a family room, five bedrooms, and three fireplaces, including one in our bedroom. There was plenty of room for Bill's parents, who lived in Denver, to move in with us when they retired. Since the house was custom built for us, we added numerous amenities and by the time it was finished it cost about $45,000.

We moved in after I finished working on *Penelope*. We rented our home in Canoga Park. Unfortunately, we spent most of our money on building the house so we had no money left to buy drapes or furniture.

The arrival of Bill's parents created another diversion for me. They liked the house except for the noises of nature. Bill's mom Mama Lou, who was used to city noise, said the crickets kept her awake. Granddad appeared to be content, though. He was a strong Baptist and was happy to learn that I knew more about religion than when we had first met.

Sadly, not long after they arrived, Mama Lou was diagnosed with bone cancer. No one told her how sick she really was. She had to stay in bed, yet she still charmed my girls, playing games and teaching them to embroider and other ladylike things I never did. I liked having Bill's parents there. They were company for my girls while I was at work.

At this point, my life seemed in order when Nellie assigned me to *Barefoot in the Park*. John was the key grip on the show. I thought I was over him, but here I was faced with my feelings again. Actually, under the circumstances, I thought I behaved very well. I was happy going to work each day, knowing I would see John. His wife picked him up each evening at the gate. He didn't drive. She wasn't about to lose him to that young hussy again.

I looked forward to working with Robert Redford again, and to meeting Jane Fonda. She turned out to be wonderful. Frank McCoy, an old timer, was her makeup man. I'd not had the privilege of working with him before. Monte Westmore, one of my favorite makeup men, was also with us. You couldn't find a sweeter man. Gene Sax, our director, was still married to Beatrice Arthur who was starring in *Mame* on Broadway.

Redford had changed - he'd become more mature and private. He looked manlier. He told me he'd taken a year off after *Property*. He sensed that he was going to be successful and he wanted to spend time traveling with his family before anyone knew who he was. They traveled for nearly a year before he began to be recognized. He returned home knowing that from now on he would always be recognized wherever he went. It was the price he had to pay for his fame. One thing hadn't changed: he still hated mascara, so he had me dye his eyelashes dark again.

Jane, married to Roger Vadim at the time, had a daughter and she enjoyed playing the housewife along with her career as an actress. At Christmas time, she made dazzling Christmas ornaments for her friends. She brought her daughter to ice skate with my daughter Laurie one weekend. Jane was a warm person, lots of fun to work with.

One morning she came to work and told us how Vadim had been writing and had left some of his work out on his desk. Meanwhile, the bathtub in the room above his office leaked water down onto the desk, ruining his papers. Instead of getting angry, he went upstairs and poured champagne into the tub. He'd decided water wasn't good enough. If his work were going to be ruined, it would be by champagne.

In the beginning, we worked on stage in the empty apartment that Jane and Bob rented when they were first married. It was thrilling to work with Charles Boyer, their upstairs neighbor. He was just as charming in person as he'd been in all his movies. He was delicate and his stand-in always watched out for him. Mildred Natwick, who played Jane's mother, was a joy to work with. She had a hair-lace wig. It looked so natural; it was one of the best wigs I'd ever worked with.

A few weeks after we began shooting, we were off to New York City. It was winter and very cold. One day as I was walking in 14 ° C weather, I looked up and saw a travel agency ad for a Caribbean cruise. I was dying to book myself on it.

We did a lot of filming in Washington Square. I loved the little park and the street next to it with all its old-fashioned houses. Our worst location was a scroungy hotel that was filthy and stunk. I put some perfume on my scarf that I wound around my neck and over my nose each time I walked through the lobby.

One evening we got tickets to see *Auntie Mame* thanks to an "in" with our director who was married to the star. We had perfect seats. Shirley, the costumer, and I went together. The music was fabulous and I embarrassed her by singing along and swaying in my seat as I listened. Shirley would have gladly moved far away from me if there had been another seat to move to.

We shot all our New York exteriors and returned to Los Angeles. The first day back at Paramount, we were scheduled to work in the apartment that had been decorated and furnished while we'd been on location. Before we started makeup, Jane decided to go look at the set to see how they had furnished it. She came back very upset. She didn't like what she saw and tried to get Hal Wallis, our producer, on the phone only to be told he wouldn't be in for a while. She sat down and I began to do her hair, the same style I'd done so many times before. But as soon as I finished, she said, "Sugar, that's just not right," or, "No, this isn't the way," and on and on until I felt like I was going to lose my mind. How could I keep making mistakes on a style I'd done so many times before? I was ready to walk out the door and disappear. I was totally confused.

Finally, sensing my confusion, Frank called me aside. "She's stalling for time so she can talk to the producer before we have to shoot the set she hates," he explained. Was I relieved?! Now that I understood what was happening, I proceeded to fiddle around for another hour until Jane could reach the producer and get her point across. Then, amazingly enough, I was able to do her hair perfectly.

We worked up until Christmas Eve. John's wife came right into the stage to pick him up that night. I guess she figured I might just take him home as a Christmas present for myself. When I saw her, I got an evil idea - after all, I'd been so good all during the film. I went over to Jane and whispered in her ear, asking if she'd go and give John a big Christmas kiss and hug from me. She threw her arms around him and gave him a big kiss. Thanks Jane. Now that the film was finished, I had no idea when I'd see John again.

On New Year's Eve, 1967, my marriage came to an end, in my mind at least. Mama Lou was now in the hospital. Bill had gone to the annual New Year's Day pool party where the guys played pool and watched football on television. I asked him to come home by dinnertime so we could all spend part of the day together. I wanted to start the New Year in a good place. But Bill never came home. At midnight I got a call from the police. Bill had been in an automobile accident and was in the same hospital in Encino as his mother.

Luckily I had a housekeeper, Maria, so I left immediately for the hospital taking Bill's father with me. Bill looked awful. His face was swollen and turning green, like a watermelon, and he needed a tracheotomy to breathe. I hated seeing him in such pain, but strange at it may seem, at the same time I hated him for making me go through the pain of seeing him that way. I was surprised by my feelings, but I couldn't ignore them. I realized in that moment that our marriage was over, at least in my heart. I couldn't take the grief any longer. It was too much. Nothing was going to change.

Bill's jaw was broken and had to be wired together. I felt so sad that Mama Lou had to see her son this way. She was in such terrible condition herself. It was a difficult time. I explained to the girls what had happened and then took them to see their Dad. It was hard for them to see him so battered.

When Bill could talk, he explained how the accident happened. He was driving home much later than he'd promised and it was dark. A car had been parked in the right driving lane with no lights on. Of course, Bill couldn't see it and he rammed right into it. It turned out that the car belonged to a man from South America who didn't have the sense to pull off the freeway when his car died. Our car was totaled. If Bill had come home at the agreed upon time, the accident might never have happened.

My situation was deteriorating. We were living in this luxurious house, without landscaping - not even grass in the backyard. Maria my maid, who was from the Dominican Republic, thought nothing of mopping the floor and throwing the dirty water out through the back door. After all, it was only dirt. Granddad begged to differ and started a huge fight. She quit. This was the day after the accident. Great. I had three kids, a husband in the hospital, and no one at home to help. I was furious with Granddad.

A couple of weeks later Bill was able to come home. His jaw was still wired shut so he had to drink his meals. I learned to fix liquid meals of all sorts in the blender. Mama Lou had returned home, too. We had a full house and luckily I had a new maid, Blanca, from Panama - a cute, plump person. But, as if my life wasn't in enough turmoil, we had another disaster at the end of January. Janie Gorton, the hairdresser who had introduced Bill and me at MGM, blew her brains out. She was an alcoholic and a strange, private sort of person, yet she had still been one of the best hairdressers ever. Her son Jack was home on leave from the Marines. Poor kid, he called Bill to help. Bill had always promised Jack's dad that he'd look after the kids if there were any need, just as he'd been helped when he was young by Jack's dad. (Jack also had a sister, Jane).

We drove over to the house. I was spooked and hoped the room she had shot herself in was cleaned up. Luckily it was. We helped Jack clean out the house. I went through Janie's things stored in the garage. It was depressing. She had saved handbag after handbag and they were full of hairpins. After that I vowed I'd never leave anything like that when I died. Ever since, I've thrown away my purses when I didn't use them any more and I never leave hairpins in them either.

After his mother's suicide, Jack moved in with us when he came home on leave. He was tall and gorgeous with bright blue eyes and very sweet. Soon he and Blanca became romantically involved which troubled judgmental Granddad: He was furious that Jack and Blanca had the nerve to sleep together in our house when they weren't even married. Finally I blew up at Granddad, screaming at his righteous judgment. He wouldn't care if Jack lost his life in Vietnam, but when Jack fell in love he condemned him.

Granddad and Mama Lou moved out after the fight. Granddad was furious with me, but it wasn't just over Jack and Blanca. He'd been angry with me since Mama Lou's hospitalization. I had tried to help him become more independent to prepare him for when Mama Lou was gone. She had waited on him for fifty years and I wasn't about to take her place. I tried to teach him to cook for himself and all he did was complain to her that I was mean to him. I wasn't sad to see him go, but I was sorry Mama Lou had to leave, she was so ill. Granddad didn't care. He just wanted things his way.

Meanwhile, more of Jack's family came to stay at our house. First his sister, Janie, with her husband and son and occasionally Jack's grandmother, Edith (who had been a body makeup woman), would stay with us. It was crazy. My life was in total chaos. At times I just went through the motions; it was all I was capable of doing. I couldn't let my feelings come out. If I had, I might have just split, but I couldn't leave my girls so I kept things bottled up inside.

Through it all, I was the only family member working. My salary had to buy food for everyone as well as pay all the bills. Try as I might, there just wasn't enough money to make ends meet. We started to fall behind on our bills. Even though the man whose car Bill hit was at fault, he had no insurance. Therefore, we had to sue for uninsured motorist insurance to get our money of which the lawyer took a third. What a raw deal!

I was working at Fox Studio on a television pilot about Custer. The only time I had to myself was at work, and I was grateful for it. Wayne Maunder was our actor. He was very nice if slightly miscast - he was afraid of dogs yet Custer always had two wolfhounds by his side. Nor could Wayne ride a horse. Mickey Gilbert, our stunt coordinator, tried to make him look good, but it wasn't an easy job.

I worked hard and created wonderful wigs, decorated with feathers and beads I'd found, for the extras. I even used fishing weights that looked like shells and stones. The wigs had to be put on very tight because the Indians were riding horses. One morning, after the first shot, I was horrified to see a wig hanging from a tree. The extra, who I never forgave, had taken out all the rubber band anchors that held his wig on. As he rode beneath the tree, his wig caught on a branch and easily slipped off. He explained to the director that it was his fault, but I was still embarrassed.

Mickey Gilbert had hired a young stunt man, Billy Burton, who was just starting in the business. Billy wanted to get enough money together to fix his teeth. It was hard to crack the stunt man's guild back then, but Billy did it. Years later I worked with him as a stunt coordinator and his teeth looked great.

Although my home life was a mess, I was happy at work. I began to notice what a nice man Mickey was. He'd talk about his wife and kids, sharing his family life. I made up my mind right then that I wanted a life like that for myself and my girls.

Jack and his Marine buddies came home for Easter and I fixed them Easter baskets. When they left they all looked so cute with their Easter baskets swinging on their muscled arms. They had a party while they were with us over the weekend. I struck up a conversation with one boy who sat apart from the others. He told me he had been trained as a silent killer. He was afraid if he had too much fun, or if he let anyone get too close, he wouldn't be able to do his job in Vietnam. I remember asking the boys what they were fighting for. They had no idea.

That spring Jack proposed to Blanca and she accepted. The wedding was held at our house a few weeks later - a Saturday so Jack's buddies could be there. Mama Lou died that same week. So we married Blanca and Jack on Saturday and buried Mama Lou on Monday. It was an intense and hectic time.

Chapter 21

BLUE
1968

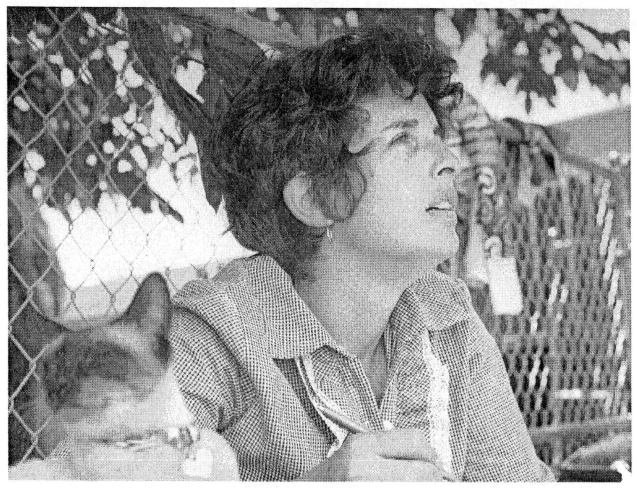

A young Ginger "Sugar" Blymyer

Life as we knew it in Hollywood was about to change. Big Business invaded us. Gulf & Western took over Paramount. Things went downhill from there and some very strange films were being made. I wasn't happy with the changes. I sensed a kind of decline in the artistic quality of our films, especially after I got my first look at Charles Bludhorn, Paramount's new executive. He was a very pale man, dressed in a suit and tie. Someone whispered "That's Charles Bludhorn, the new studio head." I just knew he had blue blood underneath that white skin. There was no humor in his demeanor.

I was disappointed. It appeared the film business was now going to be run by people like Bludhorn - business executives who only cared about the bottom line. I wondered what business executives could possibly know about making movies. How would the creative, artistic movie industry mix with the bottom-line perspective of big corporations? What was going to happen to us? What if the business partners sucked the art out of moviemaking? My fears were well grounded.

For a while, things appeared to be fine. Some very arty, if far-out, films were made, many of which unfortunately had to be shelved. This was long before the time when films that didn't make it at the box office could be sent straight to video.

Blue, the next film Nellie assigned me to, was a perfect example of the kinds of mistakes being made. Terrance Stamp, with his English accent, was cast as a blond American who was supposed to be kidnapped by Mexicans. Sylvio Narizzano, an Englishman of *Georgy Girl* fame, was brought in to direct the film. He was a good director, but didn't know much about making a western. Karl Malden and the most charming Ricardo Montalban were also in the film.

I had problems from the start. Thanks to the changes at the studio, Nellie had to justify her position as head of the Paramount Hair Department and it was a disaster. She decided to bleach Terrance's very black hair to a very light blond, in one afternoon, assuring him he would look fine for the evening. He has an important engagement that night and was wary of Nellie - with good reason. Since black hair is resistant to bleaching, it takes hours to get hair the light blond called for in the script. Nellie began to strip the black out with bleach. It didn't work quickly and only turned his hair a bright orange. It took more time and much more bleaching to accomplish the job.

Terrance was furious. He left the department and wouldn't let Nellie touch him after that. He wore a scarf on his head in the first scene that took place in a cave. I was concerned about what we would do after that when he couldn't be wearing a scarf. Unfortunately, he didn't trust me either, thanks to Nellie. On location in Moab, Utah, he found a local hairstylist who only made it worse - his hair turned green. Finally he turned to me. By the time I got the color light enough to be believable, his hair was beginning to break off.

Next we had to create the character of the wild prostitute who serviced the whole town. Nellie picked out a wig for her to wear, but the director wasn't happy with any style she created. Finally as he sat talking to the actress, I took off the wig and undid the pin curls I'd put in her own hair into to hold the wig. Her hair fell in ringlets and the director was delighted with the look. It was perfect for the part. My unconscious creativity surprised me at times.

That summer our movie crew invaded the little town of Moab. It didn't have an airport large enough for our plane to land so the pilot somehow landed in a dry riverbed and we had to climb out of the plane using a ladder. There weren't enough nice hotel rooms for each of us to have our own room, so we had roommates. I roomed with Doris, the script supervisor. We got along a bit too well - we never quit talking. I realized this wasn't going to work for either of us so I decided to search the town for a place of my own. I discovered a motel at the edge of town. It had only the bare minimum - no phone in the room, just in the office - and it wasn't nearly as nice as the one I shared with Doris, but at least I could be on my own. I needed some solitude after my crazy winter at home.

We did hair and makeup at the local high school, which was open to us during the summer. I walked to work each morning, as it was the coolest part of the day. The days were hot and the sun rose early, so I enjoyed this cool part of the day most of all.

As *Blue* was being filmed, Paramount decided to use us as a background set for another film, *Fade In*, starring a newcomer named Burt Reynolds. Everyone was sure he'd never make it. They spent many days filming around us, but I don't even remember if *Fade In* made it to the big screen.

Our company was flaky and trouble started right away. On the second day the director's boyfriend was killed in an automobile accident and the film came to a halt for a while. When work resumed the schedule was confusing. Normally at the end of each workday we were given a call sheet with our time to report to work the next day. The same thing happened on this film, but the folks in charge stayed up late into the night smoking some local weed and decided to change the schedule. Then they'd call us in the middle of the night to announce the change. After I'd been called to the office phone, a couple of times after midnight, I blew up and told Production never to wake me up again. I said I'd be at the Makeup Department very early each morning and they could pay me for any extra hours I spent there. It worked.

Gary Morris, whom I'd know since my stockroom days at MGM, was my makeup partner on the show. He was lots of fun and made me laugh a lot during the production. Thank heavens for him. He'd come up and rub my back, which he knew I loved. But as soon as I began to relax and he'd found all the tense spots, he stopped rubbing - and I always fell for it.

Joanna Pettit, the female lead, had the finest hair. It was difficult to keep it looking attractive. Sally Kirkland, who had a small part, was a peculiar woman. Her son was with her and he'd cuddle in my lap, laying his head on my chest and just stay there for the longest time. Perhaps having a mother like Sally, he needed some comfort. Eventually, Sally did some creative parts that earned her acclaim.

My friend John was working on the film, too. His wife was on location as well - ever the watchdog. I loved seeing him at work and managed to sit next to him whenever I could. I was definitely happier away from home that summer, glad to escape the madness of the past year. When Bill called and asked me if I missed him, I truthfully replied, "No."

It was so hot in Moab. Some days it seemed all I did was walk from the cooler with iced tea and lemonade, fill my cup, drink it, and be on my way back for another glass. I had a chair with an umbrella wired to it to escape from the sun. If we were working near a river, I'd set the chair in the water and soak my feet. At night after I took the wigs off and cleaned them I walked to the store for some sweet sherry and cold macaroni salad. I liked to have a drink while soaking in the tub. After soaking off the red dirt that accumulated during the day, I took a shower, dragged myself to bed, and ate my salad lying on my back. I was so exhausted. I couldn't sit up any longer. The heat really did me in.

One day Sylvio, our director, asked me to cut his hair. I'd no sooner start the process before someone called him away. I never did get it completely cut until months later when he saw me on the lot and asked me to do it all at one time.

One of our old time Paramount executives was sent to Utah to try and get the production in order. He was very nice and had been very capable of running productions through the years. But at this point he was unsure what to do. The new regime had hired people who were totally out of control and he didn't have any authority to make changes. The new executives had given free rein to people who needed lots of guidance plus there were no producers involved who knew when to draw the line and when to let it go. Drugs were also creeping into our industry during this time. There had always been alcohol around and sometimes it was abused, but as far as I knew there had never been drugs on the set before.

Terrance Stamp amused me. Once he saw that I was actually capable, he began to trust me. He complained that the makeup departments all over the world were sadly lacking in competence - except those in England. How very English of him! One day he asked me why I wore such bright colors when my bottom was so large. I replied, "Since my bottom is so big, why not cover it with a pretty color? You can enjoy looking at a pretty color instead of black or something equally boring." He quit teasing me after that.

We worked hard that summer, enduring the heat, the dust, and the lack of organization. Time passed quickly and soon it was time to return home. John's wife left a day early so she could pick him up when he arrived home. That was a big mistake. John had finally told me he was an alcoholic, but I didn't understand how it affected him because I'd never seen him drinking. The night his wife left John had a few beers with the boys. Later he came to my place and I was totally surprised. It frightened me. To see him fall apart, turning childlike, saddened me. He tried to be romantic, but it just didn't work. My dream of a wonderful evening just never materialized. I'd never seen him drunk and I hoped I wasn't the cause.

Upon our return we resumed shooting in Los Angeles at Paramount. We were told there would be a crew party the last day of shooting. Normally the wrap party would be held on another day, as we were dirty and smelled like horses and hay after working all day long. But the new regime changed all that so we had to go to the party in our dirty work clothes while the executives arrived with their wives clean and glamorous. There was no way we could really enjoy ourselves at that party.

When the film came to a close, I was still waiting to be paid for the overtime I'd earned over the summer. I received my base pay while still in Utah, but the Accounting Department hadn't been able to figure out the amount due to me for overtime until the end of the film. I also realized, too late that, though that I should have kept track of the extra hours. I'd never had a problem before so I didn't think about it. Unfortunately, I had to take what they said they owed me. I learned my lesson and would never make that mistake again.

After *Blue* I went to work for a few days on *Camelot* at Warner Brothers. The set was fantastic. It was a gigantic church. The costumes of the period were made from a material woven especially for the film. It was great fun being in Camelot if only for a short while.

One day I was assigned to work on a commercial that was shooting lingerie on the set of King Arthur's castle. The photographer amazed me. The weather was freezing and the models were wearing next to nothing, but the photographer had no sympathy. His attitude was "They make so much money that it doesn't matter if they freeze." I couldn't believe how arrogant and uncaring he was as he stood there in his warm, down jacket.

Later that month, I was called back to Paramount to do one of the first really low budget movies, an A. C. Lyles film. It was tough. We had little or no help and worked very long hours. John was working on this film, too. A change had come over him; he was more attentive to me. One day he asked, "If I ever left home, would you come with me?" Without thinking it would ever happen I answered, "Yes."

Meanwhile, while I'd been on location in Moab, Bill had met a couple called John and Joyce. He liked them and started hanging out with them while I was gone. All four of us went on a studio club trip to Las Vegas. I couldn't help, but notice Bill's attraction to Joyce, the wife. During our bus trip to Las Vegas, she came up to our seat and began to chat with us. She was holding a glass of champagne in her hand. Bill said something sarcastic to her and she poured the champagne right on him. Bill laughed and seemed to enjoy their play, something he seldom did with me. I had a hunch that there was an attraction between them and hoped I was correct. It dawned on me that maybe this might be a way out of my marriage. I wanted it to be over, but just didn't know how to end it.

A few evenings later, I found my way. Not that it was wise, but it was a way. John called. He had left home and at the moment was in the bar next door to Paramount. He reminded me of my promise to come if he ever called me. Even though it was very far from my house, I kept my promise to be there. I explained to the housekeeper I might not be back that night and wrote Bill a letter telling him where I was and that I was leaving him. . Off I went, my heart beating rapidly. I had no idea what would happen.

I arrived at the bar and found John drunk. He told me the $400, he always kept in his wallet for security purposes, was gone. His wife must have taken it. We needed a place for the night and he knew of one just down the street next to Western Costume. What a dive. It was far worse than some of the sleazy movie sets I'd worked on. I paid for the tiny, bare room. As I entered that room, reality hit. What on earth had I done? Would my children like John? Would he like them? What would happen to my life? I was scared as could be. Wasn't this what I'd wanted and hoped for? Wasn't this the man I'd loved for two years? Now I was with him and I didn't know what to do. Be careful what you ask for. You just might get it.

I was still working on the film and continued to go to work each day. John's son worked with us, too. Once John began to drink, he was incapable of sobering up and someone had to replace him at work. I fixed up the dump and made it somewhat attractive. Nursing him, I got to know him at last. He told me that his wife was ten years older than he was. She'd "robbed the cradle". He described how he had delivered his son, John Jr., how his wife had put him in the hospital for his drinking problems, that he'd had a crush on Marge Champion - a wonderful dancer - years before. He may have been a romantic man at one time, but it seemed his wife had squelched it out of him.

His son seemed glad his Dad was having some fun at last, but I knew that John was getting worse and I was worried about him. I didn't know what to do so I took him to my father's doctor who immediately put him in to the hospital. I was relieved. This wasn't the romantic interlude I'd pictured in my dreams.

At the hospital he shared a room with four other men. Seeing him so shaky with the DT's, I demanded they give him medicine to help. I think he was rather proud to have this young woman taking care of him, and he tended to show off a bit. One day he said to his roommates, "I left my color television and my $125 shoes for this woman." I was horrified. After all, I'd left my girls, my home, and everything and here he was thinking about a color television and some expensive shoes.

I wondered where it was all going to end when he decided it would be best to return to his home when he left the hospital. At first I was heartbroken, but in the end I felt a sense of relief. During the time I spent with him I realized that he was completely dependent upon his wife. She had babied him and taken all the responsibility for the relationship, and for his life, as well. I couldn't have fitted that bill, nor did I want to. I saw John a few more times at work after that and later I received a letter from him suggesting that we might get together again on location sometime, somewhere. By that time I'd finally had enough. I had learned an important lesson. Better things began to happen in my life. We remained friends although we never worked together again. His son told me that for years afterward, he was not allowed to say, "Pass the sugar." Instead he had to say, "Pass the coffee sweetener." His buddies on the set used to sing him the song, "Sugar in the Morning, Sugar in the Evening," just to drive him a little crazy. Looking back, I realized we did each other a great service. I was his mid-life crisis romance and he helped me escape my failed marriage. It may have seemed like a strange way to do things, but it worked out.

I went back home, Bill moved out, and eventually moved in with Joyce and her two boys. After our divorce, they married and he adopted her two sons and they had two daughters together. We remained friends and I was grateful to Joyce for coming along.

Chapter 22

THE BOSTON STRANGLER

It was 1969. I was only thirty-three and by that time I felt I'd had enough sorry predicaments to last a lifetime. I realized they were mostly of my own making; I couldn't blame anyone else for the distractions I created for myself. Along with that, I had come to the realization that I no longer wanted my life to be full of such turmoil. Although I enjoyed change and challenges, lately they overpowered me leaving me exhausted. As I took stock, I began to notice how the movie business allowed me (and everyone else in it) to live life as if it was a fantasy. We now call this denial. It had caught up with me and it was time to deal with it.

It was wonderful having Christmas with the girls. The tension that was usually present when Bill was around had disappeared. Although I was alone and short of funds, I felt great. I only bought gifts for my girls. When they woke up at 6:00 a.m. on Christmas morning, there was nobody was in a bad mood to fuss at them on this happiest of days. A miracle occurred, too. My old cat that had disappeared six months before reappeared early that morning, meowing to be let in. Perhaps she too sensed a change in the household and decided it was time to return.

Since I wasn't giving out presents that year, I invited everyone to Christmas dinner, even Bill and Joyce. It was a happy occasion. Up until then, even in childhood, holidays had been a strain in one way or another. But this holiday was super.

I was lucky enough to have hired a new housekeeper, Rosie, who actually spoke English. She was sensible and dependable and that made me feel secure because I needed to get back to work. I had a feeling that the good part of my life was going to begin now that I'd taken responsibility for it. I just didn't have a clue as to how that was going to happen. One never does.

I went to work at Fox and helped out on the television show, *Lost in Space*. Maggie Sullivan, head of hairdressing, asked me if I'd be able to go work on *The Boston Strangler* on location in Boston. My old friend Dorothy White (now Byrne), who I'd met in cosmetology school, was supposed to work on it, but suddenly she was unable to go and Maggie needed a replacement right away. I hadn't even thought about leaving my girls to go on location, but I really needed the work. It would be for three weeks in Boston, late January to early February. I called Bill and he said he'd help with the girls while I was gone and the girls didn't mind. By this time they trusted me to come home no matter where I went.

I made all the necessary arrangements for the house, packed all my cold weather gear plus the Marine issue they gave us through the Fox Wardrobe Department. It was heavy and bulky, but appreciated nonetheless. I also borrowed a dressy coat from my sister. It was a dark-blue pea coat-like wool, with a red fur collar. I loved it. Underneath it I wore a brilliant pink tent dress. What a combination! At the airport I encountered Sydney Pollack's secretary, a former New Yorker. She took one look at me and said, "Sugar, keep your coat buttoned up. Don't let anyone see that dress." I took her advice never exposing the dress.

Most of the crew was already at the Lennox Hotel in Boston, right in the heart of the city. They had come earlier to prepare. The Lennox Hotel was comfortable. My room was nice and warm and I could even set my bottle of wine outside on the windowsill to chill as long as I didn't forget it and let it freeze.

I was working with Whitey Snyder again because Tony Curtis was playing the "Strangler". Tony was very happy. He'd just fallen in love with his next wife-to-be, Penny. He'd also had some hair transplants. When he came into Makeup, he announced, "Sugar, be careful with every one of my hairs. If you make a mistake with even one hair, I have a sharp shooter up in the rafters who will get you." I didn't know if he was serious, but I was very careful, nonetheless.

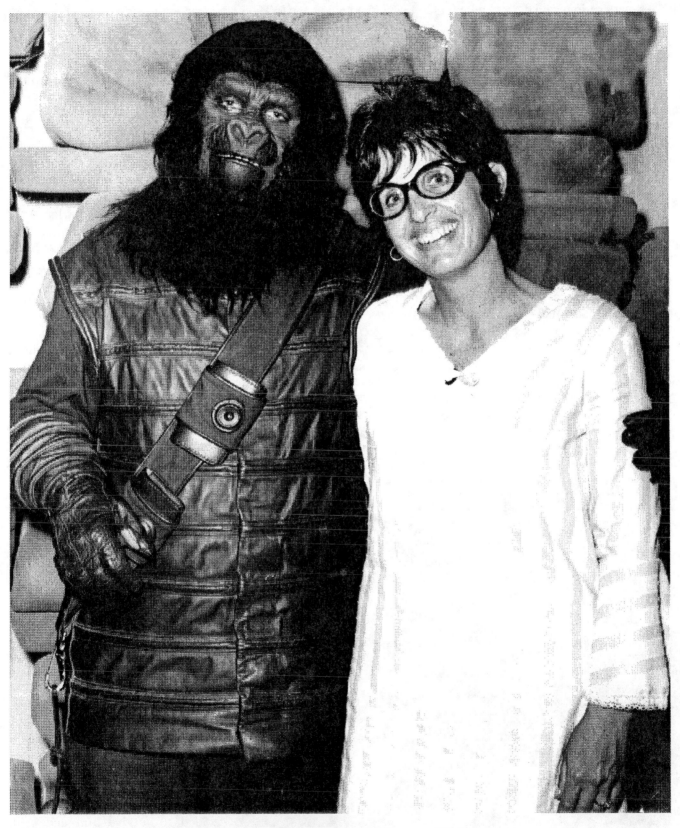

Sugar and friend, *Beneath the Planet of the Apes*

During the production meeting for all the department heads, I noticed a fellow sitting close to Dick Klein, the cameraman. I didn't remember seeing him before. He was tall with short, blond hair and the bluest eyes I'd ever seen. He looked very serious and didn't smile much. I wondered who he was. He wore a cameraman's eyeglass on a chain around his neck.

Richard Fleisher, the director, had an aversion to hairstylists. He didn't want me on the set unless it was absolutely necessary. From time to time there would be a note on the call sheet stating, "No hairstylist today." It hurt a bit, even though I knew it wasn't personal, it was just his way. I didn't want to spend the location stuck in my hotel room so we finally convinced the director that somebody had to mess up the hair on the dead bodies. Since Whitey wasn't about to do it, I was finally allowed to go to work with the rest of the crew.

The Boston Strangler was a horrifying true story, but it was also very interesting. I talked with the policeman who had worked on the actual case. He was doing research for us and became our advisor. We were shown actual photographs of the strangler, Albert De Salvo, before he confessed and then photographs of how he looked afterwards. It was astonishing. He appeared to have dissolved into a vegetable after he faced and processed what he had done.

We worked all over Boston in the places where the murders had actually taken place. One day we were in a graveyard. I was completely bundled up in my cold weather gear, even wearing a facemask. The man with the light blue eyes I'd seen at the production meeting turned out to be the gaffer. He asked me if I'd move some electric equipment for him. I said, "Sure". My feminine voice surprised him. I was so bundled up he thought I was one of his guys. We burst into laughter and he apologized. Even though I'd gladly have helped, he didn't want me to. We began to talk and he asked if I'd sit with him at lunch.

He surprised me. As we ate lunch I realized that his cool demeanor masked a very sweet man. We were joined by Joe, the East coast makeup man, and J.J. who was B.J.'s (Natalie's New York makeup man) brother. He also practiced law. During lunch we laughed a lot, exchanged food, and had a great time. Afterwards, the gaffer (who had introduced himself as Pat) and I took a walk. I noticed that he was sort of clumsy, like me. Who wouldn't be in all those clothes? Pat asked if I'd like to get together that night. I said, "Why not? Seeing as I'm already finished, I'll pick up a bottle of wine for us."

For the first time in my life, I was really free. I was about to be divorced and had no ties. It felt like the perfect time to let go and have a good time on location. I wouldn't be hurting anyone, or be untrue to anybody. Patrick came to my room later that night. We were so silly and I was so happy. I told him all about my life and my affair with John. He kept trying to be romantic, but I held back. Much later, he explained that it was a hobby of his to try to bed all the women in all the crafts on a crew. Just one night stands, nothing serious. I was in the Hair Department and he thought I might be interesting for a night. He didn't know what he was in for.

The next day at work he was friendly and we had fun. But on the way home from work he was in a car in front of me and I could see he had a girl sitting on his lap. I was really disappointed and also glad I that hadn't slept with him the night before. I would have felt humiliated. I had to remember I was going to have fun on location, not accumulate problems as I had in the past.

That night, I went to my room feeling let down. Later, Pat called and asked if he could come to my room and talk. He explained that the girl had actually been using him to get to Dick, the cameraman, and she wasn't at all interested in him. I decided to forgive him and said, "Sure, come on down."

From then on we were

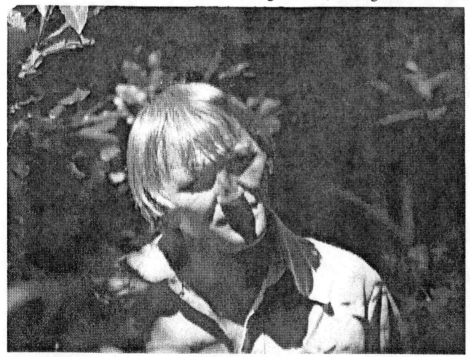

Young Pat Blymyer

inseparable. We walked through Harvard Square on our day off, drank half yards of ale in glasses so tall we had to sit on high stools. I didn't even like beer much, but I drank it with him. It was such fun. We went to dinner at the Half Shell, one of the best seafood restaurants I'd ever eaten at. That evening Pat sat there with tears in his eyes he was so happy. He told me he was married, but not at all happy in the relationship. He always dreaded going home in the evenings. He didn't realize he could have such fun after work. He'd been born in West Virginia and was an elegant hillbilly, actually still innocent in many ways.

I allowed myself to be completely taken in by his charm. One night there was to be a crew party at someone's apartment. I figured he'd invite me, but he talked me into staying home. The next day I had plans to go to Sturbridge, the old village, with J.J. so I agreed.

At breakfast with J.J. the next morning I told him that I hadn't gone to the party because Pat talked me out of it. J.J. clued me in and explained what Pat had done. Obviously he was keeping me out of circulation while he looked around. Upon hearing that, I went back to my room to get my coat and dialed Pat's room. As soon as he answered I began screaming at him about what a rotten trick he's played on me. When I finished yelling he quietly asked, "Do you always talk so loudly on the phone in the mornings?" I slammed the phone down, but laughed to myself.

J.J. and I had a great time at Sturbridge. It's a replica of a small town built about two hundred years ago. Most of the buildings were brought there and reassembled. J.J. told me to dress nicely and to wear high heels. It reminded me of B.J. telling me to dress up for the streets of New York. So there I was walking through the snow, my feet freezing. When we got to the path leading to the schoolhouse, the snow was so deep that I had to take my shoes off and go barefoot. I entered the schoolhouse and sat warming my feet near the wood stove for a long time. Next time, I swore to myself, I'd wear snow boots no matter what J.J. said. All in all it was a great day. I felt that I had gotten a real taste of New England. When I arrived back at the hotel Patrick, who appeared to be a little jealous, met me. I guess he deserved it.

One evening as we were waiting to be shown to a table at the hotel restaurant, Pat went into a telephone booth and proceeded to call his parents in West Virginia. Everyone called them Mammy and Pappy. Soon he handed me the phone asking me to say hello. I was shocked because he was married. Later, he explained that his wife looked down on his parents because they were from West Virginia while she was from Playa del Rey and had gone to USC. "Big deal", I said. His folks were so sweet on the phone even though they must have wondered just what their son was up to.

While I was having such a wonderful time, Whitey and Margie, the costumer, were happily engaged in a romance, too. They had gone out together years before, but had broken it off because Whitey was married. They were so happy to be together again.

Pat and I spent all our free time together and location just sped by. The night before we were set to leave, another party was planned. This time I wasn't about to be left home alone so I went right up to Pat and asked him if he'd be taking me. If he weren't, I'd find myself another date. He took me. It was a wild party, all of us packed into a space meant for much fewer people. I put my coat on the floor, leaving my glasses in the pocket. We talked, danced, drank a lot, and said our good-byes. When I retrieved my coat, I found that my glasses had been stepped on and one lens was cracked right down the middle.

The next morning as I waited to board the plane I contemplated the changes in my life since my arrival in Boston. I started out quiet, ready to keep to myself and stay out of trouble. Now here I was with a hangover, cracked glasses, and sad that my location romance was over. Quite a start for the "good part" of my life. Pat and I had been booked on different planes on our way home. Still I kept looking around the airport hoping to see him. No luck. The studio limo picked me up at the airport and dropped me at the Makeup Department. I put my hair cases away and talked with Maggie for a while about the location while waiting for a friend to come and take me home.

As we were driving out of the studio, I saw Patrick standing on a street corner. He looked so sad and alone waiting there for his mother-in-law to pick him up. I was sorry he had to go home to an unhappy family situation. I felt good knowing I was going to a hassle-free home. The kids and I were happy to be together again. They'd been fine in my absence, of course, and I had talked to them each night on the phone. We spent all that weekend together and settled into our new life without their father. It suited us all.

Monday, I was back at work at Fox. Patrick was just as happy to see me as I was to see him. Cleo, our script supervisor, was such a romantic. She wanted the two of us to be together so she'd come up to me and say, "That boy really loves you." Then later she'd say to Patrick, "That girl really loves you, you know." She kept this up on a daily basis.

Patrick and I were more involved than I wanted to admit. I had planned just to walk away from the affair. After all, it was just a location romance, wasn't it? But it just wasn't working out that way. He stole kisses at lunch, held my hand, and looked at me with such love in his eyes. I simply couldn't resist this young man who had come into my life. It was fun coming to work knowing he was there. I had my own drama going on behind the scenes.

I missed him on the weekends and was always anxious to get back to work on Monday. I began to realize that I wasn't being fair to my girls, that the relationship with Pat was a repeat of John and me. At least this time I wasn't trying to escape from marriage and I was in love with someone who loved me in return. But he was married with two children. Why couldn't I have fallen for someone who was single? I had really overestimated myself, thinking I could turn off my feelings once I got home.

Once in a while we'd go out for a drink after work and talk. On one such night, when we left the bar near the studio, we found a chain across the parking lot entrance. I panicked, thinking I might have to drive him home - not a good move. Much to my relief, I was able to lift the chain just enough so he could safely drive out. This little incident reinforced my feeling that the relationship wasn't working, that I was being foolish just as I had been about John. It was hard, but I had to admit it was the truth.

After one particularly lonely weekend, I told Patrick that I needed to talk with him, alone, after work. "Okay," he said. "We can meet in the park across the street." Later, as we walked around the park, hand in hand, I told him just how I felt. Our relationship couldn't work. I'd just gotten out of a situation like this and it was a lesson I didn't want to forget. I told him I didn't want him to leave home for me. I might not be "the" person for him. I knew I wasn't the cause of his marriage failing, he was unhappy before he met me; our affair was just a symptom. But if he ended his marriage I wanted it to be because he really wanted to, not because of me.

We walked along slowly. We both felt so sad. Finally we kissed goodnight. Just then a car drove up and the headlights shone brightly on us. Normally someone would have turned down the lights, but this happened to be Pat's wife. She had never come looking for him before. What a coincidence! At first she didn't recognize us. In fact, she thought we were rather romantic, that is until her kids yelled, "Hey, that's Daddy!"

As soon as Pat recognized the car, he walked over to the car and they talked for a while and I tried to disappear into the bushes. Finally, he came over to me, took me to the car, and introduced me to his wife. I was shocked. Pat was such a handsome man, tall and thin. But his wife was a short, dumpy, fat, blonde woman with a face that reminded me of a pie pan, with curly hair all around it. She looked at me with hatred, which I understood. She asked me if I knew he was married. I nodded. She asked me if I knew he had children. "Yes," I said. I felt very uncomfortable. I didn't remember what else was said, but I left as soon as I could and drove home in a state of confusion.

Pat came into work the next day and told me he was now on trial at home. He decided to give his marriage a chance, since he had never taken it very seriously before. For her part, his wife was trying very hard to win him back - she hadn't put much effort into the marriage either. Now each evening she made hors d'

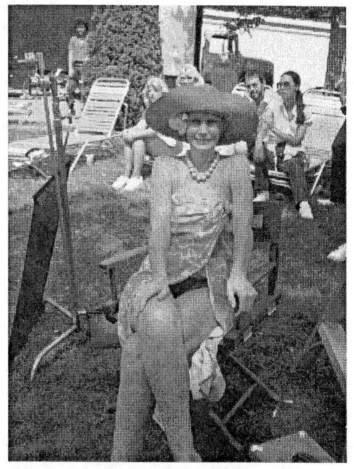

Sally Kellerman

oeuvres for him, something she had never done before. One way to Pat's heart was definitely through his stomach.

Occasionally his trial period turned into a comedy. One morning he arrived at work with a toothpick stuck in his big toe. It had fallen into the shag rug. He had to go to the studio nurse to have it removed. I chuckled. Another morning he came in with a different story. He'd put his wife on a grading system. The night before, he had given the kids a bath and used up all the towels. Later, when he went to take a shower, there were no dry towels. She got a 'Z' for the day. I couldn't believe she would even put up with that sort of treatment, although I did think it was hilarious. He entertained me with stories about how in the past he'd tried to drive her crazy. He'd do things like put the top up on the convertible when she had left it down, or he'd put clean clothes back into the washing machine. His home life sounded like a circus. One wonders why he didn't think of divorce.

A few years before, he had arrived home one evening so drunk that he couldn't find his key. His wife opened the door while he was leaning on it and he fell in at her feet. Instead of apologizing, as he lay on the floor he looked up angrily and said, "I'm gonna give you one more chance to straighten up." At least he hadn't lost his sense of humor.

We saw each other at work, but things had cooled down. Not our love for each other, rather our contact. One weekend, he had to fly up to San Francisco to scout a location and he said he'd fly back early so we could spend the day together. I picked him up at the airport and took him home with me for the first time. He met my girls and they proceeded to get acquainted. They liked him a lot - after all, he was nearly a kid himself in many ways. At one point he'd set his wine glass down on the table beside the couch and Tanya knocked it over. I didn't get angry or yell. I just cleaned it up. That impressed him. I loved having him in my home and he liked being there.

A couple of weeks later, I was sitting at home in the evening when the phone rang. It was Pat. He simply said, "Can I come home? I'll explain when I get there." I replied, "Oh, please do." That was it. He moved in.

My life felt nicely settled. Now I could get back to concentrating on my work, messing up the hair on the dead bodies for *The Strangler*. Sally Kellerman arrived, my one live body, the one the strangler missed. She was a crazy lady, so exuberant and vivacious.

Henry Fonda came to work with us. Always one of my favorites, I admired his quiet charm and friendly disposition. I had worked with his daughter, Jane, the previous year and one day I told Henry that I thought Jane was so lucky to have him for a father. At that point all I really knew about him was what I'd observed working with him on a couple of films. I knew nothing about his past. But as I made that remark, his eyes seemed to fill with tears. Many years later, I read a story of his life and finally understood why he reacted in such a manner to my remark. When his children were growing up, he'd been a much different person than the one I met. He made life difficult for them and they had suffered. Nevertheless, my impression of him was of a wonderful, warm, loving man. Perhaps we all change as we grow older.

Whitey had been so happy with Margie while they were on location, but now he had returned to his loveless, lonely marriage. They saw each other at work, just as Pat and I had done. Margie would never have asked that he leave his marriage, so me, with my big mouth, I started in on him. Each morning I'd come in and announce how nice it was to have Patrick to go home to each night. Whitey would say, "Keep talking, Sugar." Eventually I did say something that made sense to him - I said he wasn't being fair to his wife. If he remained in that marriage, much longer, she would be too old to go out and make changes in her own life. It was time to release her. His children had all grown up. He'd already had a heart attack (which I believed was symbolic of his broken heart). Finally he said, "Get me a lawyer." I did. After he and Margie got married, they moved to Washington State and did live happily ever after. Whitey died in the spring of 1995. Margie was devastated by his death, but at least they had those happy years together.

Tony Curtis needed a false nose to look like the character of the strangler. It changed his pretty boy look to something a bit more sinister. It's always difficult to get the texture of a false piece of skin to match the real thing. Unfortunately, Whitey had to leave a couple of weeks before the end of the film. He was replaced with Jack Baron. Poor Jack. The nose became a disaster. It just didn't seem to work. The color and texture didn't match his own skin. Each day was torture for Jack. Dick Kline, the cameraman, didn't have the confidence in Jack and made it very difficult for him.

The Boston Strangler was shot in panels with lots of bright white sets. The result was six or so panels of different scenes on the screen all at once. Pat had been a gaffer on *The Monkees* and had a wonderful time experimenting with all sorts of lighting on that crazy television show, but this was his first film as a gaffer. Although Dick was wonderful socially, he became a bear on the set when it came to gaffers. But Pat learned how to work with him. He'd put a lamp in a place where it was likely to be needed, but would move just a little bit when Dick called for it. Dick never noticed Pat's tricks, but he did wonder how Pat could get the lights in place so quickly.

Pat was the youngest man ever to become a gaffer and the old timers at Fox resented him. Normally an electrician didn't become a gaffer before he was in his forties. Pat had been only twenty-five when he began as a gaffer. It was tough for him, but in the end he got the job done and the film looked stunning.

One night while working on the back lot at Fox, the word came that Martin Luther King had been killed. Everyone was stunned and just like John Kennedy's assassination, I never forgot that night. What was our country coming to?

We finished *Strangler* on location in San Francisco then Pat and I went on a vacation, our first ever. It was perfect. We drove here and there, swam in hot pools, and enjoyed the desert and our time alone. Then we had to go back to work.

I hadn't wanted to work on the first *Planet of the Apes* - it just sounded so hokey, but after I saw it I was enthralled. The story and especially the artistic work of the makeup artists thrilled me. So I was happy to go to work on *Beneath the Planet of the Apes*. I was one of the many extra hairdressers on the film. We reported to the Fox Ranch at five o'clock in the morning and wrapped the ape people's hair before they got their makeup applied. Next they ate their breakfast before their faces were made up. The next step was to apply the mouth appliances and for the rest of the day everyone wearing an appliance had to drink their meals through a straw.

After Makeup finished with them, we added hair. It was an intricate process and very messy. I was always covered with the dark-brown makeup they used on the apes. We worked long hours and Frank Griffin, head of the Makeup, was always yelling and very difficult to work with. It wasn't easy.

The extras were more fortunate than the actors. They had whole ape masks to wear in the background that could be removed so they could cool off. The actors were stuck inside the appliances all day. At the end of the day it took a long time to remove the hair and makeup. Then we had to clean the hair lace of the wigs and get them ready for the next day.

One morning during this film I worked the longest day ever - reporting to Fox Studio at half past three in the morning. The people in this particular scene lived underneath the earth and had no skin and one could see all the veins in their skulls. We had to wrap their heads so the makeup men could put on bald caps and then apply the veins on the top of the bald caps. It was a time-consuming task and they looked fairly disgusting.

My days were long, but my evenings were charming. Pat wasn't working. I'd call before leaving work so he would know when I'd arrive. There he'd be, waiting for me in the driveway, freshly showered and shaved, dressed in clean clothes and looking just great. To top it off he'd have a cool glass of white wine waiting for me. I couldn't ask for more, but there was more. He'd give me a big kiss and hug and when I went into the house, I'd find my bath drawn, with rose petals floating in the water and love notes, too. It was phenomenal. I'd never been treated so sweetly before. The kids were happy, too. They loved spending time with him. The housekeeper was charmed and even the dog loved him.

There was one problem, though. Pat was jealous. An emotion I never had to deal with before. Here I was 170 pounds, four years older than he, with three kids. Now, who on earth was going to steal me away? I explained how I had worked with all the crew guys for years and I knew how to behave. He said I just didn't understand men. But he loved me so much he thought everyone saw me the same way he did. It was funny to me, but serious for him.

To add insult to injury, I got a call from Robert Redford. He was staying at the Bel Air Hotel and was going to have some photos taken. He didn't want mascara and his lashes were pale. He asked if I could dye them for him before the shoot. Of course I would. I took off the next afternoon for the hotel. Bob greeted me and I unpacked my supplies. I had him lie on the bed and I put a towel over him so I wouldn't spill anything on him. I was, as always, nervous as I applied the tint. He lay there with his eyes closed, not moving. The phone rang and I answered it. No one was on the other end of the line. A few minutes later the phone rang again and I had to answer it. No one again. It happened a third time before I finished tinting his lashes. Finally we were done and I said goodbye.

When I got home that afternoon, I told Pat about what happened with the phone calls. I thought it was really strange. Confessing, he said, "It was me. I didn't want you alone in a hotel room with Robert Redford." In spite of his being upset, I began to laugh and laugh. "I can't believe you. I've been alone in hotel rooms with many actors and nothing bad has ever happened. I can't understand you." He in his own defense replied, "You just don't understand." For years after that we never saw a Robert Redford film. I didn't feel like making waves.

During the filming of *Apes* I just had to ask Charlton Heston a question: "After being Moses, and now being the last man on earth, what would he do to surpass that role?" He laughed and replied, "I truly don't know." Does the NRA surpass Moses in his mind? I wonder?

While *Apes* was being finished at Fox, *Hello, Dolly* was in the planning stages. Maggie asked me if I wanted to be one of the main hairstylists. I backed off because I didn't feel comfortable with some of the people involved on that particular film in our department. There were some very red - neck hairdressers and it upset me to hear them air their prejudices. I didn't want to spend months with them so I told her I'd help with the extras, which worked out well.

One day we had a big call and I was called to the phone with terrible news for me. Jack Gorton, the Marine who had lived with us and married Blanca, had been killed in Vietnam. I broke down in tears. Many hairdressers on that call had known him as a boy because they knew his mother, Janie. We all cried together that day. What a waste of lives caused by that stupid war over something the boys never understood.

Chapter 23

GAILY, GAILY

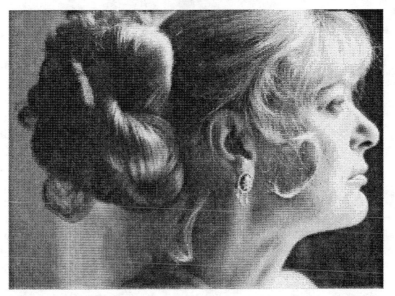

One of Melina Mercouri's hairstyles in *Gaily, Gaily*

Now that Pat and I were together, I didn't want to be parted for months. I was trying to decide whether or not I wanted to work on *Hello, Dolly* when Pat got a call from Dick Kline. He wanted him to be his gaffer on a film called *Gaily, Gaily*. I decided *Hello, Dolly* was out and called the department heads on *Gaily, Gaily* to see if there was an opening for me.

Naomi Cavin, one of my favorite people, was the head hairstylist on *Gaily, Gaily* and head of Makeup was Del Armstrong. They were both great to work with. I called Naomi to tell her I really wanted to work on the film and explained why. I told her I didn't care what I did, I'd be happy to be at the bottom of the ladder, I just wanted to work on the film. Being a romantic, she immediately found a place for me. Thanks Naomi.

Our hairstyling crew included Kathy Blondell, Lyndel Kail, Carla Hadly - a buxom redhead in her forties - and me. It was a wonderful mix of people. The plus was I was happy to be working on the film with Pat - otherwise I might not have seen him for months.

Naomi was the embodiment of femininity, tall and slender always wearing the most beautiful rings, and attractive clothing. Men just seemed to gravitate to her. One day I asked her how she managed to look so good all the time. She gave me great advice: never buy one piece of clothing at a time. If there was only one piece of clothing she liked, she looked for something to go with it before buying it. I thought of all the single things hanging in my closet that didn't go with anything. I have tried to follow her advice ever since. Naomi was also nice and our whole crew of hairstylists responded to her. We had lots of work to do, but it was never too much, not even when the sweat was running into our eyes. It was my first experience of Chicago and the summer was hot and humid, living up to the city's reputation.

Gaily, Gaily took place in the early 1900s in Chicago. It was about a small portion of writer Ben Hecht's early life. Hecht, portrayed by Beau Bridges, who arrives in Chicago, meets some prostitutes, and ends up living in a whorehouse. Melina Mercouri played the madam. Brian Keith also starred in the film. It was a huge production directed by Norman Jewison. He was a lovely man and I could sense that he really enjoyed creating the film. Ray Aghayan, the costume designer, worked directly with the art director to coordinate the clothes with the sets. Their creative ideas - all combined - did wonderful things for the look of the film.

After work we socialized and had great fun. Pat's electricians were quite compatible with the hairdressers, so we all went out to dinner as a group. One evening, in particular, stands out. Pat and his boys were already two sheets to the wind, having indulged in a bit of beer before we left for dinner at a Mexican restaurant. His boys were Timmy Griffith, his best boy; Gary Holt, who was very short; Bob Fillis, who was six foot six; and big Pat Marshall, whom we'd named "the Golden Bear". It was a wild group.

Immediately after we sat down at the table the guys ordered six pitchers of Margueritas - and they ordered more all through dinner. I began to wonder about the bill, but didn't say anything. We had a gigantic dinner and when the check came the total was overwhelming. The guys passed it around the table, exclaiming about the amount. Each pitcher of Margueritas cost ten dollars. These guys were used to California prices that were less than half that.

I became uneasy when they got up from the table, looking around at the pictures on the wall and said, "Well, well, we might just take some of these pictures with us for those prices." I didn't know these guys very well, but they didn't sound like they were joking. I threw our share of the bill on the table and hurried Pat out of there. I didn't want to end up in jail. They did calm down and paid the check, but from then on I preferred to go out to dinner alone with just Pat.

Kenneth of New York was designing Melina Mercouri's hair. He was famous for doing the famous. Someone had to go to New York, see the design, and learn how to execute it for the film. Naomi decided it should be me, which pleased me. I had certainly moved up from the bottom of the ladder.

The production company booked me a plane and into The

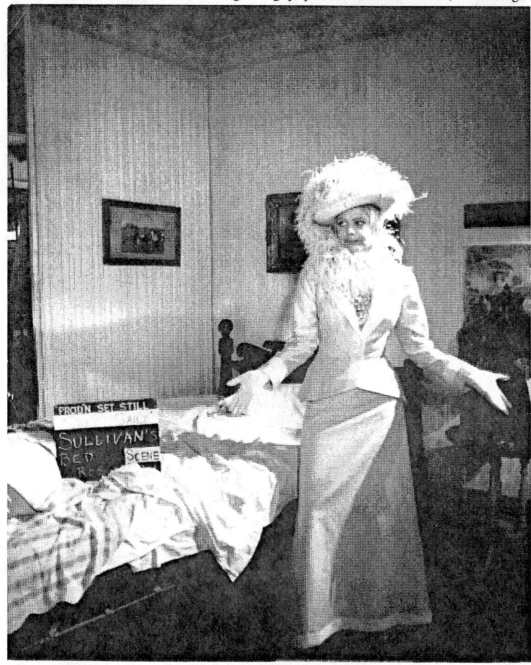

Melina Mercouri, *Gaily, Gaily*

Americana Hotel. I took off for New York on my own. It was the first time I'd been there without a film company to watch out for me and plan my transportation once I was there.

After checking into my hotel, I went to Kenneth's salon. What a huge establishment - floor after floor of women being pampered. I met Melina and took an instant liking to her. Kenneth sat Melina down in his chair and began to design the hairstyles. The whole process took place over a few days. All his designs were photographed and he showed me how he set the hair.

Sometimes while waiting for Melina to arrive, I went upstairs where the hairstylists worked on hairpieces that belonged to people who came in to get their hair done for special occasions. One day a hairpiece belonging to Jackie Kennedy came out of the drying oven with a kink in the back. It had been carelessly set and the kink had dried in it. I offered to fix it with my curling iron. I heated it up and did a little smoothing of the hair and soon the kink was no more. The hairstylists were so grateful and I was proud of myself. I felt as though I had a tiny connection with Jackie.

I called Dianne, my young friend in New York. She said she'd come visit me at my hotel. In the meantime I went out and bought all the things I needed for Melina's hair work once I got back to Chicago. My arms loaded with packages, I began to look for a taxi. The hurrying crowds kept knocking me into the streets. It was humiliating, dragging all those packages, unable to find a cab. Finally, a cabby took pity on me and picked me up. I was so relieved. That evening, my friend came to visit me at the hotel. She had just turned sixteen.

When I returned to Milwaukee, my status had changed. I had to go to work when Melina went to work. I missed my group of friends, but Melina was a treat. Leo Letito, her makeup man, was a tiny man with strong beliefs. He'd stand poised like Jesus on the Mount exclaiming his religious beliefs. He said he'd been wounded in the war and had a metal plate in his head so he had to be careful to hold his temper. If he became angry, it was impossible to control him. He always carried a gun, which concerned me.

Our first day of shooting with Melina began with her riding in a horse and carriage down the streets of Milwaukee. The 1910 early - Chicago set was lovely, filled with people and street vendors, with lots of commotion and bustling. Beau was about to meet the madam for the first time.

Leo decided to put lifts on Melina. He thought it would make her look more attractive. Lifts were supposed to make a woman look younger. Each morning gauze strips were glued to her cheeks, and then we pulled them tight with rubber bands and fastened them to the top of her head. Her hair covered them. Personally, I didn't care for the way it made her look; it gave her apple cheeks.

Kenneth had designed long, long curls to hang down in front of Melina's ears. (Shades of Sydney Guilleroff). But her hair was very fine and the curls didn't hold because of the warm humid air. I kept using hair spray to keep the curls from going straight. She was wearing a hat so the rest of her hair stayed just fine, but those strands just drove me crazy as they blew across her face during the scene. I kept spraying, hoping to keep the design Kenneth had created.

As if that wasn't enough, her lifts kept snapping and falling off. They just wouldn't stay glued to her skin. Leo would take her back to her dressing room and re-glue them, but soon after the scene began they would snap again. Guess who was the villain? Me. We finally realized that every time I sprayed her hair, the alcohol in the spray loosened the glue. Finally Leo solved the problem and we were able to get the shot. After that, I cut the tendrils to a manageable length and would hold my hand under her hair if I had to spray.

At the end of each day Norman Jewison, our director, always showed dailies for the whole crew. This way we got to see all the work we shot the previous day. It was a ritual and food and drinks were served. Often Norman would get caught up in meetings and he would be late, but we just sat and enjoyed the food while we waited for him. It was our mealtime anyway and we were served well. After seeing the dailies, we were ready for bed - our days were very long.

Pat and I were each allocated a room and we kept them both so we would have two bathrooms and be out of each other's way in the mornings. On weekends, Pat's boys would sometimes borrow our extra room. (Most of the crew shared a room.) Different guys in anticipation of getting lucky used to borrow our extra room and I laughed when I saw its condition the next day. Sometimes it was left very neat, but other times it was all topsy-turvy. Everybody had their own style of lovemaking.

There were two very pretty, young girls hanging around the set who called themselves Peaches and Cream. I had the feeling they wanted to land one of the crew in matrimony, or perhaps they were just looking for adventure before getting married and settling into an ordinary life. I never did know for sure, but the crew guys were quite attractive. Maybe, just maybe, one of them would propose.

Sometimes working with Melina was an ordeal. Not because of anything she did to me, but because she was the most emotional person I'd ever worked with. She was from Greece and her country was going through some very hard times. Many of her friends were in prison or in hiding. It seemed that each morning she would get a call about another disaster. It was as if she was supposed to save them, but she was banned from Greece because of her politics and couldn't go home. She was filled with such sadness.

Each morning Anna, her cook and friend who traveled with her, prepared my favorite Greek coffee in a little copper pot. It was sweet and strong. I bought myself one of those pots so I could continue having that coffee even after we finished the film.

When Melina wasn't working, I worked at the fairgrounds in Milwaukee with the rest of the crew. It was our base camp, a huge place. One of our makeup men, Jack Stone, who was quite character, was working with us. I'd known him since I was twenty, working as a stock room clerk at MGM. He'd gotten very strange since then. For example, during the Cuban crisis he dug himself an air raid shelter and wired it so nobody else would be able to get into it. He loved to take things from the studios. In fact, it was rumored that his garage was full of stuff he'd pilfered through the years. I'd see him walking along with a package all wrapped and ready to mail. One day I asked him if he was stealing the whole fair ground, piece by piece, and was it going to collapse around us. He laughed.

Brian Keith brought his son, who was about ten, with him to the set. He was a hot ticket and would get into just about everything. Pat's boys decided to teach him a lesson; they were bad. They showed him how he could stick his finger into the electric sockets and nothing would happen to him. Of course they had the power off. Then, after they had him well trained, he stuck his finger in a socket and the guys turned on the electricity. The kid got a good shock. It was really mean of those adults, picking on such a sweet little boy.

We had the 4th of July off. The company planned a picnic at a lake and bussed us to the site. It was lovely and cool, but there were no restrooms so we had to use the woods. By the end of the day, we were all sunburned, tired, and dirty. That evening after we had showered, we sat around the pool. I was sitting next to Pat when he made a remark that inspired me to take my foot and push his chair into the pool, with him in it. That started a near riot. The whole crew joined in and soon everyone was in the pool, clothes and all. Pat Palmer, our unit manager, was furious because his wife, who was pregnant, had also been thrown in. She thought it was great fun, but he was furious. Pat Palmer never learned to play. He was much too serious.

The next day my Pat began itching in his private parts. He couldn't figure out what it might be, so off he went to see the doctor. When he came home, I asked what the doctor had said. He told me that while the doctor was examining him he asked him if he fooled around. Pat said, "No, but I don't know if my girlfriend has." I threw my purse at him.

Actually it was poison oak that he'd gotten the day of the beach party while peeing in the woods. To add insult to injury, I'd washed his clothes with plenty of bleach to get the dirt and oil out. Some of the bleach remained in the fibers. So when I pushed him, clothes and all into the pool, the chlorine added to what was already in the material and only made matters worse.

Poor Pat, we called his disease Poison Ivy of the Vine. He had to soak in a solution, wrap himself in gauze, and then he covered it with a baggie. He had to take a pan to work and soak himself a couple of times a day. It was a good thing he wasn't modest. In fact he was so proud of his production he demonstrated it to the guys. Guys are weird sometimes. It took him a long while to recover. Later I told Pat that if he didn't think my love for him was true, after this ordeal he must realize it was.

Our next location was Dubuque. We filled a bus with beer and off we went. Anytime this crew had time off, everyone partied to their limits. Dubuque was so pretty with its Victorian architecture. Our motel was sort of grungy, but it was only for a couple of days. There was a porch where we'd sit in the evenings and muse about what it would be like to live in a small town like this. I thought it would be great. Pat grew up in the small town of Beckley West Virginia and he remembered how much fun it had been. That day a small seed was planted for our future.

A day later I was sent back to Los Angeles with Melina's hairpieces, to work with Ray Aghayan. I was sorry to miss the big picnic scene in the park, but Pat took photos of it. I didn't want to leave, it was such a lovely place and I was reminded of the time I was sent home from Kentucky while working with Natalie.

I took all my hair equipment to Goldwyn Studio and set up the Hair Department. Then I decided to scope out the set and went down to the stage to see the whorehouse. It was absolutely beautiful. What a treat it was to be able to see it before all the equipment was moved in. The set had stained glass windows, with rubies in the center that had been rented from churches. Ray Aghayan our costume designer had coordinated all the costumes with the furnishings and it was extraordinary when it all came together. So much goes into sets, but usually nobody really sees the total picture. I was happy I had.

Melina and the crew arrived in Los Angeles and we started filming again. Melina and her husband were talking about going on a civil rights march with the Black people. They were both into trying to make things better for people.

One morning after I did Melina's hair in a beautiful up-do, she came back from a rehearsal all upset. "Change my hair, it must be down," she moaned. "Why?" I asked. She explained that she was going to be standing on the balcony and the shot was going to be done from way down below. People shot from that angle look most unattractive. She figured having her hair down would help. She was right. In fact, when I saw the film I noticed that even Beau, who was so young, looked pretty bad when shot from that angle. It made his chin look heavy. Shame, shame on the cameraman (or whoever decided on those shots). Once again I longed for the old cameramen I'd worked with, those artists who wanted to make people look beautiful - and knew how to do it.

Melina invited us to her house for a Greek meal. Anna cooked for us. We saw a Garbo film and had a wonderful time. Pat was in heaven with all the good food. Melina was a great hostess, so friendly and generous. But she exhausted me. Her life was in such chaos that it rubbed off on me because I felt for her. I absorbed her frustration, sadness, and her despair at the loss of her friends.

Eventually, Pat got upset because I came home nearly totally exhausted every night. He was ready to have me quit. Of course I wasn't about to. But I did need to learn how to listen without letting it affect me. I loved the education I was getting from her about world affairs, though.

I liked working with Ray, our designer. He was from the Middle East and told me about his life before he came to this country. He loved his work and was so creative. His suggestions were always helpful. I learned to listen to designers over the years, but some hairstylists resented any interference. I felt that if a suggestion was helpful, I'd use it and if not I'd just listen and do what I felt was best.

One scene in the film stood out for me. It took place in the main salon where everyone was gathered for a party scene. Melina stepped out on the balcony and called everyone over. As the lights were lowered, she held up a beautiful box and then opened it. The box was full of butterflies. In theory, they were supposed to fly out and all around the room. But only a few butterflies flew out. The other butterflies clung to the velvet on the sides and bottom of the box, ruining the dramatic effect. What happened next would never be allowed today. The only solution anyone could come up with was to cut the feet off the butterflies so they couldn't cling to anything. They flew right out, when the box was opened the next time. Wouldn't anyone try to get away from such butchers?

Gaily, Gaily was a long, wonderful production, full of amazing sets and scenes. Chicago in 1910 was an exciting place to be. On the stage, they recreated the Chicago Grain Exchange. There were so many extras that we cut hundreds of people's hair. I think all the craft members in Hollywood were working that day. Pat had so many electricians, and he was really proud of his work. It was the biggest set he had lit in his career.

As the film drew to a close, Melina finished early. She gave me a beautiful pair of enameled earrings she had ordered especially for me from a Greek artist. As she said goodbye she began to cry. I was uncomfortable and said, "I'm sure that we will see each other again." I didn't want to cry, too. Melina exclaimed, "I can't believe you Americans, you never show your feelings. What's the matter with you?" By then I was feeling amused and did not want to cry anymore.

Many years later, I spent some time in Greece and began to understand what she meant about emotions. My tears fell easily when I was there.

Chapter 24

BOB & CAROL & TED & ALICE

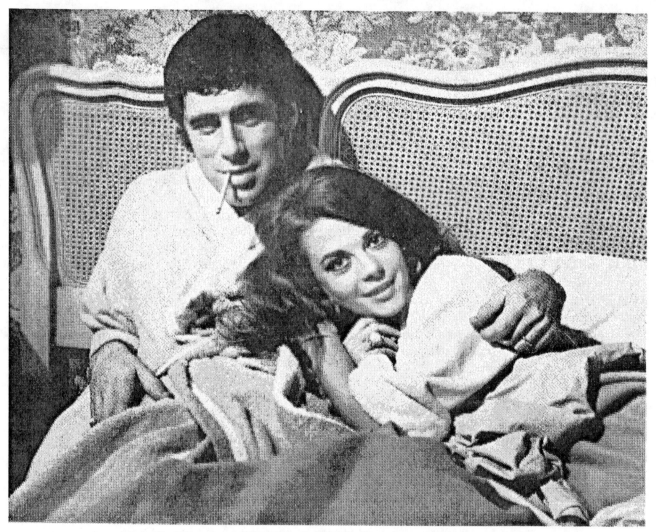

Natalie Wood and Elliott Gould, *Bob & Carol & Ted & Alice*

During the summer we filmed *Gaily, Gaily*, Pat and I moved back into our home in Canoga Park. Neither Bill nor I had been able to keep up the payments on the house in Agoura, so we let it go for foreclosure - I never thought of putting it up for sale. Pat, the girls, and I returned to our old neighborhood and the girls were in seventh heaven. They loved Patrick and they loved being back in the neighborhood with their old friends. I realized they had wanted a real family life and now we had one with Pat.

We had a great time treating Pat in special ways because we appreciated him so much. We would gather round him and give him a shave. He loved it. Taurus people love pleasures of the flesh. He took photos of us all in general and especially tons of me. They were in black and white and he enlarged them and hung them everywhere. Looking back at myself in those photos, I looked young and very happy. The whole family was on a honeymoon then and it was a very joyful time in our lives.

We had a swimming pool at our house and on weekends Pat's friends would show up and enjoy the pool and play with the girls. In the meantime, I was content to be curled up with a good book. I was so happy that Pat loved playing with the girls. I was never very good at games. I was better at discussing life with them.

One of our sets on *Gaily, Gaily* was filled with plants and trees. When the set was finished and struck, the green man who supplied all the plants, offered Pat as many trees as he could use. Pat decided to have a tree planting party and invited all his friends to it. That weekend twenty-five trees were delivered to our house and I bought two kegs of beer. Pat's friends arrived, shovels in hand. All day they dug and planted, dug and planted. At the end of the day we had a barbecue and a swim in the pool. It was such a success. If all the trees had survived, our yard could easily have become a forest.

Our life at home was fun. We had lots of parties with Pat's friends and my girls were really happy. It was the first time I was able to have the kind of family life I wanted. Pat had brought us all together. As time went by, all of us began to travel to locations together. Our kids were part of the crew when we were on location and got to see and do many things around the movie set that most kids never did. To quote one of Pat's friends, "Growing up around Pat and Sugar was like being raised in Disneyland."

My divorce finally came through. It only took about seven minutes, but Pat's was taking longer. One day his wife's lawyer called me in for a deposition. Pat was out of town scouting locations so he couldn't go with me. Despite being accompanied by Pat's lawyer, I was uncomfortable when I entered the office. I had no idea what would happen. I was shown to a table and had to sit across from Pat's wife, a faded, unhappy woman who just wanted revenge. She glared at me, but I didn't respond to her anger. I was asked questions like, "Did you promise to be there for Pat if he left?" I answered, "No." Evidently she'd found some letters I'd written to Pat and they questioned me about those. Fortunately, I hadn't incriminated myself in those letters.

The final question to me was, "Did you know that you were causing this woman mental problems?" I looked directly at her and sweetly answered the lawyer, "To be truthful sir, anyone who is five foot two and two hundred and thirty pounds obviously had problems long before I came along." I was proud of my answer and even Pat's lawyer was proud of my coolness. That night when Pat called I told him what had happened at the deposition. He laughed and confessed he was glad to have been absent from the occasion.

In the meantime, Natalie had a new beau, Richard Gregson. She spent time with him in England. It was getting serious, and she wasn't interested in working much. I was so happy she had finally found someone to love. Richard was an agent and seemed very taken with her. I always wondered whom Natalie would settle down with. Though so many men

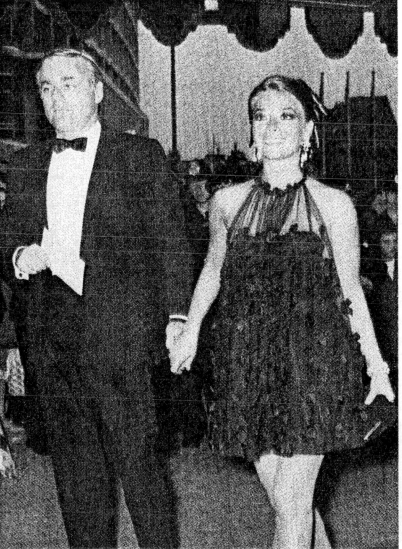

Natalie Wood and Richard Gregson

cared for her, I'm sure it ran through her head whether they loved her, her image, or her income. It isn't easy, being beautiful, famous and rich. There were many parallels in our lives. As I was meeting and falling for Pat, the same thing was happening with Natalie and Richard.

In September, I got a call from Natalie's agent announcing that she had a new project - *Bob & Carol & Ted & Alice* at Colombia Studios. Paul Mazursky was the director and her co-stars were Robert Culp, Elliot Gould, and Dyan Cannon. They sent me a script and by the time I finished it I was totally disappointed. It just didn't seem to be Natalie's kind of story, but who was I to decide? It actually turned out to be a great success and brought Natalie back into the public eye in a big way. In fact, as we began working, I quickly began to realize that it was my kind of film. It was about the relationship between two couples that were trying to make their lives more interesting in a spiritual way. They become influenced by therapy sessions advocating natural, spontaneous behavior, which made for a very interesting story.

Paul Mazursky and Larry Tucker had written the script. They were like the odd couple. Paul spent a lot of time at Esalon in Monterrey doing research. Larry was a huge fellow who even had to have a special chair made to hold him. He'd never been to Esalon. He said that stuff scared him. So although they both wrote the script, Paul did all the research.

In the late Sixties things were entirely different. People weren't into therapy, or encounter groups, or even twelve step programs like they are today. In those days most folks considered the kinds of programs held at Esalon outrageous. Only cutting edge, far out people were into that sort of thing, but I loved it. It was my cup of tea.

The first day of shooting we drove up Angeles Crest Highway to a mountain retreat just outside of Los Angeles. It was very early and most of the neighborhood houses were all tucked in and cozy, with hardly a light on. I began to wonder why on earth I'd chosen a profession that got me up in the middle of the night. We drove up winding roads, into a pine forest. I was surprised anything like this existed so close to Los Angeles.

The center where we worked was a great place. Paul, our director, knew his stuff. The script came alive and it all became something believable. I loved all the scenes showing the processes people went through, the naked women sunning themselves, the people doing Tai Chi exercises, the encounters, the deep breathing. I was ready to go to a place like this myself. They pounded pillows, learned to deal with feelings, not thoughts, in a loving atmosphere. It was the beginning of what is happening today.

When most people learn new ways, they want to share them with others. It improves communication. That is exactly what happened in this film. But it upset the balance the characters thought they had achieved in their lives, disturbed their "comfort zones".

The costumes were great - love beads, hip huggers, Nehru jackets, and men sporting long sideburns. Natalie wore her hair long and straight, the longest I'd ever seen it since I'd known her. She always had to flip it out of her eyes. It looked so pretty. Her lips were glossy and she was as beautiful as ever.

Natalie was also in love. Each evening she waited for a call from Richard, who was in London and eight hours ahead of us. She loved his attention and letters. She met Pat and liked him and was happy for me, she knew how I felt because she was experiencing the same thing.

One morning Elliot Gould came into Natalie's dressing room and while I was doing her hair he asked me if I ever did anyone else's hair. I guess he was asking for Barbra Streisand. They were still married at the time. I didn't know what to say. I knew that Barbra was a perfectionist and had a habit of using a hairstylist for one film, only to fire her at the

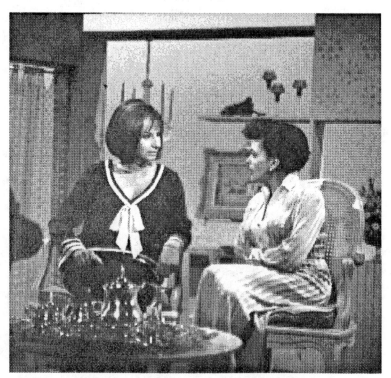

Barbra Streisand and Judy Garland,
The Judy Garland Show

beginning of the next one. I didn't want to be fired and I doubted I could please her. But I totally admired her so I said yes, but I never pursued it.

Years before, when I was working at CBS on the *Judy Garland Show*, Barbra had been the guest star. I had already discovered her talent and loved her records, but the makeup man was not acquainted with her. Barbra had her own style. She had realized that she wasn't the normal Hollywood beauty. When she did the makeup her way, she looked great. The makeup man kept trying to make her look beautiful in a more conventional way. It didn't work and he was frustrated. I finally explained who she was and about her unique style. He relaxed a bit. The best part of the evening was when Judy Garland and Barbra sang together. Judy Garland was on her way down health wise and not as exuberant as she had always been, but she came alive while she sang with Barbra. The electricity just crackled between them. It was thrilling. It was wonderful.

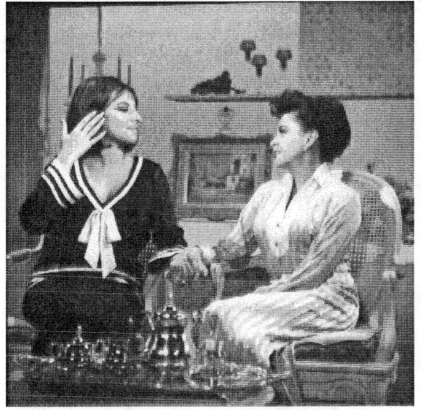

Barbra Streisand and Judy Garland,
The Judy Garland Show

I had a great desire to ask Elliot Gould if Barbra ever sang to him. Just imagine, wouldn't it be the most wonderful thing to have her sing to you? When I asked him, he became angry and felt insulted at my question. I guess they weren't getting along at that time. I never did get an answer. Later I told Natalie how he had reacted and asked her if asking a question like that was out of bounds. She laughed and told me it was his problem, not mine. She had done so much work on herself by this time that she was well aware of people's reactions and why they had them.

I'd never worked much at Colombia, but it was Pat's old stomping ground. He'd done the *The Monkees* series there and had worked on lots of other series that were filming at the time including *The Farmer's Daughter* starring Inger Stevens. He even confessed to me that he spent a night with Inger and liked her a lot. He had been delighted to work on *The Monkees* where he got his start as a gaffer, with all the darling little girls. He used to make stars in their eyes with his lighting. I met lots of his friends from his past. It was a wild crew that hung around together when he worked there. He'd often visit me at the studio and enjoyed running into his old friends.

In the meantime Dick Kline, the cameraman, was asked to do *Dream of Kings*, a story about a Greek family in Chicago. They wanted me to work on that film too, but that meant that I would have to leave Natalie a couple of weeks early. I mentioned it to her, and once again she was wonderful. "Go ahead and take the job," she told me. "My hairstyle is so simple someone else can do the last couple of weeks for me." I took the job and left two weeks early when the film went on location to Las Vegas.

Chapter 25

DREAM OF KINGS

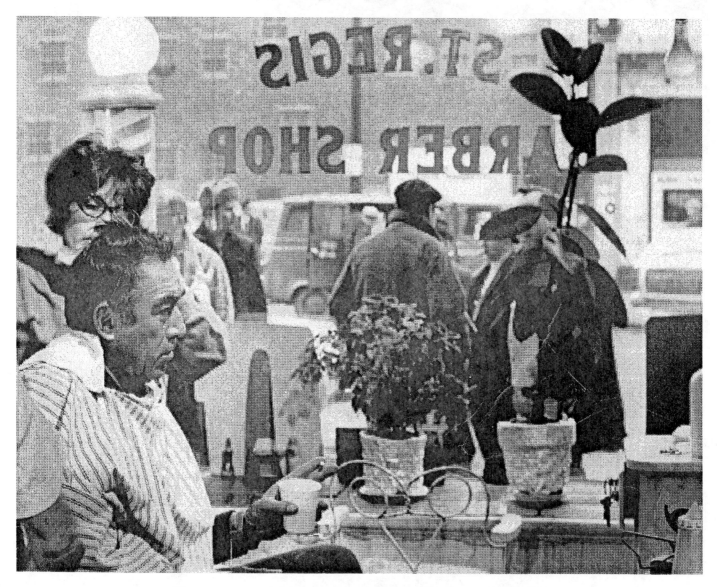

Sugar styling Anthony Quinn's hair for *Dream of Kings*

Anthony Quinn and Irene Papas had already been cast in *Dream of Kings*, but there was one more main part for a young woman that finally went to Inger Stevens. When Pat called me on the phone, I casually mentioned that Inger would also be working on the film. Then, being really bad, I asked if he thought she'd remember him. He was embarrassed. It was sweet. I wasn't jealous. After all I hadn't known Pat when he had slept with her. It was before my time. I thought his response was very funny, but I decided I probably shouldn't tease him anymore and I was sure he regretted sharing his experience. But, nobody's perfect.

When I made my deal for that film, I did so without thinking of the money. I just wanted to be with Pat. Later I realized I could have asked for more because the unit manager confessed that he always tried to get our deals down even if in the end he had to give us what we wanted. I kept that bit of information in mind for the future. I was where I wanted to be, which was what mattered.

Anthony Quinn was a big powerful man, full of energy and could be scary at times. I could imagine he might have a quick temper if he wasn't pleased and I certainly wanted to avoid his anger, if possible. Irene Papas, the Greek actress, was lovely. Inger Stevens was perfect. She was warm, sexy, and easily communicated her feelings. We became friends immediately.

Once again we went on location to Chicago only this time it was much colder. Our first location there was on Halston Street in Greek Town. This was very different from my experience with Melina on *Gaily, Gaily*. We were working on the streets and it was so cold that we were always being offered Ouzo by the restaurant owner where we worked. He knew how cold we were standing outside on the street and Ouzo warms one wonderfully. It was great working in Greek Town because there were restaurants everywhere and we could eat to our hearts' content between scenes.

Most of our filming was done out-doors. When it was edited, the film had a feeling of really being in Chicago. The interiors would be done at home in Los Angeles. One night we worked in a cold, windy area where Anthony Quinn was waiting to catch a bus. He needed to look cold, which didn't take any acting. He picked up some newspaper and put it inside his jacket next to his chest. During the shot, he got colder and colder and began to feel sorry for himself. He was out working in the cold when all his friends were in his warm dressing room. I offered him some Ouzo, which he appreciated. I sensed he was feeling like a little kid and wanted attention. It also warmed him up.

We flew home to Los Angeles just before Christmas and began working on Main Street in downtown Los Angeles - the pits of L.A. The restaurant where we worked was just ghastly. As the lights came on for the scene the interior of the restaurant heated up and became hotter and hotter. In fact, it was so hot that the grease on the air vents began to melt and ooze along the pipes. Cockroaches crawled around everywhere. One electrician almost threw up when he opened the walk-in refrigerator. The smell was horrible. Nobody ordered any food in that place.

Thank goodness, it wasn't necessary for me to spend much time inside there. Instead, I stayed outside and consorted with the drunks and bums - we didn't call them street people at the time. When they came up to me asking for a quarter for a bottle of wine, I lectured them on the effects of alcohol. They learned to stay away from me. I think I reminded them of why they left home. There was one exception though. One man, seemingly well educated, said he wouldn't talk to me if I talked with all those other drunks. He was one of them, but he assured me that he only drank at special times.

Pat was actually so sickened by the filth, the poverty, and the bums that he became ill and had to stay home until we finished that location. I never saw that happen to him again. His senses just couldn't stand it.

We began to film interiors at Selznick Studios, a small studio where *Gone with the Wind* had been made. It was dusty and worn, but still had a friendly feeling to it.

Danny Mann was our director. He loved doing really long rehearsals and we'd have to sit on the set and be quiet the whole time. He wouldn't even allow us to read which surprised me because reading really kept me quiet. So we all sat quietly and prayed for the scene to work.

Every morning I'd go to Anthony Quinn's room to dress his hair. He was balding at the dome and told me he never wanted to see a bit of that skin on the screen. First of all, I sprayed his hair and bare head with Streaks and Tips. It worked well and he was pleased. But a few days later he came in and said I had to do something different. His wife was furious with him because all his pillowslips were turning black. Of course he could have washed his hair each night, but that didn't occur to him. Next, I used an eyebrow pencil to fill in the spaces, which seemed to work better except that he was so impatient he never allowed me enough time to do a good job. I was always stressed, trying to finish in time. He reminded me of my father who had also been impatient and intimidating.

Inger was a nice woman and this was a difficult period for her. A few years before, she and Anthony Quinn had an affair. She was young and had become pregnant with his child. He sent her to Mexico for an abortion. When she returned, he was with someone else. She tried to take her life, but since then she had done lots of emotional work to deal with it and move on. Strangely enough, she had just finished therapy, and it was at this point, she was offered the part. It was a real challenge for her to work with Tony in a film that was so similar to her own past experience. One of the major scenes in the film was the one that bore a similarity to her own life. It took forever to get it right. They rehearsed it for more than two days. We weren't allowed on the stage until it was done. It was cathartic for Inger. She had described Tony as a steamroller, but now she felt able to deal with him. For her sake I hoped this was true. On the home front, Pat and I bought an old Volkswagen camper. This was when people were putting flower stickers on cars. Our Volkswagen was faded and shabby, but instead of buying stickers we cleaned all the paint out of our garage and used it to paint our own flowers on the car. We painted beautiful, bright flowers all over the car. We invited all the neighborhood kids to join in the fun. Then we put the rest of the paint in the camper and took it to work so at lunch time the crew could add their efforts. It was a beauty. There wasn't another van like it in existence.

We only had one scheduled day off for Christmas that year, but Anthony Quinn did us a great favor - he got sick. The day's shooting had to be canceled so we had the weekend to recover from our Christmas festivities.

When the film came to an end. I was sorry to finish working with Inger. I had grown to love her. She was so cute, never mentioning that she knew Pat before or that anything had happened between them. At the end of the film, she gave me a lovely gift and said to give her love to Pat any way that I wanted to. He liked that.

She died only a year later. Many people felt it was suicide, but I have difficulty in believing it. She seemed so sane and wonderful, like she had done the necessary work to live a full life.

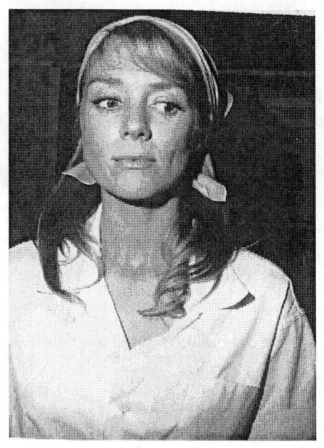

Inger Stevens, *Dream of Kings*

Chapter 26

GRASSHOPPER
Life Changes, 1969

During the filming of *Gaily, Gaily*, Dick Kline, our cameraman, met a beautiful Haitian/ French woman named Jacqueline. Our return to Chicago for *Dream of Kings* gave him time to fall in love with her, and by the end of the film they had made plans to get married in the spring. Dick asked Pat to be his best man and he offered to pay for Pat's trip to Chicago for the wedding. Pat said he preferred to take the cash so the whole family could drive to West Virginia. That way the kids and I could meet Pat's parents and then fly up to Chicago for the wedding.

Ever since Pat and I had met, we'd been working constantly. I welcomed this trip. I also wanted to meet Mammy and Pappy. I'd spoken to them on the phone and they sounded like wonderful people. We took our flowered bus to our friend Terry Marshall who knew everything about Volkswagens. He told us we needed to replace the engine before our trip, so we did.

We figured it would be best to start out at night. It was only March, but the desert was still very hot and we wanted to avoid the heat. We packed all five of us into the bus and off we went. We hadn't driven more than a couple hundred miles when the engine began to chug. Pat had to keep blowing sand out of the engine all night long, nursing the camper along through the desert. At dawn we were parked outside a mechanic's shop waiting for it to open. We discovered that although Terry had changed the engine, he had neglected to change the spark plugs.

The trip was almost perfect. It rained each night, just like in Camelot, and the mornings brought freshly washed landscapes. We did have to stop each day for some repair or other, but we finally made it to Mammy and Pappy's house in Beckley, West Virginia. What a welcome they gave us. They were so happy to see Pat, and I loved them both immediately. Pappy was quiet and very nice. Mammy was vivacious, full of energy and had a wonderful hillbilly accent.

We called Dick and told him we had arrived and then we made our reservations for Chicago. Now we had time to look around the countryside. With Pat, I realized how important family life actually was to me. I was ready to change my life. I was tired of the movie business. I never really felt at home in L.A. I wrote to New Zealand to get information about immigrating. They replied saying that we would need $50,000 or the ability to do something the country especially needed. It seemed impossible. As we drove through the beautiful mountains of West Virginia, my mind was wandering looking for a place I could call home. I fell in love with the countryside filled with trees and mountains. I began to picture myself in a house with a front porch and rocking chairs, where we could sit in the evenings. I wanted my life to be more peaceful.

Just as a lark, we went looking at homes here and there and everywhere. The prices were so cheap. We were amazed. We traveled up and down hollows and through the mountains. One day we saw an advertisement for a house in Amigo and decided to check it out. The toothless old man at the store directed us to take the road up a hill. But first we had to go under a huge coal trestle where they cleaned coal, up a rutted, bumpy road, and then a mile and a half up a narrow road that wound up a mountain. At the top stood a big, lovely farmhouse. It was well worth thinking about. We left the kids with Mammy and Pappy. We flew to Chicago and met Jacqueline's charming family. They were a loving group of people and quite well - educated. Jacqueline spoke seven languages and her grandfather had been on the supreme court of the United Nations. Dick was fortunate to find such a terrific wife. Pat was terribly nervous in his role as the best man. He was sweating; sure he'd drop the ring, but finally made it through the wedding without a disaster. He was relieved when it was all over and we were on our way back to West Virginia.

We had more time to spare. I didn't have work and Dick was on his honeymoon. He told Pat he would call him when his next project came up. We were enjoying ourselves, so we stayed on in West Virginia where the kids enjoyed their first snowstorm ever. We decided to buy the farm - the one on the top of the hill. We paid $6,500 for one hundred and fifteen acres, which included the house, the barn, and outbuildings. We leased the surrounding five hundred acres for five dollars a year. For those five dollars we had the farm rights. The coal and timber rights were leased already. We left a hundred-dollar deposit and hurried back to Los Angeles to get the rest of the money together. We still had bills left over from our divorces, so we needed to get back to work.

I didn't have a project yet so I was doing day checks, daily calls here and there. Pat and Dick were set to work on a film called *The Grasshopper* starring Jacqueline Bisset and Jim Brown. In the meantime I got a call to do a film with Dick Van Dyke called *Cold Turkey*. It was about a whole town that quit drinking alcohol. I was going to do a screen test for it the next week, so in the meantime I decided to surprise Pat and drive up to Las Vegas where he was shooting. I packed up the three kids, and two of their friends in the camper and off we went. What a mistake that was. We descended on Pat in the middle of the night and he wasn't terribly happy to see me, especially with five kids. But he got over it and we changed motels so we could all fit in. A few days later I had to fly to L.A. for a day so I could do the screen test.

Clark Paylow, the unit manager on *Cold Turkey*, called me in Las Vegas, to ask me to bring back some of the little one ounce bottles of booze. They didn't sell them in California, and they used them in the film for nips. He asked for a hundred of them. I bought them without realizing how heavy they would be. I had to haul them back myself, seeing as I couldn't put them in my luggage. By the time I arrived at the studio that morning, my back hurt. Clark Paylow, true to his name, always tried to get things in the cheapest way.

I had a wonderful time with Dick Van Dyke that day. He was moving to Arizona and I told him about our plans for moving to the farm. I ended up turning the film down because I wanted to be with my family, but I did entertain the idea of buying a camper so we all could stay in it on location in Iowa where the film would be shot. We could have actually pulled it off, because soon after that Dick had some differences with production and was let go from *The Grasshopper,* freeing up Pat.

While I was in Las Vegas, I met Jacqueline Bisset. What a beautiful human being. She was so nice to all the kids. I hoped I'd be able to work with her some day. Jim Brown, her co-star, was gorgeous to look at. He walked like a Leo, very sexy. It was hard to equate the way he looked with the news that came out about him throwing a woman off a balcony. Whoops! Guess his beauty was only skin-deep.

In Las Vegas, the guys started having a great time working backstage with the bare-chested ladies, but in time they began to get bored and started eyeing the girls with the bikinis. Guess they liked the mystery better than the bare facts.

The lead nude dancer named Pat took a liking to "my Pat." Perhaps I had a tinge of jealousy. I didn't think Pat would fall for her, but I wanted to make sure. I wanted him to remember what he had at home. I was in a thin phase, in fact the slimmest I'd been since I was a teenager. I looked quite good, if I do say so myself. One night after the kids had all gone to bed I stripped down to nothing for Patrick and danced naked on our bed. I reminded him that all I had was really mine. No Styrofoam breasts for me. He loved that and laughed and laughed, enjoying my little bout of jealousy.

We still had our flowered bus and one day I was driving in town, when a policeman stopped me. He was quite surprised to see who was in the bus - Dick's wife, Jackie, and a lot of kids. He had expected to see a bunch of hippies. Lamely, he said, "A bus like this was just reported in a bank hold up." I knew it was a lie, but I said, "Isn't that remarkable. Why on earth would someone rob a bank with such a recognizable vehicle?" He excused himself quickly and left. I was sure they didn't want any hippies in Las Vegas. If you didn't have any money to gamble away, you weren't welcome

The kids had fun. One evening we were out till midnight looking into the heavens as men were landing on the moon. One day the kids were asked if they would work as extras sitting on the merry-go-round at the hotel. They were excited and so was I until lunchtime when I learned that they were not going to pay the kids, or feed them either. Pat was furious and let Production know. Soon we were invited to lunch.

After Dick Kline was replaced and the new cameraman brought his own crew, Pat's crew thought they would show the new cameraman what a great crew he was losing. The last night they were there, they literally ran across the desert with all the huge lights doing things in an amazingly short time. They wanted to show up the new crew, who were due to arrive and in no way could have kept up that pace.

Chapter 27

BABY MAKER
Summer 1969

My big project that summer was getting our house sold. We had to come up with $6,500, minus our $100 deposit, by the beginning of August. We made it, but we also had to sell Patrick's beloved 1955 Thunderbird. I don't think he ever forgave me for that.

I went back to day checking at Fox Studios where I was assigned to work on a television film with Suzanne Plechette. I was delighted to work with her again. Typical of television productions, no provisions had been made, either in the budget or in the schedule, for me to get a good hair lace wig made for Suzanne. This became a problem because a major element of the story was that her hair color changed back and forth from platinum to black. To make matters worse, her own dark hair was supposed to be the wig in the show, so we had to use a cheap wig to simulate her "real" hair. It was a difficult situation, but I tried to work as best as I could.

Things went okay until one night when the director decided to have her drive with the top down on her convertible - while she was wearing the platinum "real hair" wig. Of course when the wind blew the bangs back, her own dark hair was visible. It was ridiculous. If I'd had a hair lace wig, I could have covered her own hair and the lace would have made it look real. The cheap wig made this impossible - there was a straight line right where the wig hit her forehead. The director didn't seem to care and neither did anyone else. They just asked me, "What can you do?" I replied, "Quit, I guess." There was no way I could solve the problem.

As it turned out, a week later I did quit. Pat had met a new cameraman, Chuck Rocher, while doing commercials. Chuck was hired to work on *Adam at Six a.m.* starring Michael Douglas - his first starring role, I believe. Michael was very young, but already his star appeal was showing. We all liked him. The movie was going to be filmed in Excelsior Springs, Missouri and Pat had to leave immediately. Not wanting to be left behind, I quit my show.

Tanya, Xochi, our cock-a-poo, Daffy, and I accompanied Patrick on the plane to Missouri. I was so happy to be going with him and it was great for the kids to have the experience. Laurie, my oldest daughter, decided to stay at home, so she wouldn't have to change schools.

Excelsior Springs was a little old-fashioned town. The department store even had those tubes you put money in to be whisked along the ceiling to the office where they made change and returned it through the tube. The town was named for the hot springs that attracted people for health treatments. There was a big hotel where you could take the treatments, drink the beastly tasting water, and leave feeling much better than when you had arrived.

We stayed in a motel near downtown. The day we arrived I took the girls to the old grammar school to enroll them for the next three months. The first day of school Xochi got a stomachache that lasted for three days, and then she began to enjoy herself. Tanya fit in immediately.

Pat enjoyed working with Chuck. Dick had always been mean to his gaffers at work, though he'd be charming to Pat when they weren't working. But Chuck was nice all the time and he was creative, too.

Things were beginning to change in the production departments of the film business. One of the newest ideas, a production van, came from a little Armenian man, Fouad Siad. Usually the electricians, the grips, and the Camera Department each had their own truck. In this new van each department had its own area. The van also included a makeup room and a rest room. I'd first seen it demonstrated on *Dream of Kings*. It was a clever idea, but there was great resistance to it from all the crafts. The movie business is actually rather old-fashioned and doesn't take to new ideas easily.

For this show Fouad had sent his double-decker bus. The crew could actually ride in top of the production van.

It was quite an impressive sight as it drove into the little town - the first double-decker bus. Johnny Jenson, now a cameraman, was the driver. One day he forgot he was driving the double-decker and drove into a gas station with a roof over the pumps. Wrong move. Disaster. Finally, after facing a great deal of resistance, the production van has now become commonplace. Fouad sold out for a huge profit before all that happened.

Fall in Excelsior Springs was beautiful. I'd walk downtown and enjoy the cool, crisp weather knowing that next year we'd be settled on our farm in West Virginia enjoying our own fall. I liked having the time to go to the school when something special was happening. I had never been able to do that before. I didn't have a car so I bought myself one of the shopping baskets little old ladies use so I could carry my washing or groceries. Daffy would prance happily along beside me as I walked through town. In the evenings we gathered with the crew, all the kids and Daffy joining in. It was a delightful time. I just knew I'd love life in a small town.

As our house had already been sold, we went home to stay at my mother's house when the film was completed. I began to visualize (although I didn't call it that at the time). I'd read some books about creating what you want to have in your life by picturing it. I pictured myself in a bathtub with feet, like the one at our farm, but I found out a few weeks later that visualization has to be very detailed.

We moved to a tiny place in Lennox owned by Pat's friend, Terry Marshall, the man who helped us with our camper. We called Terry's place the Chicken House as it had originally been a chicken coop. Guess what? It had a bathtub with feet. I had to laugh at myself. From then on I tried to put more details into my visualizing, trying to make it more accurate.

Before moving to Lennox I had not been aware of that part of town even though I'd lived in Los Angeles my whole life. It was probably the roughest area in Los Angeles at the time, beneath the LAX airport. It was so loud when a plane came in to land, we'd have to stop talking until it landed. At night we heard helicopters searching for criminals, shouts, and sometimes gunshots. Still, we felt very safe because a high fence surrounded our little house. The gate was always locked with a combination lock. The girls enrolled in school and seemed to enjoy themselves making new friends. When it was cold, we made a fire in the little Swedish fireplace in the living room. It was our only source of heat. Actually we had a lot of fun living there. Terry and his brothers and many relatives often dropped in. Terry's garage, next to our place, was the hangout for all the "boys". Life was very simple. Mostly I was thinking about our move to the farm.

Chuck Rocher was offered another film, *Baby Maker*, which was a story about a couple that hires a girl to have a baby for them. James Bridges, a sweet man with long, wild, black hair, directed it. Colin Wilcox played the wife unable to have a child and Barbara Hershey played the girl. I loved Barbara. She was wonderful, down to earth, and fun to work with. I believe it was her first film. She was going with David Carradine at the time and we all wondered why. Barbara was so cute. She had a scene where she had to dive naked into the pool. It took her a long time to get up the nerve to do it. She was worried about what her parents would think about her taking her clothes off for a film.

One night we all went to a light show - my first. It was fantastic. Who needed drugs? The lights made me high. A beautiful German Shepard/Collie mix hung around the set. He did not seem to have a master, so we took him home. We named him Timber. He lived with us for the rest of his life. I think he hated being a street person; he took to us as if he belonged with us forever.

Other things began to disturb me. I smelled pot fumes coming from under many of the dressing room doors. It made me angry. I know that if I drank on the job I wouldn't be able to do my job well. So I wondered how in the heck these folks could do their best work if they were high. Perhaps it wasn't any of my business, but that's how I felt. I loved the business and wanted it to continue. I didn't want it to be destroyed by drugs. Still, it didn't seem to pose a real problem right then like the cocaine habits that nearly ruined the industry later on. But it was the beginning of the drug scene. Before that time we sometimes went after work and had a couple of drinks. With the entrance of drugs, everyone became very secretive.

We bought a big Ford truck with a stake bed to take our stuff back to the farm. Pat's crew helped us build a cabin for the kids and animals to ride in. We felt like the Beverly Hillbillies, going east. Everyone on the set was thinking up ways for us to make a living back there. One driver, the wrinkliest person I'd ever seen, told us it would be great to raise worms. He explained the process. I opted for something else, but appreciated his sincerity.

Jim Bridges, our director, was a lovely human being and we were all pleased to work with him. He had learned that the producers were afraid of him, thanks to all his wild hair. I saw him years later, when everyone else was sporting long hair, and his hair was quite short. He explained that he liked to appear the opposite of fashion.

Colin Wilcox was an organizer. She got us all together one weekend at Martin Sheen's house to try and get a production company going. It sounded like a lot of fun, each of us taking a job we didn't normally do. I opted to be a producer type and raise money. We thought we'd all live together in a big house in Northern California while we worked on the project. It sounded great, but it never came to fruition. We all just went our own way.

As we finished that film, reality set in. We were totally changing our way of life, giving up on the movie business. That was okay because the business was changing. Producers didn't appear to care about the quality of our work any more and with the exception of films like *Baby Maker* it just wasn't much fun either.

Chapter 28

THE REAL MA AND PA KETTLE

The events in the following few pages took place over a two-year period - an interlude that gave me enough experiences to fill another book…

I threw myself wholeheartedly into our new adventure thinking it would continue for the rest of my life. I have always loved jumping head first into the unknown, then finding out how things work as I go. I guess you could say I was obsessed.

Our friends and families simply couldn't understand why on earth Pat and I would want to change our lifestyle so radically. They were concerned that we had no concrete plans for making a living on the farm, and I think they were worried about our sanity. Of course we did have a few ideas, like a summer vacation farm for kids. We knew we could return to the world of movies if necessary, or even just go to Los Angeles for the winter, but that was as far as our plans went. The only thing that mattered to me was getting out of Los Angeles. The only thing that mattered to Patrick was making me happy.

Off we went in our big stake bed truck stuffed to the gills - Ma and Pa Kettle come to life. Actually, I was a bit more attractive than Marjorie Main and Pat was bigger and certainly more handsome that Percy Kilbride. We had no idea how many similarities the future held for us.

It was still winter when we arrived in West Virginia so we moved in with Mammy and Pappy for a while. Pappy reminded us politely that this was only a temporary situation. Their house was small, the perfect size for the two of them and an occasional guest. Five extra people and dogs stretched it beyond the limit.

We knew we needed a four-wheel drive vehicle. Our big truck would never make it up the hill to the farm in the snow. We found an old Scout at a price we could afford, but even then it was difficult going. Tanya was so frightened as we struggled up our road, slipping and sliding, that she was ready to go straight back to Los Angeles. In the past, the road to the house was the main road, but it had since been rerouted through the hollow down below.

Within a few weeks we were settled. The coal company built our enormous old house in the early 1900s. It was a simple, two story, white clapboard structure with a cellar full of huge bins that were used to store the apples that used to grow in the orchard. We had plenty of room and spread out, enjoying ourselves.

I was in my Pollyanna mode with visions of perfection and beauty all around the farm. I pictured myself getting up each morning, putting on a starched, puffy-sleeved dress, and walking out to the sparkling clean stall to milk our cow. I imagined beautiful, friendly animals wandering around the farm, and our crops growing fruitfully. Our children would be healthier with all that clean, fresh air and homegrown food. We even named our place Happy Hills Farm. Reality, however, turned out to be very different.

As the snow melted we could see that the place was a mess. The huge orchard we had planned on pruning so that we could make money-selling apples was too far-gone to be brought back to life. There were dead car bodies everywhere and we had to pay someone to tow them all to the bottom of the hill where we planted vines hoping they would eventually grow and hide the bodies. Ours wasn't the only property with more than its share of old junkers. I began to call West Virginia the Dead Car State.

The old cement garage where I planned to have my milking shed was full of discarded car parts and the chicken house next to it was filled with old chicken droppings. Shoveling all that chicken shit caused me to cough for months. Every project took so much effort we were often overwhelmed. I was only thirty-five years old and had plenty of energy, but it was still difficult.

Laurie, Tanya, and Xochi started school right away. Pat drove them to the bottom of our mountain early in the morning and the school bus picked them up. On the first day, Laurie, who was immaculate by nature, wore a long, gray coat to school. By the time she got home the bottom of it was filthy with coal dust. The thing that amazed my girls most was the one bus stop where twelve kids rushed out of a door and climbed on, nearly filling the bus. It was one family. My kids, especially Laurie were overwhelmed.

Our barn was a beautiful post and beam structure that sat on the hill above the house. We decided to become "real" farmers and get some animals. First we found a beautiful hog that Mammy bought Pat for his thirty-first birthday. The hog was already bred, so we had piglets in our future. Our next investment was twenty-six sheep and a couple of guinea hens. The sheep were Pat's real challenge and frustration. The day they arrived he sat in the field with them just like David, the shepherd in the Bible. He made sure that no neighborhood dogs would harm them, not realizing yet that our neighbors were miles away. I brought him lunch in the field.

We planned on bunking the sheep in the chicken house that we had prepared for them. At day's end Pat opened the gate to the field and began to lead them to the chicken house. They followed him for a while, and then walked right on past him, out through the gate, which he had forgotten to close, and into the forest beyond. How frustrating! Disappointing! After he'd taken such good care of them all day. He filled a bucket with corn and walked to where they had settled in the forest, calling, "Sheepie, sheepie". Over and over again. No response. Eventually he threw the pail down and yelled, "You can rot in the forest for all I care," and stomped into the house. At that moment Pat could have happily shot each and every one of them, if he'd had a gun.

Xochi, who was only five at the time, picked up the pail Pat had thrown down and began tapping it and calling the sheep. Lo and behold, they responded to her gentleness and followed her out of the forest, back through the gate, and into the chicken house where they were safe for the night. We always remembered to close the gate from then on. Chickens, ducks, and horses all followed, each with its own new frustration. What on earth did we know about farming? Not much - but we were learning.

We planted our garden on top of the hill beside the barn where others had planted in the past. Then we had to carry water up the hill for the plants. I learned and the next year put the garden below the house so I could use a hose. We decided to plow an acre and plant potatoes. We tried to find someone who could plow the field for us, but they were all busy. One man offered us a plow suggesting we attach it to the jeep. That way I could drive slowly while Pat held the plow; it would be just like using a horse and plow. Wrong. It might have worked if Pat was a marathon runner, but there was no way I could drive the jeep slowly enough for him. I had no idea I was going too fast for him and didn't realize I had nearly wiped him out while he tried to keep up. Luckily the jeep stalled and Pat stumbled up to the window, red-faced and panting. He was sure he was going to have a heart attack. We gave up on that idea.

For some reason, in the beginning, I didn't notice the huge piles of slag left over from coal mining that lined the roadside. Some of it caught fire and now smoked all the time. When we first looked at the farm, I focused on the good things. Now I would walk around and see bare mountains where the coal had been stripped away. The coal companies were supposed to reclaim the land after mining, but they never did.

Our Scout broke down on a weekly basis, one window never closed, and the exhaust pipe fell off repeatedly because of the potholes and the bumpy road that the coal trucks demolished. Thanks to that open window, I ended up covered in black coal dust whenever I drove anywhere.

We decided to apply to the welfare department for a license to open a vacation camp for kids. They sent us to Charleston to see about the requirements. It was discouraging. We were told we would have to add fire escapes and block off the top floor with a firewall. We simply couldn't afford to comply with the regulations. But the welfare department had another idea for us. They suggested we become a home for kids just brought into the foster care system. They would stay with us while welfare decided where to place them and we'd be paid $200 a month plus another amount for each child. It sounded like a feasible idea.

Meanwhile, summer was approaching and the hay was getting high. Our neighbors, the Lily's, who lived above us on the mountain, offered to cut our hay if they could keep half of it. This is what they did for the former owners and it sounded fine to us, too. Early one summer morning we met in the top field and got started. We had a great time cutting, raking, and baling hay. Then we sat down to a huge midday dinner - fried chicken, mustard greens, and fresh milk all topped off with an apple cake. By the time I finished eating I doubted I could move, let alone go back to work. Actually, we worked until dark and after a bath fell exhausted into bed, all sunburned and scratched, but happy and content. I was worried about Laurie. She was depressed and hated the farm and our way of life. I was very happy myself, despite our problems and I wanted her to enjoy herself. There was nothing I could do though. She hated everything about the place. That summer she went back to Los Angeles to stay with her father and Joyce. I missed her terribly, but I also felt it was best for her. Xochi, on the other hand, was Pat's right-hand man in black brogan boots and overalls. She handled the animals and kept Pat happy. Tanya was happy and easily made new friends.

Pat was having a tough time. In the movie business he was used to carrying around a light meter and pointing to other people to do the physical work. Here, he had to do it all and it wasn't fun for him. He was born to be a pointer, not a doer. One day he decided to be creative and build us a huge dining room table. He chose some old, very thick, almost petrified rough wood boards and laid them out to nail together. The wood was like concrete and the nails just wouldn't go in. I heard him cussing outside and when I looked through the window, I saw him throw his hammer into the bushes. He was feeling like a total failure.

I walked outside when I heard him and shouted, "You can light a set beautifully. Even a great carpenter couldn't light a set like you do. It's okay not to know how to do everything perfectly in the beginning." He calmed down eventually and built a wonderful, huge table that had slanting sides. He used round logs for legs and there were always carpenter ants munching away on those legs. It was great fun watching things roll off the table when we weren't careful.

Eventually the welfare people showed up. One woman thought it would be a perfect place for an official foster care attention home, but the man who took the kids to court put the kibosh on the idea declaring we were too far out of town. He didn't want to have to drive so far. We were bummed. The welfare department was desperate for homes, so they suggested we take in foster kids. We would get $60 a child, but not the $200 extra. Like the naive fools we were, we agreed.

Our first arrival was Mike, fourteen, and possibly a thief. It was us or juvenile hall for him. He was happy to be with us, but Xochi became distressed as he tried to take her place as Pat's handyman.

Next they gave us a family of six: Bobby, fourteen; Donna, thirteen; Sharon, twelve; John Henry, ten; two little girls, eight and six. In addition, we had Gary, fourteen, just out of a mental institution, and Ann who was sixteen. Her parents had dumped her at the welfare office.

We were quite a household. Tanya was thrilled to have so many friends. Most of the kids chose to sleep in one room on the first floor near Pat and me. All the little ones, including our girls, shared the bunk beds. The older kids each had their own room upstairs. My girls had never shared a room before and now they were all sharing their bunks with another child, sometimes sleeping head to foot. It was great.

We bought an old truck to carry our new family. It was dark green with a bed in back for us to ride in. There was no other way to transport a family of thirteen. We were really the "Kettles" now.

The day that Mike arrived, our water ran out. Upon investigation we discovered our spring was low. No water was coming into the house. It was awful. We dug deeper and deeper hoping the spring would fill with water, but no luck. Here we were, a family of thirteen and no water. So we collected it from rain barrels and Mike and Pat bought big plastic bottles, which they filled from a spring down the mountain for drinking. When we could, we went to the swimming hole to bathe, Ivory Soap in hand.

We put bottles of water on the front porch where the kids brushed their teeth, spitting over the rail. Luckily we had an outhouse. The kids were great about it, but I suffered. Water had always been my refuge when I was tired or depressed. Now a nice hot bath was out of the question. We heated water and poured it into the bathtub for the kids - four or five kids to each bath-load of water. Pappy felt so sorry for me that he installed a new water heater in his house so whenever I went into Beckley, I could take a nice, hot bath. Bless him.

What a problem laundry was! Pat, now a school bus driver, took the kids to school, and then came back up the hill to pick up the dirty wash. On the average there were eighteen to twenty loads a week. We drove as fast as possible into Beckley and almost filled the whole Laundromat. It took hours. What a horror story. For years after that I couldn't enter a Laundromat without a great depression coming over me.

The rains came and because of the strip mining, there was lots of flooding, as the bare, unplanted cliffs didn't hold water. I was furious at the irresponsibility of the coal companies. Buffalo Creek had a dam that burst that year killing the people who lived below it. It was a real tragedy and I grew angrier and angrier, ranting and raving about how the coal companies walked all over people.

One spring day a huge bulldozer crawled up our mountain road and stopped on the property below our house. The driver informed me he was looking for coal to strip. The coal company had the strip-mining lease; we only had the farm lease. I was so upset, each day I walked down to where I could hear the bulldozer to see if they had located a vein of coal. I prayed they wouldn't. Luckily they only found a narrow vein, not worth their time to mine. I thanked God. I had been prepared to lie down in front of their machines to prevent it from ruining our land if necessary.

I decided to run for House of Delegates. I had bitched and grumbled about the strip mining, now I needed to do something. I figured I was at least as smart as half the people who lived in the state. I also decided to run for school board. I knew very little about politics, but gave it my best. Needless to say, that wasn't good enough. I think I might have managed to win the school board election, but never the House of Delegates. I was just too honest. Pat listened to me as I talked on the phone to someone from the strip-mining coalition. When they asked my opinions about stripping, I replied, "Your empty cliffs condemn you." Pat remarked, "You'll never get elected if you are that honest." He was right. I didn't. Years later many of my ideas about reclaiming the land have been realized. I was ahead of my time.

We were slowly going broke. $60 a child went so quickly, it didn't pay any of our bills. Pat's bus driving job brought in some income. It was amazing how he could drive that bus all the way up to the farm on that narrow road. He brought it home each night so the kids wouldn't be able to steal the gas. The local kids figured if the bus was out of gas there wouldn't be any school.

Most of our foster kids eventually ended up going back to their homes. Mike was the only one left with us. Nobody wanted him.

The second year we got our first milk cow. Once again my imagination and reality just didn't match. The cow resided in the apple orchard. I didn't have my starched outfit to wear when I milked her. Instead I wore old jeans and boots and carried her feed in a pail. When the flies bit her, she switched me in the face with her tail. The rich milk was great, though.

All told, I was quite happy being a farmer and foster mother, even though it was the most difficult thing I'd ever done. Pat felt differently. He'd about had it. We were almost broke so when he got a call to do a movie job in Pittsburgh he was ready to go. We only had Mike by this time and he opted to work in the tobacco fields that summer. It worked out that we could all go to Pittsburgh.

I made arrangements for someone to live on the farm and take care of the animals. Pat was already on location so we drove up. I hadn't given any thought to returning to the film business so I had let my union dues go. I wanted to be a farmer forever. The production company asked me to work on the film for a few days so I called the union and asked the business agent to find out what I needed to do to reinstate myself. The agent wouldn't tell me, he just kept repeating that I had to read this or that regulation. I was angry when I eventually found out that all I had to do was pay my back dues.

While in Pittsburgh, we all lived in one motel room, but I found myself enjoying it. There were actually good restaurants and I could stay clean all day. The kids were in heaven. By this time Laurie had returned and decided that our way of life was preferable to the strict one she had to live with her dad and stepmother. In fact, she decided the way we lived was quite the stylish life. What a difference a year made.

The film, *Going Home*, starred Robert Mitchum, Jan Michael Vincent, Sally Kirkland, and Brenda Vaccaro. I loved Mitchum. I remembered getting his autograph when I was seventeen. He still had that wonderful, animal sex appeal. One afternoon he invited us to his room at the motel for a chili party. He had a chunk of pot and almost everyone was partaking of it and enjoying themselves. I almost apologized for not smoking, but he said to quiet my screechy voice and relax, it was okay not to smoke.

As we were sitting there, people would drive by and look in his window. After a while Mitchum got tired of it and decided he'd moon them. The next time a looker drove by, he dropped his drawers. We were hysterical with laughter. It was fun being around him when he was relaxed. He was bright, funny, and truly one of the boys. The girls liked him a lot, too.

I went to the set a couple of times and once ended up working as an extra. I wasn't thrilled about it, but they were short of bodies. So for the first half of a very cool morning I stood in a lake with my pants rolled up while the water seeped upwards until I was soaked. After lunch they had me lying on my stomach on the beach, elbows bent, my face in my hands, while Mitchum walked by. By the end of the afternoon, my elbows were raw. All of this was for only fifteen dollars a day.

One week they worked in an old, unused prison. The warden's deserted apartment was wonderful, and it had a huge bathtub, the biggest I'd ever seen, probably imported from Europe. I tried to buy it for the farm, but no luck. The prison was a gigantic place with lots of buildings. It had been self-supporting in its day. Inside there were rows and rows of cells, level after level. At one point, someone pulled a switch and all the doors closed with a huge clang. The sound was so jarring and final, that it has remained with me ever since. I still think it would be a good idea to take kids into these kinds of places to see what it would be like. Perhaps it would help them refrain from breaking the law. It certainly impressed me. I believe that today they do take kids into jails as a deterrent.

At the end of our stay the company threw a party at a Greek restaurant. The lovely belly dancer carefully danced up and down our table, gracefully keeping her toes out of the eggplant. The food was delicious and the whole experience was fun. I realized I was going to miss this back at the farm.

Before we left for home, Mitchum did a wonderful thing for us. He knew how badly we needed a new truck and an old one had been used in the film. Somehow he figured out how to get it and gave it to us. It was a lovely gesture and we were grateful. Our rolling stock wasn't in great shape. Pat drove the new truck home.

Chapter 29

HEX
Fall, 1971

After a taste of life in the big city, our return to the farm was a real let down. I wondered if my dramatic change of career had been too harsh on the rest of the family. I was having second thoughts now that we once again had to face the problems we had left behind. I felt as if a huge weight had descended upon my shoulders once again.

It was a pain always struggling to pay our bills, or not being able to pay them at all. Like Mammy always said, "Money isn't the most important thing in life; it's just so unhandy without it." Before our move to the farm Pat and I had always worked on films bringing in whatever income we needed or wanted. My dream of living on the farm hadn't included a way to make a living. I just assumed it would work out, but obviously it hadn't.

Not long after our return to the farm in August 1971, Pat got a call from Chuck Rocher to go to South Dakota to do a low-budget film called *Grasslands*, a weird little film set in the 1920s, released years later as *Hex*. We were delighted for the opportunity to take off again.

We needed a suitable vehicle and found an old, khaki-colored, telephone company van. It wasn't very pretty but was exactly what we needed. We didn't paint this one with flowers, but we did decorate it a bit by painting Happy Hills Farm on the front tire cover. It looked nice and added a bit of color to the otherwise drab vehicle. We named our van Vanessa; vehicles should always have a name.

After making arrangements for someone to watch the farm, off we went, stopping in Pittsburgh to pick up Denise, a girl Laurie had become good friends with while we'd been on location there. There were six of us in the van plus two dogs and each night we stopped at a motel and booked two rooms, except for the night we couldn't find a motel. That night we had no choice, but to sleep in the van. It was cramped and then there was a thunderstorm that night which made for an amusing adventure.

We arrived on location in South Dakota and made our home in an unusual place called Swift Bird, located on the Sioux Rose Bud Reservation. It had been built by the government as a Job Corp. center for the Sioux. The nearest town was Gettysburg, nearly twenty-five miles away. It was a perfect set-up. There was a cafeteria, schoolrooms, an auditorium, and lots of deserted buildings. Crewmembers with family were allotted a trailer; singles had to share a trailer. There was a huge kitchen where a caterer served meals to the crew if they didn't want to cook themselves.

Our trailer was long, with two bedrooms and a small, plywood storage shed off the side. We gave the kids the inside rooms and Patrick and I made the shed our bedroom.

This was the first time I'd lived in such close quarters with the whole crew. Usually we stayed in a hotel on location. When we wanted privacy, we could go to our room and close the door. This was more like a Kennedy Compound.

Leo Guerrin, our director, was a strange man whom nobody liked very much. He always looked grubby and had a long ponytail full of huge knots and mats. I'd imagine throwing him into a hot, soapy tub and making him soak - after cutting off that matted ponytail. Scott Glen, Gary Busey, Keith Carradine, Robert Walker, Jr., Tina Raines, and Hillary Thompson were the actors in the film. Scott, Gary, and Keith later went on to successful careers. It was great fun knowing them early on.

Dan Haggerty was the animal trainer for the film. We loved being able to watch him and his assistant at work. This was a great beginning for Dan, too. He later went on to become Grizzly Adams.

Every evening we all gathered in the gymnasium, sitting on mattresses spread on the floor while we watched the dailies. Everyone seemed to be smoking pot and the room filled with smoke. It didn't bother me, but it annoyed me that people kept offering it to me. They wanted me to smoke just because they were smoking. When I turned the stuff down I was belittled. I wasn't a prude; I just didn't want to use drugs. Strangely it was a good experience in many ways. I talked to my girls about smoking pot. I explained what it was and asked them to notice how it changed the personalities of the adults who smoked it. I didn't want the kids to be afraid of what was going on. I think that the fact that they were around it gave them an awareness of what drugs were like. It squelched their curiosity so when they grew up, they never had a drug problem, for which I'm grateful.

Pat was the gaffer on the film, but one day he was given a small role in the film. He liked the idea of sitting in the back of this old antique car acting the part of a hillbilly, which was a natural for him. After he had done the scene a couple of times, they still had to do it over and over. He became bored and fidgety. He was ready to go back to gaffing where he could relax. He did look very good up on the screen, though.

We were going to be on location for a long time so I enrolled the girls in school. Tanya and Xochi were in grammar school and went to the Native American school that was nearby. The teacher was great and they made friends easily. It was different for Laurie and Denise who had a long drive to the nearest high school in Eagle Butte. The school was dirty, dusty, and unattractive, but there was no other choice. Unfortunately, the Native American kids were mean to them, maybe because they were outsiders. The other kids considered them hippies, which they were, compared to the folks who lived in South Dakota at that time.

Although I didn't understand it, South Dakotans were prejudiced against the Native Americans. They looked down on them and considered them lazy and good for nothing. Maybe they resented them because they got government money. Anyway, by the time our girls arrived, the Native American children who had been on the receiving end of this prejudice seemed willing to pass the treatment onto strangers. It surprised me. One day Laurie came home and told me someone had hit her. I was furious and took the girls right out of school. No way was I going to say they needed to learn to defend themselves. From then on they studied at home.

The grammar school teacher was a very special person and I loved talking with him. He explained how it wasn't only the white man who took advantage of the Native Americans, but often more powerful Indians who were greedy and did not look out for their brothers, but mistreated them.

I had the great privilege of spending time with Henry Crow Dog, the Spiritual Leader of the Sioux who lived on the Rosebud Reservation. He had been hired as a technical advisor and lived in our compound. Henry was disappointed because he was seldom called on for advice. The crew considered him more of a good luck totem.

We became great friends. He would ride with me when I went shopping and I listened intently to his soft voice as he shared his wisdom with me. He told me how music is like a spider's web, drawing us into it with its mood. He also told me how the druggies tried to pull things over on him and the other Elders, trying to procure drugs from the Native Americans who could use them legally for religious ceremonies. The druggies were sure the Indians were so naive they wouldn't figure out why they wanted to buy the drugs. Wrong.

Henry explained that in his religion each person had to purify his mind and body before he ever smoked or ate a mushroom. They did this by spending time in the sweat lodge. This way when they received a vision, it was clear - not confused and distorted, as were most of the drug-induced hallucinations the unprepared non-Indians experienced.

One evening a Black Panther Native American arrived. His name was Lloyd. He was an angry young man. I believe he was killed during some of the violence that followed same years later. When I met him, Lloyd already had many scars. He proudly showed me the scar on his hand where his thumb had almost been severed.

One afternoon when I was relaxing in the tub, Henry and Lloyd came over for a visit. They asked for a drink and as I wasn't ready to get out of the tub. I told the kids to give them a couple of glasses and a bottle of whatever they wanted. Big mistake on my part. They drank until they were drunk. When Henry left, he fell down the stairs and hurt himself slightly. Lloyd, on the other hand, roamed around the compound all night knocking on our door yelling, "Someone is after me." Finally we yelled back, "Who?" Lloyd replied, "Indians!" We sleepily growled, "Well, you're an Indian. You can deal with them better than we can." We rolled over and went back to sleep. The next day Henry's wife came to get him and took him home. Lloyd left, too. Sadly, we never saw Henry again.

Even though I didn't work on the film, I felt like I was part of the crew. The actors became friends with the kids, even the dogs made friends. Keith Carradine had a big, yellow lab named Sun. He stayed with us when Keith was working. Gary Busey and his wife, Judy, had their baby Jake with them. Laurie became best friends with them and the friendship remains to this day. Early in the mornings, I'd look out the window and see Scott Glen and Robert Walker, Jr., making strange movements while slowly moving about. I'd never seen Tai Chi before.

On weekends we all got together at Bob's Bait Shop, across the river from the reservation. We enjoyed great steaks and generous drinks. It was the only restaurant close by and we were fortunate the food was good.

Xochi made friends with a little Indian girl in her class and she invited her to spend a weekend with us. While I was waiting in the car to pick them up at the bus stop, I saw little boys poking a puppy with sticks. It made me sick, but I didn't know what to do. I was in a different culture and didn't know if I had the right to tell others what to do. I would stop them now, but that day I was afraid to and so I didn't. I still feel bad when I think of it.

Next I took Xochi and her friend to the girl's house. I thought I'd be polite and go in and meet her mother instead of waiting in the car. The house was an awful mess and as I walked in the woman tried to straighten things up, pushing stuff under the bed and rushing about. Uncomfortable, I said I'd wait in the car. Twice that day I'd blundered, not knowing how to act. It was strange, what was proper for me wasn't at all comfortable for others here in Indian Country.

Xochi and her friend did have fun together at our place. And through her friend we discovered two darling dogs, my favorite kind - fluffy, stocky, medium - sized, and oh so cute. They were named for alcohol, Booze and 3.2 (alcohol rating). I was told they were destined to be someone's dinner. Later that winter I bought them and we took them back home with us.

As usual, our trailer became the center for everyone to gather. Even the dogs all came in, walked down the hall, took a drink from the toilet, and trudged back out, leaving muddy foot prints behind, The dirt in South Dakota was a terrible kind of dirt or mud they called gumbo. It stuck to the dogs' feet and was tracked everywhere. Once Pat asked why our trailer was always so dirty when everyone else's was so neat and clean. I explained how "his" friends and their animals preferred to spend their time at our place, drink our water and our booze, and leave their own places clean. I'm not sure he got it.

Because we had the kids, I cooked every day. Leo, the director, was prone to come by and lift the lids of the pots on the stove and inhale the aromas. I liked that about him. What I didn't like were the mats still growing out of the end of his repulsive ponytail.

One day the weather changed drastically. The wind blew so hard I swear I could have flown if I made myself wings from the sheets. A few days later it snowed and everything froze, even the water in our trailer. We had to use the plumbing in the main buildings. Shooting became a problem as well. The landscape was not supposed to be covered with snow so we had to return to Los Angeles to finish the film.

This presented a problem for us. We had driven to location in the van and now Pat had to get to Los Angeles immediately. The rest of the crew was flying so they had no problem. We packed up and put Denise on a plane for Pittsburgh. We made a bed in the back of the van for the kids and the four dogs, and took off that night. It was so cold driving that we all cuddled up to the dogs giving new meaning to Three Dog Night - they were great heaters.

As we drove down the highway, we had to watch for the herds of deer and elk that slowly gravitated across the landscape. The herds were hungry because the snow had covered their food. I realized that many of them would die due to lack of food and began to understand that hunting actually helped by thinning the herds.

It took us a couple of days to get to L.A. I wasn't looking forward to returning. We spent the night in Las Vegas and took off early. As we approached Los Angeles, we saw the brown smog bank appear. We stopped at a store and bought a bottle of strawberry wine to ease the pain of having to return to what I now thought of as Smogville. We drank the wine and sang our way into town.

Actually, it was fun to see my mom and sisters and Patrick enjoyed seeing his friends. I worked for a few days on the film now that it was being shot at Fox Studios. They hadn't had a hairstylist on location.

One afternoon Keith's dog, Sun, disappeared and for some reason and the guard at the gate called me. I told Keith, but he was doing a scene and couldn't leave. Sun was such a wonderful dog and I didn't want anything to happen to him so when Keith asked me if I would take his car and look for him, I agreed. Luckily I spotted Sun fairly soon. He came right over and got in after I opened the door and called his name.

One night Clark Paylow, our unit manager, had us to dinner. As we were eating, I heard a little sound. I went to the back door to check it out and there was Daffy, my pregnant little cock-a-poo, whimpering. She had given birth and she was carrying one in her mouth. I found another pup on the lawn and another in the gutter. Now we had eight dogs.

Film over, we hugged and kissed all our relatives and friends, packed up the van, and headed home again. Two adults, three kids, and eight dogs. The trip was fun until we hit Durham, North Carolina. We had planned on visiting some of Pat's old school friends from Beckley. As we pulled up to our motel, the engine belched out some strange noises and blew up. What timing. At least we had friends to visit. We left the animals at his friend's home, except for Daffy who cried so much when we tried to leave her that we had to sneak her and her puppies in and out of the motel in a cardboard box. It took us five days to get a new engine in the van then we left for the farm in time to be home for Christmas.

Chapter 30
BACK TO HOLLYWOOD
1971-72

Coming back to Happy Hills Farm was in a way, a let down. Yet a part of me was happy to be home. Pat's mom and dad joined us for Christmas. For our first Christmas here we had tried to find our Christmas tree in the woods, but finally had to wire three scrawny ones together to get a tree that looked okay. This year we bought one. It was a great relief to be able to afford to buy presents for the kids.

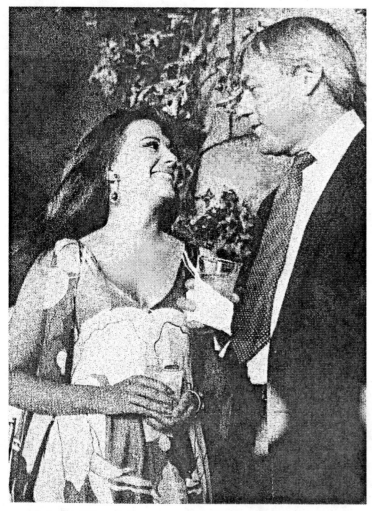

Natalie Wood, happy with Richard Gregson

Yet it seemed, almost immediately, we were out of money again. We'd paid off all our old bills and already new ones were coming due. After Christmas, Pat got a call to go to Los Angeles to work on *The Harrod Experiment*, a very sexually advanced film for the times. He decided to go, but had to borrow money from a friend to buy his ticket. We had never been so broke in our whole life.

I was in tears when we parted. I had no idea when Pat would be able to return. I was on the farm all by myself; my dream of a life together had disintegrated. I wondered how I was going to cope, but actually I did pretty well. Our sow had piglets and I built a pen for her and the piglets, cussing my inability to use a hammer and nails all the while.

Each week Pat called to tell me he had deposited $50 in our account for groceries and such. I went shopping each week after the call and for entertainment that winter the kids and I baked lots of cookies.

Two boys arrived from South Dakota to stay with us for a while. They were a real help with Pat gone, but eventually they tired of the life on the farm and left for home. One day before they left, the exhaust fell off the van while we were driving down the road. Gary, one of the boys, said, "Just get it fixed." I burst into tears. "I have no money to get it fixed."

To make matters worse, Pat's film kept getting postponed and I became more and more lonely. It was ironic in a way. For the first time in my life I had let myself become dependent on someone and when he left I became a total wimp. I was surprised at myself.

Pat returned a couple of months later, at which point we had a long talk. We had to admit there was no future for us on the farm. We simply couldn't bring in the money we needed to pay our bills along with Pat's child support without working on films. It meant we would either be separated or constantly on the road.

As luck would have it, an opportunity came to work on a picture for the Evangelist Billy Graham's Film Company. It was called *A Time to Run*. Once again, we found someone to live at the farm. We left all our dogs behind except Timber, our German Shepherd/Collie, and Michelle, a piglet whose name was derived from the script we had received for the film. Michelle was to be a joke gift for a couple Pat had met and become friends with on his last sojourn in California. He knew they would be happy with her at first, before they realized how large she would grow. Their son was going to love her; his mom was going to get a real, big surprise.

Off we went, once again in our Happy Hills van. It was quite a trip with the piglet. She followed Timber everywhere. She even used a litter box when she had to go to the bathroom. I was worried about getting her over the California state line, but Michelle was perfect. We covered her head and tail and she slept through the whole procedure. She looked just like a little black and white dog sleeping among the children in the van.

After we arrived, we moved back to Lennox where Pat's friend, Terry, had an apartment for rent next door to the chicken coop where we had lived before. We took it. The girls made the garage into a bunkroom for themselves.

I was very tired and weary and disappointed that my dream had failed. But I was ready to get our finances in order and knew the only way we could do it was for me to get back into the film business.

While I'd been living the life of a farmer, Natalie Wood had married Richard Gregson and given birth to her first daughter, Natasha. She hadn't done any films. In fact, the next time I worked with her, she was divorced from Richard and remarried to Robert Wagner.

We reported to Billy Graham's Studio, World Wide Pictures in Burbank. It was quite a place. There was even a chapel for prayers before production in the morning. I was the film's hairstylist, but I wasn't needed every day because, in those days, men didn't use hairstylists so I only worked when the women did. The makeup man was Charlie Blackman.

A Time to Run was a simple film and even though I was rather tired at times, it felt oh-so-nice to be working again. The tiredness got to me. I didn't know what was the matter with me, but I was beginning to sense something was wrong.

We went to Santa Barbara on location and stayed at a lovely hotel on the ocean. On the weekend the girls came up with Terry's wife bringing Michelle, the piglet, with them. Michelle was a real hit with everyone. She roamed the beach, whereas the dogs had to be on a leash, and horses were banned. She rode the waves and got sunburned. One evening while I was walking her, a woman came up to me and asked, "What kind is that? How large will she get?" It never entered my mind that she didn't know Michelle was a pig until I saw her shocked face when I answered, "About 700 pounds." Then I realized she thought Michelle was a dog. Everyone on the beach had fun with Michelle and wanted her to return the next weekend, but by that time we were through with the location and on our way home.

We filmed a huge love-in on top of a hill. Hundreds of young people came dressed in hippie attire. Our kids were there, too, and Michelle was in heaven being petted by hundreds of people. Eventually we had to give Michelle to Frank Raymond, a camera assistant who had become a friend. He took her to Yosemite where he had a place for her to live. She grew bigger and bigger and was very content there.

When the picture finished, I decided to do something about my weight and energy, so I went to Dr. Harper, a weight loss doctor. He gave me shots made from the urine of pregnant women and put me on a 500 calories a day diet. I'm sure that on such few calories I would have lost the weight without the urine shots.

Pat got a call to go to Dallas, Texas to do one of the first all Black films, *A Book of Numbers*, directed by Raymond St. Jacques. We were off again and Dallas was great, but so very hot. We moved into condos and rented some furniture. The nicest thing was our friends; Matt and Barbara Leonetti and their children lived there, along with Warren and Sally Bateman and their kids, and Frank Keever, the grip, and his family, too. We had our own little community.

The kids were happy, Pat was happy, and I was trying to cope with my diet. I got shots from a nearby doctor, but I just didn't feel right. I couldn't remember anything; I was listless, and even jealous, which I'd never been before. Something was terribly wrong. I was relieved I hadn't been asked to work. I don't think I would have been capable.

On our way back home to Los Angeles we stopped for the night at a crewmember's lake cabin. Pat and I slept in the van and I ended up with at least three hundred mosquito bites from my knees down. I was in misery. We stopped at Carlsbad Caverns and I walked through the caverns barefoot. The cold ground felt so good on the bitten soles of my feet.

Upon my return home, I went straight to Dr. Harper. Lo and behold, in my absence he had discovered the cause of my problem. I had hypoglycemia - low blood sugar. I was so relieved. I wasn't crazy. Nobody had ever told me about hypoglycemia, but the test I was given proved it was causing my problems. The discovery changed my life. Even before this latest episode, during much of my life, my energy level had been low. I had often wondered if I was always going to feel so dragged out during my whole life, but I coped by just pushing myself. When I complained to my doctors they just said, "You're too fat," and gave me more diet pills. (This was when they prescribed Speed to lose weight.) Now that I knew what was wrong, I began to study nutrition, take vitamins, and eat small meals more frequently. I realized that while sweets made me feel better for a while, they were the worst things I could eat. At last, my body responded to the proper nourishment and I began to heal. I also learned that stress contributed to hypoglycemia and I certainly had been under enough stress while living on the farm.

That September we went to Tucson where Pat worked on *The Soul of Nigger Charlie*. I was still not working, but I enjoyed our stay at the Tucson House. The kids attended school there and I found a doctor who advised me to take vitamin E to raise my blood pressure. I was still healing. We spent Thanksgiving in Tucson.

When we returned to Los Angeles, we moved out of Lennox to a much nicer place called Saugus. It was right next door to our friends, Warren and Sally. It was a tiny, funky house that shook when the train went by. It was far better than our Lennox apartment and much safer, too. We named it Tortilla Flats. The kids enjoyed sleeping in the house once again and we didn't have to lock the gate every time we entered the yard.

That December Bill Fraker, the cameraman, offered Pat the opportunity to work on a film called *Day of the Dolphin* being filmed in Miami and the Bahamas. The hitch was that no families could go because there were so few accommodations. I told Pat to take it, but he didn't want to be away the five months it would take to do the film. Finally the production company realized it was too much to ask the crew to be separated from their families for such a long time. The decision was made to allow families. Immediately Pat said, "Yes."

Chapter 31

DAY OF THE DOLPHIN

We knew *Day of the Dolphin* would be a very special experience. It starred George C. Scott, his wife Trish Vandeveer and was directed by Mike Nichols. The location of the main set was paradise - Abaco Island, in the Bahamas.

Our first location was Miami. We stayed at the Coconut Grove Hotel, where the girls quickly learned to use room service and impressed the waiters with their orders for delicacies like chocolate mousse.

Our lives were extremely different now. Last year we had been as broke as could be, on the farm in Appalachia, the poorest region of our country. This Christmas, we were in Miami, staying at the newly-built coconut Grove Hotel, going out to Joe's Stone Crab for dinner. I loved watching the rich people in the restaurants. They drove up in their fancy cars, dressed to kill, jewels adorning their wrinkled necks. Living that sort of life would never even occur to my friends back in Amigo, West Virginia.

One morning in Miami, the casting woman asked if I'd attend a casting call for extras. She was short of people. I didn't want to be an extra, but she was my friend, so I went. I was chosen and I had to laugh at myself. We shot at the Miami Woman's Club - a very exclusive place. The day of shooting, I found myself lunching with many wealthy women. When the conversation turned to me, I shared the story of our adventures on the farm. I told them about our pig and surprisingly the old ladies began to share stories of their earlier lives, growing up on farms. They really enjoyed my story. Perhaps I was the snooty one.

New Year's Day was stifling, hot and humid. I felt strange walking the streets wearing shorts. I longed for snow. The day after that, we took off for Abaco and the sight of the turquoise water beneath us, took my breath away.

Abaco was an out island and the airport was tiny. We checked through the small immigration office and were quickly off to our destination: Treasure Key Hotel. The complex included a large hotel, condos, and lots of amenities. The air was warm, the foliage lush, but not as tropical as I had imagined. It was truly paradise - our own little Lost Horizon.

We checked into the hotel and were shown to a small condo on the beach side of the hotel. It was perfect. The girls could walk to the beach and we were close to the hotel, the market, and our friends. Part of Pat's crew stayed in Marsh Harbor, a town on the other end of the island closer to the set, about thirty miles from Treasure Key. They had rented houses by mail before we arrived there.

We stayed in the beach condo for a week, and then were notified that we had to move to another condo near the golf course. At first I was disappointed because it seemed so far from the center of things. It was actually better and we ended up with our own little community out there, nearer the English school where the girls were enrolled. This condo was perfect, much larger, with two bedrooms, one for us and one for the girls.

Abaco was a very special island. There was no crime at all. We left money on our dresser and the maids would never touch it. Our kids could hitch a ride and not worry about any harm coming to them.

Pat was having a super time. He loved working with the dolphins. In contrast, I was lonesome and getting depressed. I was used to working, but here the maids cleaned my room, the kids were in school, and I had nothing to do. I couldn't even go to the set because no visitors were allowed. I didn't know what to do with myself.

Fortunately, I met a woman named Linda who owned a little beauty shop at the hotel. Although she owned the place, she needed someone to run it. She wasn't a hairdresser. When she found out who I was, she asked me if I'd be interested. Interested! I was overjoyed to be part of something, I said, "Yes." She showed me the shop, and it was nice and compact, next to the production office. I was able to be close to the crew, but also on my own. I could work while the girls were in school.

I opened for business and Linda became my shampoo girl. It was amusing having the owner work for me. Thanks to the beauty shop, I became part of the local winter community, meeting the wealthy women who lived in Connecticut in spring and fall, Bar Harbor in the summer, and in the Bahamas in the winter. Quite a lifestyle!

Many of the people who came to my shop were from the States. They were thrilled that someone with my experience was available to do their hair. Most of the time they just wanted something simple. It was more difficult to please the local ladies who wanted their hair backcombed and sprayed so it would last them a week or more. This was hard because my training was to keep hair on the natural side.

The wives of the crew would come to have their hair done, too. They were often in such a hurry, I'd remind them to relax and be on "island time". I also invited the Black folks who wanted their hair done to come in. I knew I had a lot to learn about doing Black hair and I figured this was the time to do it, but I also wanted them to feel welcome. Unfortunately, Linda didn't agree and because she was very prejudiced, she made them feel uncomfortable. Her attitude was embarrassing. Hardly any of the natives wanted to face her.

My friend Dorothy White, now Byrne, was working on the film. She reminded me how to give good perms, as they had been her specialty before she started working on films. I became an expert at perms and people from miles around came especially for them.

I never knew how my day would go at the shop. There were a few appointments, but mostly people just dropped in. It all depended on the weather. If the seas were rough, appointments were canceled, but on nice days I was bombarded. It was great though. I earned fifty percent of the income plus tips. Linda hoarded her American money because she couldn't take much Bahamian money out of the country.

On Mondays, my shop was closed. I'd do the weeks shopping at the market in Marsh Harbor, about thirty miles away. Prices were high on the island, but the hotel groceries were outrageous. We had purchased a group car, an orange and black heap. Eddie Butterworth, Natalie's makeup man, lived out there, near us with his new wife, Ginny. She and I would do the grocery shopping for all the others who were working. We had a ritual. Upon our arrival in Marsh Harbor we stopped at the Conch Inn for lunch. First we'd order a Goombay Smash, the best drink I've ever had, made of pineapple juice, coconut rum, orange Curacao, white rum, and a raw egg. We had to have at least a couple of them, then, after we were pleasantly "smashed" we'd wander over to the grocery store and do our shopping in a haze. We'd drive home, sobered by then, and we would wait for our husbands to come home. Ginny taught me how to be a location housewife.

There were lots of parties and because the men worked short hours, we often went out dancing and drinking in the evenings. The local men loved to dance, too. They'd arrive dressed to impress in their polyester suits and colorful crocheted hats. Those suits looked as if they were so hot. The men asked us to dance and we accepted, but only the fast dances. We saved the slow dances for our husbands. It was too hot and sticky to dance close to someone we didn't know. Our favorite song was "I Can See Clearly Now" done Bahamian style.

Near the hotel was a delightful little snack bar called This Must Be the Place. We sat there in the evenings and watched the boats come in and tie up for the night, while sipping a few Smashes. The kids played outside. George C. Scott, the star of the show, brought his two German Shepherds with him. They were wild. They appeared to like people, but chased and attacked anything else. One evening George's driver came to our house for dinner along with the dogs. They were just fine and friendly. Yet the next Sunday, when I visited the empty set, they were driven crazy by the dolphin teasing them. That dolphin seemed to know how to get their goat. It swam back and forth in its tank confusing the dogs no end. One day the dogs ate the upholstery and steering wheel of George's limo.

George was having a hard time during the filming. To put it politely, he was difficult. He often drank a fifth of vodka in the morning and would simply lose it. Sometimes he disappeared for hours. Sometimes the crew was glad he did. He was very successful and at that time I couldn't understand why he needed to do that.

Mike Nichols was very considerate. He brought his own gourmet chef to location to cook for the crew. They didn't appreciate it; they just wanted meat and potatoes kind of food. Eventually there were two lines for lunch, one gourmet, and one plain. Patrick loved the gourmet food; his crew thought he was crazy.

Because we were on an island, almost everything had to be imported making it expensive to live there. One evening a crewmember, who was quite short, had too much to drink and decided to cut the legs of the furniture in his condo to fit his size. Big mistake! The hotel manager was ready to kick him out. Even though he offered to pay for the furniture, it took weeks to replace the furniture and he had to pay dearly.

Pat bought me a Honda motorcycle for transportation back and forth from work. Each morning I'd fill my basket with my lunch and putt off to work. It was very convenient. The only problem was the midges that would bite me even when I was moving. I hated them.

One Sunday we took off for Green Turtle Cay, a nearby island. We got off the boat and began walking around the island looking for drinks for the guys, but nothing was open. We stumbled upon a small inn, way off the beaten path. We walked in through the door and Pat met a man to whom he took an instant liking. In the course of their conversation the fellow indicated he wanted to sell his inn. Pat thought it would be great fun to run a small hotel on the island. The only problem was that the ex-wife still owned half of the inn, whereupon Pat decided he'd leave me and marry the ex-wife, put the inn in his name, divorce her, and run the hotel with me. Needless to say, I didn't think much of that idea.

The innkeeper was generous and filled Pepsi cans with scotch for the guys and we went on our way. While winding our way toward town, we walked through a backyard where someone was giving a haircut and not doing a very good job of it. I walked up and asked if I could help. The woman, getting the cut, recognized me and said, "She runs the beauty shop. Let her do it." I finished the cut and she looked good. By the time we reached the center of town the New Plymouth Inn was open for lunch and we sat there enjoying the breeze and the conch salads. I wouldn't have minded running a hotel on that island.

On another nearby island, Man of War Cay, they made canvas bags, jackets, and other items of canvas. The folks who lived on Man of War Cay were a bit different. Many had more than five toes on each foot. Apparently there had only been five white families living there so inbreeding was common. One day a man from that island came into my shop wearing thongs. I was sure he wanted everyone to know he had five toes, not six.

One morning Dorothy, the hairstylist, was sick. Del Acevedo, George's makeup man, called and asked me to come to the set for the day. There was nobody else that could replace Dorothy. She was the only hairstylist. I panicked because I had appointments that day and I began to wonder who I should serve. My film training kicked in and I canceled all my appointments. When I got to the set, I was told I wasn't needed after all. I was furious with Del. His only remark was, "Well, you didn't have to come."

One Sunday the girls and I went to visit the set, meet the dolphins, and see the house that had been built there. I lay in the hammock on the porch and began to feel that I might be able to live that sort of life. I didn't know if I'd get island fever, but I was willing to take the chance.

After three months our stay on Abaco came to an end and we moved to Nassau for more shooting. I was sad and so were the kids. Our time on Abaco had been idyllic. I had considered remaining in Abaco and continue to run the shop, but finally decided against it.

What a difference! Nassau was tourist town. We flew on the Flamingo Special and in the beginning, stayed at the Sonesta Hotel. It was pretty and full of wonderful things for the kids to enjoy. It was also very expensive. Nassau was a big city and people's attitudes were very different from Abaco. The local's anger and frustration with the tourists was palpable.

Laurie, who had opted to stay in Los Angeles, finally decided to join us and we were expecting her when she called, stranded in the Miami airport. The travel agent hadn't bought her a round trip ticket and she needed one to get into the Bahamas. She was seventeen and very capable, but still I worried. In the end, my sister went to the airport at four thirty in the morning to settle things and Laurie finally arrived after spending the night alone in the airport.

A few days later we moved to an apartment at Delaport Point. Now I could cook our meals, which pleased me. Pat traded our motorcycle for a larger, more powerful one and we liked that better, too. That was until one day when Pat came home early because the sea was too rough for shooting and we decided to take a tour of the island on the motorcycle. A tour meant stopping at lots of bars for lots of drinks. I loved riding behind Pat on the bike because I could feel the changes of temperature as we drove along and smell things I never noticed in a car. We stopped and explored an old deserted, unfinished hotel.

We ended up at the Barefoot Bar in downtown Nassau where we mingled and had more drinks, while we talked about the problems between the Bahamians and the English. (The Bahamas would get their independence next year.) For some odd reason, I surmised that Patrick had too much to drink. Of course, "I hadn't," so I decided I'd drive home. It was a little iffy driving on the opposite side of the street, but all was fine until we got right to our driveway. I downshifted and all of a sudden the bike quit, throwing me forward and my eye hit the handle bar. Pat fell on top of me and barely got a scratch, but I ached all over and got a real doozy of a shiner, all swollen in shades of purple and yellow.

Bill Fraker, the cameraman, invited us to dinner the next night. I was embarrassed about my eye. He calmed me at dinner saying, "Sugar, look around. All these women have fancy dresses, lots of expensive jewels, but nobody has such a colorful eye as you do." I was grateful for his kindness and relaxed and enjoyed the rest of the evening.

I was still embarrassed about my eye when I went to the market. I need not have been because after seeing my shiner, the women there remarked that I must have a great husband, he kept me in line. Oh well!

After that I had no desire to ride the motorcycle again. It was so much more powerful than our other one. It scared me. There was too much traffic on the road and we had to drive on the opposite side of the road like in England.

We were getting ready to return home and Pat wanted me to sell the bike. I had to go downtown to do it and I dreaded it. Pat wanted at least $400 for the bike, but I was such a wreck by the time I got to the shop, I would have happily taken fifty dollars for it. I got $375, which was fine, and took a taxi home.

Initially we had planned to return to West Virginia at the end of the film, but our plans had changed because there was a job possibility so we headed back to California. We all wanted to return to those fantastic islands as soon as possible.

Chapter 32

THE AFFAIR AND MRS. SUNDANCE

After months on our lush island paradise in the Bahamas, our dusty little Tortilla Flats shack in hot dry Saugus, California felt dry and barren. Our neighborhood boasted a few trees and some grass, but we longed for the lushness of the Bahamas. We felt flush with money left over from the location and our income tax return had been more than $5,000. The movie business was slow and seeing as we were in such good shape financially, we decided to enjoy our time off.

The girls returned to school and in many ways it was great being home. While we waited for the phone to ring offering us a new job, we continued to overindulge in the "good life". Each morning after the mail came we'd look for a new place to go for lunch with our next-door neighbors, Warren and Sally. Although I was having fun, all the drinks, wine, and rich food weren't helping my health.

Every doctor I met, as long as they were into a natural approach to preventive medicine, pointed out that I had to take responsibility for my own health. It was finally sinking in. When I ran the beauty parlor in Abaco I took lots of vitamins and noticed I had more energy. It was no longer such an ordeal for me to keep up with everyone else. My back had started to ache while I was in the islands so now I decided to find myself a chiropractor. Terry Hovey was my choice and what a find he was! He helped me make profound lifestyle changes. I found I was ignorant in so many ways. After I told him about all the great rum drinks I'd enjoyed over the past few months he said, "No wonder you're having problems. No more Goombay Smashes for you." He said "rum makes you dumb". Then he laughed and said, "You must eat fresh, healthy food, eat simply and take supplements". My education about food and nutrition had begun.

Ever curious, one afternoon, Pat, and I decided to go to a porno film. My first. I'd never seen one. We chose, *Deep Throat*. I was blown away! I never expected to see anything like that on the big screen. It was mind-boggling. After seeing that film I was ready to go to another. I wanted to see if they were all that amazing. Pat called me a pervert. We never went to another porno film.

In June, Bill Fraker called Patrick about doing a film that would be filmed in Madrid, starring Robert Ryan. We decided to take the whole family on this adventure. We moved out of Tortilla Flats, packed our van, and headed back east to West Virginia to visit Mammy and Pappy and to check up on our farm while we were there. We traveled across the northern route of the country. We drove through South Dakota and stopped at Bob's Bait Shop, where we'd had so many great steaks on *Grasslands/Hex*.

We drove to Detroit where Pat had work on a commercial. We stayed away from the city center, at a snooty motel in the wealthier part of town. Unfortunately, no animals were allowed in the motel so we sneaked our dogs in through the rear exit, and out again in the early morning. That was fine until one night the fire alarm went off suddenly. Gas was leaking from the radiators so the firemen rushed us out of our rooms. We panicked at first, but quickly regained our cool, quietly got the animals out, put them in the car, and came around to the front of the motel. Everyone was outside dressed in pajamas and bathrobes. It changed the atmosphere. All the snooty people who usually ignored us common folk were friendlier dressed in their nightwear. It didn't last long, though. After the scare was over they changed clothes and returned to their former, snooty selves. Maybe clothes do make the man.

Pat finished the commercial and we continued on to West Virginia, anxious to see the farm. What a mess it was! Disappointed, I spent lots of time cleaning it up, but it was fun for the kids to be there again. Pat was depressed about the place, it was costing us money and we were never there.

While waiting for Pat's tickets to Spain to arrive, disaster struck. Robert Ryan died. The project in Spain was canceled. What a blow. Luckily for Patrick, Bill Fraker had a commercial in Monte Carlo, so he flew off to Europe. The rest of us stayed in Beckley with plans to meet Pat in New Jersey where his brother, Mike, lived, before returning to Los Angeles.

Mammy and Pappy decided to come with the girls and me to New Jersey so they could be with their other son, Mike. I put a mattress on top of all the suitcases in the back of the van. This was where Mammy, the girls, and the dogs rode, proving, to my mind, how much Mammy loved her sons. (Mammy didn't like animals much, but she didn't complain). Pappy sat up front with me. We put the cat box under his seat and fortunately the cats had good aim when they used it. Pappy was so fastidious, but he didn't complain either. We did write some unusual Lysol room deodorant commercials during that trip.

We made it safely and there was Patrick, fresh as a daisy, bursting to tell us all about his wonderful adventures in Monte Carlo. He went on and on about the wonderful time, the great food he'd had completely forgetting that he'd left me to do all the work. I really didn't care. I was furious with him. He told us about the Hermitage Hotel where he stayed, about meeting the King of Monaco and Grace Kelly, the wonderful meals, gambling, and his trip to the Italian coast. Finally I had to laugh at myself. Normally I would have been happy for him he'd had such a good time and finally I realized that I felt left out and jealous.

In the meantime I got a call about a job with Natalie Wood. Natalie, now divorced from Richard Gregson, was back together with Robert Wagner who had been her first husband. I was so happy for her. I remembered her telling me one time that she didn't know how she could ever get along with any other man if she couldn't get along with R.J. as she called him. He was so very nice.

This was the first time Natalie had done a Movie of the Week. This film was called *Love Song*, later renamed *The Affair*. Natalie played a crippled girl, opposite Robert Wagner. She brought her baby daughter, Natasha, with her to the studio. Natasha was a wonderful baby. She and I played for hours in the dressing room.

We moved back in with my mother while Pat, the girls, and I searched for a place to live. We quickly found a little house way up on Sierra Highway in Newhall. It was on thirty acres and reminded me of our farm, without trees. I was so happy to have a home again. I knew by now it wasn't my style to be a gypsy. Traveling while I was working was fine, but I wanted a home for my kids and a place to put down roots when I wasn't roaming the world.

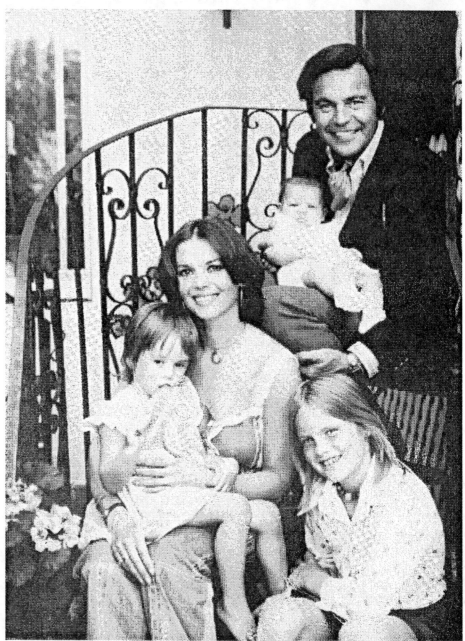

Natalie Wood, Robert Wagner and their family

Once we settled into our house, I relaxed. Natalie had such a great haircut that my job was easy. She was often nervous during the filming. Her dad was ill and she was worried. She'd always been closer to him than to her mother.

I was feeling good. It was nice to get back to work. My absence had been too long. I was now making seventy dollars per day, very good money at the time. Natalie played a rich woman and they filmed in beautiful surroundings. We worked in classy locations, no back alleys on this one. Eventually we worked at the Hope Ranch in Santa Barbara, a choice location. I got to know Robert Wagner; it was the first time I'd worked with both he and Natalie together. At the time, the movie business was so busy that they were using permits (non-union) people. Pat's brother, Mike, had been trying to support his family working at a lumberyard in New Jersey. It was a struggle. While we'd been in New Jersey, Pat had felt generous and wanted to buy Mike a motorcycle as a gift. I had suggested that he save the money for something that would be more important to Mike. Little did I realize how soon that would come up. Pat needed help at work and they were using permits. He sent Mike a plane ticket so he could come out and help on commercials. Mike began making a hundred dollars a day. He was hooked. He went home, packed up his family, and moved to California.

My career began looking up again when Rolf Miller called me to work on a Movie of the Week, called *Mrs. Sundance* starring Elizabeth Montgomery and a young fellow, Robert Foxworth. Lizzie was a terrific person who had been born on the same date as my dad. Just like Daddy, she loved the races and always had her own driver, Joe, who drove her in the Bluebird - a long, blue limo. Her agent, Miltie, took care of her business affairs. Rolf, her daughter, and I had all been born on June 17. What a coincidence.

We worked together and we got to know each other and became close friends. Lizzie had an ex-husband who was much older and no fun at all. He had produced *Bewitched* so they still had business between them and whenever she had to have anything to do with him she became so stressed. It seemed strange to me that this beautiful, successful woman wasn't really enjoying her life. There was much loneliness there. She began to have fun with her co-star, Bob Foxworth. It wasn't romantic, at first, but there was lots of laughter and an attraction seemed inevitable. I told her about my romance with Patrick and how I hadn't realized how perfect it was to have a friend for a mate until it happened. Perhaps she was already falling in love with Foxy, as we called him.

Before I ever worked with Lizzie, I always noticed how terrible her hair looked on *Bewitched*. After I started working with her, I understood why. She wasn't vain at all and just didn't want to spend much time getting ready for shooting. I had to do her hair quickly before she got bored and decided to do something else. It was always a challenge to keep her hair looking good; it was so fine and took lots of upkeep.

We worked at Twentieth Century Ranch in Bronson Canyon where I'd worked on *Blue*. The cave we had used as a set on *Blue* was all boarded up. We flew to Lone Pine, shot, and flew back the same day. Lizzie liked her film family and we all grew close.

Lizzie was competitive and intelligent. She loved games, especially the quiz show, *Password,* which she played often. Each time we went with her we earned two hundred dollars for the afternoon's work. Not bad for 1973.

After finishing *Mrs. Sundance* we immediately began another film at Universal, called *A Case of Rape*. It wasn't the same without Foxy and Lizzie was displeased with her co-star. We all missed Foxy, although he did visit. We wanted it to end quickly.

I reported to Lizzie's brown-shingled house at 6:00 a.m. It was a beautiful home and cozy as could be, I could have moved right in. Her bedroom was fanciful, full of flowers and at least a hundred little pillows on her bed. I was absolutely charmed by her taste. We'd have breakfast together and after I got her ready for work, we hopped in the Bluebird and off we went to where we were filming for the day. I enjoyed those times together. I felt sorry for her, too. Sometimes she'd come home from work at night and there would be no dinner even though her grocery bills at Jurgensons were sky high. Her help appeared to be enjoying themselves, eating high off the hog, most likely ransacking the cupboards for food to take home. I wanted to call them on it, but it wasn't my place. I felt terrible. Lizzie was so generous and they were taking such undue advantage of her.

Lizzie loved to serve caviar and sour cream to her guests at work. She always had the best and most expensive caviar one could buy, at least $75 an ounce. I tasted it once, but didn't feel it was worth the money. She loved playing backgammon and burned the wonderful smelling Rigaud candles in her trailer.

The movie was difficult, especially when it came to the rape scene and the examinations afterward. Lizzie was very sad and had a difficult time. I could sense how humiliating it must be for women who actually had been raped. We finally came to the courtroom scenes, which were boring as those scenes can be. The close-ups in each scene just dragged on and on. We finished filming just before Thanksgiving.

After the Thanksgiving holidays, I got a call to work on *Day of the Locust* from Lyndel Kail. It was a dreary movie about Hollywood, the sets were huge, but dimly lit, and it was depressing to spend all day working in the gloom.

Jerry Lewis commercials kept me going until Christmas. I liked Jerry most of the time, but that weekend before Christmas he showed up very late for work. This was so thoughtless and we were unable to do our last minute Christmas shopping even though we'd been promised we'd be out early. Jerry wasn't my favorite person that day.

On Christmas Eve we went to see *Day of the Dolphin*. I was in tears. I always cried during animal films, but I wasn't crying about the animals. I was remembering and wishing life could be like it had been while we'd lived in the Bahamas. It was so idyllic.

That same day I dropped off a present for Lizzie at her house. My sister had made her a beautiful velvet patchwork pillow. What on earth did one buy for someone like Lizzie? Her home was so beautifully decorated for Christmas. Garlands were wound around the banister leading upstairs and every room was completely decorated. There was even a merry-go-round horse in the bar. Even though it was sunny California, it felt like Christmas in her house.

Chapter 33
THE DAY OF THE LOCUST

The year 1974 began quietly. I assumed that was how it was going to continue. I was fooled. We were spending more than $1,400 a month, keeping up the farm, child support, and our own living expenses. I'd made a resolution to lose weight; I figured a 70-pound loss would do it. I had become a mother figure and I was tired of it. I wanted to change.

I day-checked on a television series at Fox Studios called *Chopper I*, a story about helicopters, of course. At night I'd arrive home all dusty and dirty from all the dirt spewed up as the helicopters landed with all its brave cops. Pat was in Hawaii working on *Death Wish* with Charlie Bronson, doing retakes and having a fabulous time. He seemed to be getting all the prime opportunities. Was I jealous? Perhaps.

In the middle of January I got a call from Tomorrow Entertainment about doing a Movie of the Week, a story starring Maureen Stapleton. She is a fantastic, beautiful person. It was a joy to work around her. She was so warm and humorous. We worked on Third Street, an older area of Los Angeles with charming neighborhoods. I loved the little houses, so many of them with Victorian touches. Between shots, I sat out on the curb and imagined what it would be like to live there. I'd think about how I'd fix up this house or that. Actually it wasn't what I'd call a safe neighborhood, but it did have lots of character.

I was now very interested in natural healing, and I was always offering advice about vitamins and herbs. I was Mother Earth, whether I wanted to be or not. One afternoon we were standing around on the set when Joe Odessa, the gaffer, began to tell us about his second wife who drank a lot. Even though he was a quite good drinker himself, he was having a dreadful time living with her. Maureen was sitting nearby listening to our conversation. I suggested to Joe that he give her some vitamin B complex and a few other things. He turned to me with the saddest look on his face and said, "Sugar, I don't want her to get better, I want her to die." My mouth dropped open. I was speechless. He explained, "My last wife cleaned me out when we divorced. No more divorces for me." He was adamant.

Maureen silently took it all in. Later, nearly in tears while convulsing with laughter, she described the situation in detail telling how I was trying to be so helpful and here was this man in so much pain. She had been amazed by his reaction yet she saw the humor in the whole play of things. It was typical of me. I always believed there was a better way out of any situation.

For weeks, I'd noticed signs around our neighborhood inviting us to a seminar about Transcendental Meditation. They said that meditation could relieve stress. I definitely needed that, so I signed up the whole family. At the seminar they gave us a demonstration about how it felt when stress was released. They told us it bubbled up and out of our bodies. When it did, it felt so good. The following weekend all five of us reported to an apartment in Friendly Valley for instruction, which we each took individually. We were given our mantras and told never to reveal it to anyone.

I began meditating immediately. It was wonderful. I'd meditate twenty minutes in the morning and twenty minutes at night. It made a real difference in my life and in my energy level. If I was really exhausted during a long day at work, I'd throw in an extra meditation and it revived me.

In February, I got a call from Harvey Laidman to work on a period television pilot called *Moose*. It was one of the first of the Sixties period shows. I had lots of haircuts to do because in the Sixties haircuts were short and worn full of grease. Lorimar Productions had such success with *The Waltons* that they decided to do more period shows.

How to make the extras' hair look greasy became a dilemma for me. Everyone had clean hair at that point, but in the Sixties guys seldom washed their hair making it easy to train in the ducktails and that type of style. The grease ensured the hair would stay in place. I had to retrain the extras' hair and it wasn't easy. I used the only thing I could think of, Vaseline. It worked, but took forever to wash out. The guys would go home and wash and wash their hair and still it would be greasy. They hated it and I couldn't blame them.

One morning an extra approached me shyly with a tube of something and asked me if I would try it on his hair instead of Vaseline. It was called Groom and Clean, a combination gel with something that gave the hair shine. What a blessing. It probably saved my life. The extras would have eventually strung me up if I hadn't found an alternative to Vaseline.

As we were shooting *Moose*, Lorimar was also shooting a series called *Apples Way*, a story about people who made an alternative lifestyle choice, like we had done when we moved to the farm. Only this story didn't ring true. I talked to Harvey and told him about our experiences on the farm. He said, "Why don't you write it into a script and bring it to me?"

As soon as I finished the pilot I began to write. I sat on my bed for four days, the typewriter on my lap and wrote about our adventures on the farm. When I finished, I took it to a script service where they typed it up, making corrections in spelling and punctuation before it was printed.

I was so excited and actually quite proud of myself. I called it *The Cardboard Boxes* because all the foster kids who had come to stay with us had all their stuff packed in boxes which they stored in the closet to re-pack when they went on to their next foster home. I thought it made a good dramatic point.

I gave Harvey a copy. I was so excited; I couldn't wait to hear his response. He did read it. Now that I look back, that was a real favor. It was really amateurish, but the information was all there. The sad thing was that they canceled *Apples Way* just about the time I finished my script.

I went back to helping out on *Day of the Locust* from time to time. Lyndel did something typical of her - she gave me the most difficult job, one she didn't want to do herself. Karen Black's hairstylist was leaving and Lyndel knew I could do Karen's hair and also get along with her. Karen was difficult and rather hard to please, but I liked her anyway. Her mother always set her off. She reacted just like a child when her mother came around. But she was fine with me if a bit hysterical at times.

A couple of days after I started doing Karen's hair, I reported to work one morning and the whole crew was in tears. Wolper, a movie company, had been doing a film in Bishop, way up north, in the mountains of California. On the way to location their plane had crashed, taking the lives of so many of our friends. Rolf Miller and his brother, Bill, were among them. I was devastated. I'd known Rolf since high school. We'd taken our kids to the same nursery school and he'd gotten me the job with Lizzie. I couldn't believe it. It couldn't be true. But it was. There were so many dead remembered that day. It felt right to be among my fellow workers who also felt the loss.

Driving home that night, I was actually headed in the direction of Bishop where the plane had crashed. Saugus was north of Los Angeles. As I drove closer to my home, I began to cry. I just couldn't get over my shock and sadness. That feeling came across me every night for a week. When I'd arrive home, my big dog Timber was so sweet that he'd see me crying and climb up and almost put his arms around me, trying to console me. I just couldn't seem to stop crying.

Rolf was buried at the same place where Marilyn Monroe was buried. Kenny Chase was so kind, saying, "Remember how we always felt when our children were babies. We'd never forget that time?" I nodded. "Now that our children are older, we can hardly imagine them as babies." I nodded again. "So perhaps in time our sorrow will lessen about the death of our friends."

Rolf's wife, Mary Anne, came up to me at the funeral and I was glad to be able to tell her about the last lunch I'd had with Rolf while working on Lizzie's film. It was when they had been separated. He told me then that he loved her very much. Looking back to that day, it was as if he wanted me to give her this message. She appreciated my story and I later sent her a book about reincarnation by Ruth Montgomery.

The next difficulty came the first day I had to work with Lizzie again. Rolf would never be there again. Eddie Butterworth was going to take his place. I was relieved that it was Eddie because I knew him so well and I was worried about how I was going to handle it. Fortunately for me I had an appointment with Terry, my chiropractor. I told him I was so sad and I just couldn't stop crying. He said, "Lie down and close your eyes." He gently took my head in his hands and softly said, "Go back to the incident, to the day you walked into work and heard the news about the plane crash. Make it as detailed as possible, feel all you can remember."

I lay there and my mind went back to that dreadful day, to the horror of what had happened, and relived it. All the time Dr. Hovey was holding my head in his hands. When I was finished, he held my head a little longer and then let go. I felt a little better and asked him what he'd done. He explained, "It's like there is a secretary who files our thoughts each time we have one. She takes each one as it comes in and files it in the appropriate place in our brain. But when we have a shock it's like she has a huge armful of tapes and she cannot hold them all. She drops some of them. Then each time she walks over the tapes, in this case thoughts, she trips on them." That is what caused me to cry. The process he had done was to have her pick up the tapes and put them in the proper place. From then on each time I thought of Rolf I was sad, but I didn't burst into tears.

Eddie and I met at Lizzie's the day after that. It was difficult, but we made it through. She was just as sad as we were, but she loved doing Password so her mind was occupied. We sipped a few glasses of wine and talked about Rolf knowing we would miss him for a long time.

It was a relief when we finished the *Day of the Locust*. I liked getting to know John Schlesinger, the director, who gave me a lovely little perfume bottle. Conrad Hall had been cameraman. He was "sort of" a relative of mine, having been married at one time to one of my cousins. He always seemed grumpy and I wondered if he ever had any fun. He must have at some point, because eventually he bought himself an island in Tahiti and loved being a hermit out there.

Chapter 34

PEEPER

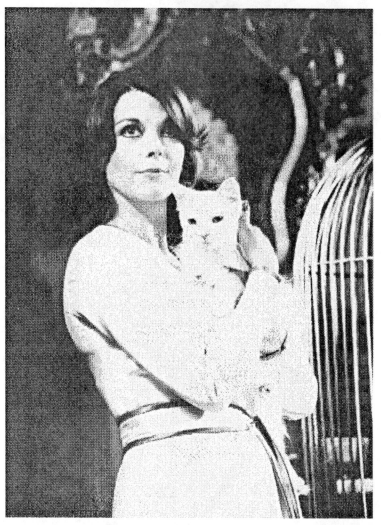

Natalie Wood in *Peeper*

My life changed in many ways during 1974. I learned to meditate and lost a great friend. It was spring and Pat was called to work on location in Livingston, Montana on *Rancho Deluxe*. It was a film about two cowboys who end up in prison thanks to their clever schemes. The film was directed by Frank Perry and starred Jeff Bridges, Sam Waterston, and Elizabeth Ashley. Bill Fraker was the cameraman.

As soon as we found out about the location the first thing we did was go out and buy a car we'd wanted, a Volkswagen Thing. It was supposed to be a copy of the German Jeep used during The Second World War. We thought it was just adorable. It was a cute orange car, orange with a black convertible top. It wasn't until after we bought it that

Ginger *Sugar* Blymyer

we realized it was extremely noisy. There was nothing insulating us from the engine noise.

We took off for Montana in tandem with Steve Wolper, a friend and camera assistant. Steve had his own car and offered to pull a trailer for us. Tanya and Xochi rode with him. We stopped for the night in Idaho and, after settling in, we decided to go to the movies. *The Sting* was playing, starring Robert Redford. I hadn't seen Redford in a film since I'd dyed his eyelashes at the Bel Air Hotel years before. At that time Pat had been so jealous I figured I'd just avoid the subject of Redford for my own peace of mind. But his jealousy had since disappeared so we went to the movie. It was a great film and I didn't say a word about Redford until we left the theater. Then I just had to. I turned to Pat and, in a very sweet voice, announced, "He's still cute." Ahh!

We drove onto Montana - a huge, spectacular state. Livingston is a small town nestled in among the mountains. It was a perfect location, especially for the crews as there were bars by the dozen, pleasing them no end. They were warned to be careful and stay out of the bars reserved for locals or they would most likely land in trouble.

Our home was the Del Mar Motel, on the edge of town, in rooms right next to Steve's. Though we had a refrigerator in our room we weren't allowed to cook in the rooms so I set up a camp stove on the table outside. Steve shared it with us. The girls loved being part of the crew again.

One weekend we went to a yard sale. As I was looking around, I discovered four stacks of a magazine called *Yankee*. Each stack was a complete year. I bought them all. Each issue was full of pictures of houses surrounded by lilacs, beautiful gardens of perennial flowers, and winding roads. I began to realize that I was homesick for New England even though I had only been to Boston once. Little did I know how the purchase of those magazines would change my life.

The kids and I loved visiting the set. It was really quite wild at times. My favorite scene was one where the guys took a big bull, known in the film as Baseheart of Bozeman, into a motel room. There stood the beautiful, prizewinning Charolais bull, so obedient, watching a western on television like he really understood what was going on. It was so funny I had to stifle my laughter while they were shooting. These bulls were so valuable that each one had his own trainer. The trainer said they would probably starve to death if left on their own in the fields, so spoiled and pampered were they.

Toward the beginning of May I got a call about a film Natalie was going to start in June. It was called *Fat Chance*, later renamed *Peeper*, to be directed by Peter Hyams. Michael Caine would star along with Natalie.

I had to leave early to get back to Los Angeles in time to start, so toward the end of May the kids and I packed up the Thing and took off for Los Angeles. This time I decided to take a route that went through Utah. I wanted to take a look at Sundance, the place Redford had made famous.

I giggled to myself on the way, wondering if I'd even tell Patrick about my side trip. He might still be jealous of Redford and not understand my curiosity. We headed toward Heber City, Utah and found the road to Sundance. It went up and up and was really beautiful. I remembered Redford telling us about a metal sculpture light fixture his friend had made for him. This friend had been quite a character. He had a hobby of stealing things out of museums and later replacing them. I got a kick out of his story and later bought a necklace the sculptor had made of horseshoe nails.

I never saw Redford's house on that trip, but I took the road to the top of the mountain and found beautiful golden aspens quaking and shimmering in the sunshine and light breeze. I never forgot the beauty of that place and fully understood why Redford had left Los Angeles with his family to live there.

Back in Los Angeles there was a production meeting on June 5 and I went in to meet everyone. I loved Michael Caine immediately. There's something about those men from the British Isles. I also met Peter Hyams, the director. He was very bright and quite a character. The first thing I noticed about him was his dark tan, and how he wore his hair carefully combed.

Fat Chance was a period film that took place in the late 1940s. Peter told me Michael's long, curly hair would have to be cut very short to fit the period. Michael was cooperative, but asked me to cut it only part way the first day so he could slowly get used to the new look. I obliged and eventually we got it short enough for it to look correct. We ordered a wig for Natalie to see how it would work, but it didn't suit her at all so we just ordered a small hairpiece that I added to her own hair.

The first night of shooting took place at the Million Dollar Building in downtown Los Angeles. What a way to begin a shoot, working all night long. The building was destined to be torn down so it was deserted, but still beautiful and suited the Forties period exactly. Michael Caine played a private eye looking for a man's lost daughter. His office was in the building.

During our first shot I realized that Peter could drive a grip to drink. A grip lays dolly track for the camera to move on and also pushes the camera dolly during the shots. I came into the room and saw the dolly track they had laid, going back and forth across the room like a puzzle. It was amazing. As they began the shot everyone was moved and scurried to get out of each other's way. My friend Don Merritt, the boom man (who held the microphone), was running behind the camera trying to stay out of the way and not trip as it moved about. It continued like that throughout the film. It was quite an operation!

We worked very long hours with Peter. He had abundant energy and hated to quit. On our first night we worked from 6:00 p.m. to 6:00 p.m. I meditated a couple of times during the night to stay awake.

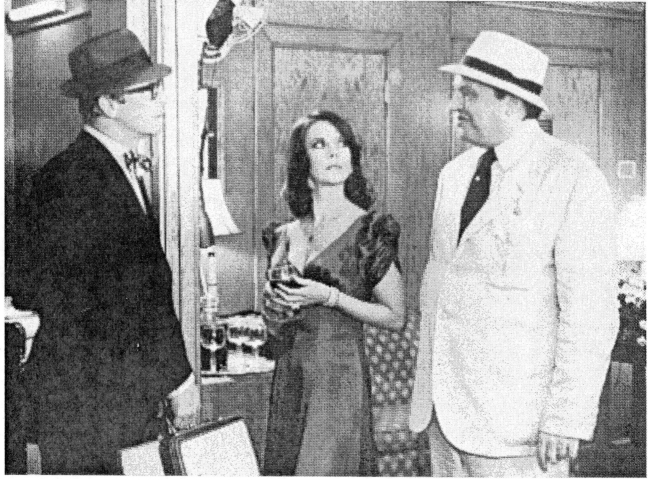

Michael Caine, Natalie Wood and Thayer David, *Peeper*

We worked in intriguing places during the film. One of my favorite locations was the Harold Lloyd estate right across the street from Elizabeth Montgomery's house. By this time Lizzie and Bob Foxworth were happily living together. One day they came over to visit me and I introduced Lizzie to Natalie. They had never met before, which was amazing to me. Lizzie was shy and she surprised me. She hesitated in going to meet Natalie. I guess my friendly nature just didn't give a person a chance to be shy, at least not with me.

The Harold Lloyd estate was huge. There was an adorable little playhouse all decorated for a child. The terrace elegantly laid out a gigantic swimming pool, and a living room with a huge organ built into the wall. One room had a Christmas tree in it that must have been at least fifty feet high. That room always gave me the creeps and I stayed away from it as much as I could. The tree remained there all the time and it had a weird smell. I surmised that someone had probably died under the tree and atrophied and nobody ever noticed the body.

Years later, when the estate had been sold, we worked there again. I went into the Christmas tree room and the tree was gone. It was actually a beautiful room. There was a lovely, delicately painted mural on the ceiling and the bad smell had disappeared.

I loved wandering about the estate when I wasn't busy. I would imagine what it might have been like in its heyday. I looked through the bedrooms with their own dressing rooms, the maids' rooms, the room above the living room that seemed to be a secret lookout for spies, and the huge kitchen where sumptuous meals must have been prepared for guests. I had endless fantasies going on in my mind.

We also shot on the ship *Queen Mary* in Long Beach as part of the script took place at sea. It was my first time on the ship. Seeing as I was far from home, I decided to spend the nights there. I went on board the ship and never left for a week, imagining I was on a cruise. The ship was marvelous with its burled wood. The grandeur of years past filled my mind with visions. I slept in the makeup room, took baths in the huge tub which even had a spout for salt water, no longer used.

One morning I woke up early to the sound of someone shouting at the top of his lungs. Looking through a porthole I saw a man jumping about yelling, "They all said they'd do it and I did it," over and over. I've always wondered just what it was he had done.

While we were on the *Queen Mary*, our unit manager was working on a deal to get us on a cruise ship in the Caribbean. Since the arrangements had been made at the last minute, we were told we'd have to share our accommodations. I didn't care, but the crew was fussing. It wasn't the way we were supposed to be treated according to union rules. But eventually it was worked out and we were set for the cruise.

We took off for Miami on July 26, stopping in Atlanta to change planes. I enjoyed a couple of Piña Coladas, felt the warm Atlanta summer breezes on my body, and felt homesick for West Virginia. I wondered if we'd ever live there again. We arrived late in Miami. After checking into our hotel, the crew gathered in the bar for a while before we retired at four o'clock in the morning. We boarded our ship the next day at one o'clock in the afternoon. I shared my cabin with two other women - Peggy Pemperton, Natalie's wardrobe woman (who took the place of Ann Landers on this film) and Marge, the production secretary. Unlike Ann, who had constantly scurried around, Peggy always looked so cool, and with her white makeup she was a wonder to behold. We sometimes referred to her as Casper the Friendly Ghost. She was quite nice if a bit prim and proper. Marge was a tall, coltish girl always on the lookout for a guy. Our room was crowded. Peggy hid her towels so we wouldn't use them by mistake.

With music playing softly, the ship pulled out of the harbor. The cruise ship was designed for total enjoyment and was lovely. I decided it was okay to be sharing my cabin; I wouldn't be spending much time there if I could help it.

The first evening we worked until midnight. I sat and talked with Dick Hart, the new gaffer - a round, cuddly, man. He recalled that Patrick had told him hairdressers and gaffers always got along famously and then proceeded to tell me about his favorite hairdresser. He didn't say who she was, but he did say he liked me because I reminded him of her. I kept trying to figure out just whom he was talking about.

The next morning I awoke very early, probably due to my overindulgence of food and drink. Seeing as I couldn't sleep, I decided to sit out on the deck in an effort to get a tan, but soon it turned gray and started to rain. Despite the overcast skies, my legs turned bright red and my toes looked like tiny, red sausages. It was our day off so we relaxed, ate delicious meals, and went to the dance that was held that night. The ocean was rough and the ship was rocking and rolling right back and forth. I danced with Dick and dramatically fell into his arms and he into mine with each roll of the ship.

Haiti was our first stop. As I walked off the ship, the cameraman, Earl Rath, reminded me that I was working. "This is not just a pleasure cruise." I laughed, "Earl, my whole life is a pleasure cruise." Port au Prince was awful, so dirty and smoky and the people were very poor. It was depressing and hard to imagine Dick Kline's wife, Jackie, having grown up in this poor country. Surprisingly when we finally left the city behind and were driving through the countryside it was quite beautiful. I decided Jackie's family must have lived in a beautiful area, not the squalor that met us on our arrival. The trees were full of red blossoms and women walked down the road balancing loads of goods on their heads. When we stopped to visit a rum factory, people gathered around our taxi saying, "Gimmie," or "Buy this," even sticking things in my bag telling me, "You don't have to pay for it if you don't want it," knowing full well I would pay for anything I kept.

By this time my legs had turned a fluorescent red and my skin was sticking to the Naugahyde taxi seat. My toes now resembled a row of swollen, red jellybeans.

After our tour I took a good nap before going to work that night at quarter past six. Jesus, one of our crewmembers, liked my hefty arms and asked if my husband was a good lover. "Why not have an adventure with me?" he asked. I made a friend of him instead of a lover.

The next day we sailed into beautiful Port Antonio, Jamaica. I bought a ticket to go on a raft ride on Ocho Rios. After lunch I went out to wait for the others in the crew who were also going on the ride. I thought I must have missed them, but then Dick Hart came along and suggested we go together which made it much more fun. We got into a raft and a man pushed us along the river with a long pole. It was so relaxing and hot and every once in a while a small boat came by with cold drinks for sale; even iced beer. I could have drifted along all day. I bought a post card to take home to show Patrick the raft we traveled in. When Pat saw it, he laughed and said, "Those rafts are quite small, both you and Dick are rather pudgy. Are you sure you behaved?" "Of course," I answered truthfully.

After the raft trip I walked to the straw market near the ship where a young fellow of about seventeen took a liking to me. He said he liked my ass and asked," Do you have a husband?" When I said yes, he quipped, "A man who likes a fat woman is a good man." I thought to myself, "I like these natives. They make me feel quite perfect."

The next morning our alarm went off much too early. Peggy and I had promised Marge the room to herself that afternoon as she had a possible rendezvous with a crewmember. When we docked at Montego Bay, Peggy and I left the ship for town. We found a woman taxi driver who took us on a tour and shopping. When it was time to return to the ship for departure, our driver kept heading away from town. She told us she was running out of gas and I was nervous about the situation, but Peggy was even more upset. Peggy hadn't approved of the whole deal in the first place. I could see our ship in the distance and began to wonder if we'd make it back in time. I also wondered how we'd catch up if they did leave us behind. As it turned out, we made it back in time. What a relief! We stayed away from our room until dinner then discovered that the guy never even showed up.

That night the stunts they performed were extremely dangerous. The stunt men were fighting on one of the lifeboats with the crew situated in another lifeboat shooting the scene. The boats hung over the side of the ship above the ocean and both boats were rocking wildly. The sea was rough and the ship was going so fast that if anyone fell overboard they would never be found. It was very tense and I was concerned for the stunt men and the crew. I didn't need to be in the boat so I stood beside Jim, the tall Norwegian officer who was assigned to watch over our crew. (The cruise ship was from Norway and the officers were tall, blond, and gorgeous. I think it paid off to have these men socializing with the passengers.) Jim told me he had a pair of trunks in his pocket just in case anyone should fall, but he said he'd probably never find anyone. The sharks would get them first. While we talked, I prayed for our crew.

We wrapped as dawn broke. Bed had never felt so good. The ship was traveling all day, so I slept until 2:30 p.m. and felt well rested that evening. Our cruise was coming to an end soon. That night Natalie let down life boats and it was exciting to watch.

Our last stop was Nassau. I had wonderful memories of my time there when Pat was shooting *Day of the Dolphin*. I wanted to take a motor scooter ride, but first I went shopping and bought some Nassau Royal, the great liquor they sell there. I rented a scooter and as I started off, I spotted John Stephens, the camera assistant, sadly wandering around, missing his girlfriend. I decided to cheer him up and told him to jump on the back of the scooter and I'd take him for some great conch salad. Later, while enjoying a couple of Goombay Smashes and the promised conch salad, he offered to drive us back to town. He confessed that I'd scared him with my driving, but didn't tell me at first because he hadn't wanted to offend me. I was quite happy to leave the driving to him. The day turned out great and I found I still loved the island.

That night was the Captain's party. We all attended the cocktail party and had a delicious dinner with all sorts of wines and we danced. Later I stood on the top of the ship with Michael Caine and his lovely wife. The wind was calm and moonlight shone on the water while lightening flashed in the sky. It was a perfect end to the cruise. It was easy to forget I was working.

We left the ship when it docked in Miami, but our flight wasn't to leave for Los Angeles until later that night. We waited in a couple of motel rooms and I thought how strange my life was. Who'd ever have thought my life would be like this. Me, the mother of three, sitting in this motel with all these men, flamingos and ducks wandering about outside, trying to get a bit of sleep before going home? The flight home was great and Patrick met me looking so handsome. I had missed him. I wished he could have gone along with me to share the fun.

I was still rocking from my week on the cruise when I woke up the next morning. It took a couple of days to get my land legs back and to come down from the high of being on the cruise.

We went back to work on the stage for a few days to pick up some scenes. What a let down. I had a new friend in Dick Hart and he eventually confessed that the hairdresser he loved was Kathy Blondell. I understood, because I loved her, too. He was still married at the time, but later divorced. Many years later Kathy and Dick rediscovered each other on a location and married.

Peter, the director, had been wonderful to work with. He appreciated everything I had done which, in turn, made me better at my job. On the last night he seemed depressed, sitting in a dressing room on the stage all by himself. I understood why he hated his film coming to an end. Directing was his life and I'm sure he wondered when he would be directing again. I hoped I'd have an opportunity to work with him again.

Chapter 35

MANDINGO

Peeper ended. I had a big let down. I hadn't made the connection yet about how the higher you go the farther you fall. For the two months I had been working on *Peeper* I hadn't thought about anything else. It was like being at a two-month party. My close relationships with friends flourished, but once again at the end of the film they dissolved as we went our separate ways. Still, I loved how I felt when I was working on a film. It was magical at times. I felt blessed, I had it all - or so it seemed. I had two families in a way, which was both good and bad. The good part was I learned to trust myself with others and just enjoy their company. The bad part being, that I often I spent more time with my film family than my real family.

Natalie, always generous with gifts at the end of a film, gave me a gold bracelet engraved with, "Thanks for Fat Chance." I went to her house to bring her the hairpieces she's used in the movie and we talked for a while. We always were close during a film and easily picked up our friendship when another film began. I gave her a big hug as I left.

Nixon resigned (what a surprise!). My mother, an avid Republican, loved him, but. I did not share her views. She and I argued about what Nixon did. Her feeling was other presidents had probably done similar things. Hey, they just didn't get caught. I said he shouldn't have done anything wrong to begin with. Now I'm not so judgmental.

During that time my mother had to be rushed to the hospital suddenly with a huge, non-cancerous tumor that had to be operated on right away. I'd finished the film so I was able to spend time with her. She had lost a lot of blood and was pale, but soon after the operation she began to look much better.

Patrick was cruising the Caribbean, working on a Bristol Creme commercial. I was working here and there, taking calls on various shows. I worked with Jan Brunson, the hairstylist, in Hollywood at a lovely old home for a wine commercial. The caterer on the show was new and actually served us healthy food - fruits, large salads, and pastas. Most of the time, the caterers for commercials were men who wanted to become teamsters. (Being a cook was one way to get into the union.) The result was that the meals had often been very basic with dehydrated mashed potatoes, canned vegetables (usually peas), and roasts, too well done. This was great.

Later that evening, while we were watching the prop men open bottle after bottle of wine and pour it down the sink Jan was called to the phone. Peter Harrold, a unit manager, was on the line. He needed a hairstylist right away in Baton Rouge. The film was *Mandingo*; a story about a slave-breeding plantation in the 1840's where passions run high. There was a problem with the present hairstylist. Jan handed me the phone "You talk to them, Sugar. I'm getting married and can't leave town." I wasn't sure I was willing to leave home either. Pat was on the high seas, my mother was in the hospital, and we were in the process of buying a new house.

As it turned out, Peter wasn't sure about me. He had to check with the makeup men to see if they approved of me. I went home confused, wondering how it would turn out.

The next day was my mother's birthday and I wanted to spend time with her. When I arrived at the hospital, she looked very old and weak. I knew it was partly because she didn't have her teeth in or her glasses on. It wasn't a great celebration, but at least she was alive and recovering. The following day, August 17, was my youngest daughter Xochi's twelfth birthday. I was now forty.

We were getting ready to move from our rental house in the country to our own, larger house on a cul de sac, not too far away in Newhall. Our finances were better, but we still had to borrow $5,000 for the down payment. As long as we kept working we felt we'd be able to pay the loan off quickly.

Peter called back to tell me I had the job if I wanted it. I would go on location to Baton Rouge and then New Orleans. It was summer so we decided Tanya and Xochi would come with me and Laurie would stay home and move us into our new home. She was just seventeen and very competent. Before I left, I went to the escrow office to sign the papers for the house. Pat would sign them when he returned. We were able to store things in the garage before actually moving in.

This was my second trip to Louisiana. The last time I was there it was very romantic - December in New Orleans. This time it was August and the first stop was Baton Rouge. It was hot and humid. I expected the charming mix of French, Creole, and the South like it had been in New Orleans. Was I ever disappointed! The spiritual vibrations of Baton Rouge were about minus one on a scale of one to ten. Baton Rouge is not New Orleans by any means.

Upon our arrival we were driven straight to the big, sprawling Belmont Motor Hotel. We were shown to a huge corner room that even had a kitchen. There was plenty of space for the three of us. The kids changed immediately and hurried out to the pool. I was told to go to the head makeup man's room. Hank Edds, a big, calm, cowboy-type man, opened his arms and gave me a hug. Jerry O'Dell, his assistant, was there, too, a short, round man gifted with the wildest, most wacky sense of humor you could find anywhere.

Hank wasn't calm that day, but he was relieved I had arrived. The other hairstylist wasn't working out and the producer was furious with her, as was Hank. There was lots of tension between the hairstylist, Del Ree Todd, and the actress and the producer just wanted peace. Del Ree wanted the hairdo to fit the period, but Suzanne George, the actress, wanted bangs. Well, bangs were just not worn in 1840, especially by stylish, wealthy folks. If things continued the way they were going, there didn't seem to be any peace in sight. This was why they sent for me. The most important thing was to keep the actress happy.

Unfortunately, they hadn't told Del Ree that they had hired me. They were going to spring me on her. I was furious. From that day on whenever I've been called to replace someone I made sure to call them to let them know before I'd take the job. At first they hid me away in Hank's room and gave me a script to read while I waited. I felt quite ill at ease. What did they think Del Ree would do? Then they took me to meet Susan and her partner at the time, the singer Jack Jones. She seemed sweet and was happy to know I'd arrived. James Mason, Perry King, and Kenny Norton, the heavy weight boxer, were in the film.

Finally they notified Del Ree and told me to report to the makeup room the next morning so she could show me how she did the hair. I was very uncomfortable, but Del Ree was quite nice. Apparently she had seen the writing on the wall and was prepared to leave. Actually that's how it usually is.

The next morning Susan walked in acting as though she was meeting me for the first time. Del Ree showed me how she did Susan's hair. It was very complicated and I stood by, watching and hoping I could remember what she had done. I went to the set with Susan and Del Ree went to her room to pack.

After my indoctrination, I was ready to make things work out, to heck with the period, to heck with my peers' remarks or criticism. There was always a feeling way back in the minds of hairdressers that we might be ridiculed when the credits came on if a hairstyle was obviously not in the proper period. By this time my feeling was, if the producer didn't care and the actress didn't care, why should I? Del Ree obviously cared too much and she got fired.

Our set the first day was a lovely old southern mansion, an elegant setting, surrounded by ancient, huge oak trees with silvery moss swinging from the limbs. Inside, the mansion was filled with antiques. The rooms still looked like the 1840's. There was a modern, air-conditioned kitchen that we used for our makeup room. What a relief. The humidity must have been a hundred percent.

There was no air on the set and the lights made the already steamy set even worse. We were filming a wedding scene and everyone in the cast was dressed in heavy costumes, sweating like horses in lather. The sweat was pouring off me, too. I was so nervous. I followed the makeup man into the set as he dried off Susan's face. This messed up her bangs so I had to straighten them after he finished. Trying to carefully back out of the set, I knocked over gobos and bumped into things. The more nervous I got, the clumsier I became.

It's always difficult to take over in the middle of a project and try to match someone else's work especially when you aren't sure what exactly you are supposed to be matching. On this particular day, Susan's hair seemed to fall apart so easily. I suspected that Del Ree had put it on a little loosely that morning as a parting gesture. I'll never know. After lunch I had time to redo her hair and it stayed just perfectly during the afternoon. I really earned my money that day. The fan blew the hair all around, sweat was pouring off everyone, including me. I nearly fell asleep in the afternoon from exhaustion.

I found that I knew a lot of the crew. Richard Fleisher, the director, had directed *The Boston Strangler*. Dick Kline was the cameraman and the gaffer was Ross Mahl, an old friend of ours. The key grip was Gene Kearney. Gene became an instant friend as he moved things out of my way so I wouldn't trip, or resetting them when I did bump into them.

The next morning I was able to do Susan's hair in the hotel beauty shop and it stayed put all day long. I now had photos so I could match her hairdo.

As we arrived on the set the second morning we were each handed a T-shirt with name *Mandingo* on it and were told to wear it. Our producer, Dino De Laurentis was going to visit the set that afternoon. The T-shirt wasn't all cotton and was uncomfortable and hot, but we wore them anyway. I was sleepy, so during my break I decided to go out on the front porch, sit in a rocking chair, and meditate. My timing left something to be desired, however. When De Laurentis arrived, there I was looking as if I was happily sleeping. At least I was wearing my T-shirt.

Meanwhile, Pat arrived back in Los Angeles with all the money we needed to close the deal on the house. He also had lots of job offers. I began to regret taking this job, but we needed the money for the house. Pat called and told me that he would decide on a project and then come down to visit us on the way to his next job.

Dick Kline's beautiful wife, Jackie, was on location with their kids. Tanya and Xochi began to pal around with them. They also met Perry King and his daughter, Weezie. Everyone was having a wonderful time. It was a real vacation for the kids. But the hot weather was getting to me and I was exhausted. It always took me a week or so to get acclimated anyway. Some mornings I wished I could just sleep all day long.

Later on in the film we would be shooting in New Orleans where there would be a huge scene with lots of extras and I had to plan for that right away. I called the union and got Alma Johnson, a tough, old-time hairdresser, who knew her period work. Luckily she was willing to come. I ordered lots of wigs, switches, and hairpieces for the extras, too. I was relieved when that was all organized. At the end of the first week I had worked sixty-three and a half hours. My paycheck was $531.93, clearing $359.01.

We filmed at another beautiful property with huge oak trees lining the path. This was the home that was supposed to burn down. We worked on the slaves who were in a chain gang that really depressed me. Of course it was only a movie, but all I could think of was how could we ever have treated human beings so terribly?

The next week we moved to our permanent set at Belle Helene, where most of the exterior action took place. The interiors would be done on stage at Paramount when we returned. What a shock! I expected this set to be gorgeous like the first set, but it was an awful mess. There were no floors, the beautiful wooden floors on the first floor had been sold and were long gone. The floors were just dirt. The weather was damp and humid, making everyone's job difficult. It rained nearly every day. All the foliage surrounding the mansion was overgrown giving it an uncared-for look. Although it was right for the film, it was a great disappointment to me.

Some of Susan's hairpieces didn't match her own hair and I had to dye them one night. First I sprayed them, which looked okay, but I didn't trust the color not to wash off with all the rain. I could just imagine the color running down her face onto her gown.

The days were long, hot and humid. Sometimes I had to work on an actor in the evening after we got home. I was exhausted holding myself together while I longed for a bath and my bed.

Patrick finally decided on a film in Montana, *The Killer Inside Me*, starring Stacy Keach. He was offered a deal he couldn't turn down - $900 a week plus one per cent of the profits of the $500,000 film. It was one of those deals that sounded so lucrative until we learned about studio bookkeeping. Nobody ever made any money on those deals, at least not the crew. But we had no idea at the time.

Pat spent a week in Baton Rouge, before leaving for Montana. One evening I came home to find him beside the pool with the girls, talking with the other wives. He said he was going to enjoy being a location wife. He rented himself a car, joined the other wives at the pool and cocktail parties, and every evening he was all cleaned up and waiting for me when I got home all sweaty and tired. He was having a great time and I was getting a kick out of having a location wife. It was nice to have everything all done, like the wash and the kids all looked after.

One evening we went out to dinner at Jack Sabin's, a well-known restaurant. We pulled up in front of the restaurant and there were five men sitting in chairs out front, all dressed in white jackets. We assumed they were the parking attendants, so we stopped, expecting one of them to get up, open our doors, and park the car. But to our surprise, they all pointed in unison, "Just park right over there." I couldn't stop laughing, but Pat, being a Southerner, remarked on how lazy Southerners really are. I wouldn't have touched that one. Our dinners were mouth-watering - lots of spicy Creole food, oysters stuffed with crab and lobster.

I could hardly wait for Sunday. My love cooked breakfast for us and that afternoon we went to the movies and saw *That's Entertainment*. We went home and crashed. It was just what I needed.

Pat left at the end of the week for Butte, Montana. I wasn't alone though, because the kids were there and they were having a wonderful time with all the other location families. I was feeling low a lot of the time and I wondered about it. Usually I was able to make the best out of whatever was handed to me. Maybe it was because I didn't have close friends like I'd had on the last film.

James Mason and his wife entranced me. We would sit on the set's verandah and talk. He'd tell me about living in Switzerland and how he and his wife traveled a lot. He was interested in nature, especially birds. I'd loved him since I was young and it was a treat getting to know him. He was truly as sexy and attractive as he had always been.

My other favorite was Kenny Norton who played the "Mandingo." He was beautiful and a sweet person with a childlike enthusiasm for life. He loved my girls and they loved him. He often spent time with them when he was off during the day. He'd sneak around outside our room, peeking in the windows. He gave Tanya a "Billy Jack" hat he had bought for himself. The kids also enjoyed time with Perry King and his family. We all had a good time together. Once again the hotel became our home and we had become a film family.

Finally the weather began to cool off. My mood improved a bit and my weariness began to disappear. One morning as we were driving to work we heard hurricane warnings on the radio. The girls were back at the motel and I figured they'd be looked after, but I still wanted to be with them. Why on earth were we going to the set? It was near the river and according to the locals, the tornadoes that come with hurricanes follow the river. It was crazy to be there and I was frightened. Here I had dodged earthquakes in Los Angeles only to be caught in a hurricane in Louisiana.

Movie companies are notorious for not giving up a day of shooting no matter what and this company was no different. We worked, although nobody could concentrate. The wind picked up and everyone was nervous. There were twelve-foot tides in the river. Hurricane Carmen was heading our way. Finally, coming to their senses, Production told the grips to cover and tie down the little slave cabin that had been built in back of the mansion. We wrapped at noon and headed back to the hotel.

We rode back to the hotel in a bus and could look down into the cars heading out of town. They were packed full with necessities and all heading in the opposite direction from us. I couldn't blame them. I'd been in New Orleans just after a hurricane year and saw what damage it could do.

We reached the hotel, I found the kids and we hurried across the street to the little grocery store. It was very crowded. We bought canned goods and a can opener, things that didn't need to be cooked in case we lost power. We went back to our room and filled the bathtub with water, all the time listening closely to the radio for news of the hurricane. We taped the little panes of our windows so that if they broke they wouldn't shatter. We moved the girls' mattresses, sheltering them from the windows. We had taken as much precaution as we possibly could.

We gathered with our friends outside. Fred Broast, the first assistant, was married to a French woman, Dauphinais, who was a great cook. She prepared soup and invited us all to dinner. We sat outside for a while watching the clouds whirling in the sky. When it appeared they were no longer moving in our direction, we went inside and poured ourselves a glass of wine as she ladled out sumptuous soup. I hadn't wanted to drink before just in case the hurricane hit, but finally the wine and the good company wore me down and I began to enjoy myself. The kids were having fun, too. They loved the excitement.

We finally went home to sleep. In the morning the radio said that the storm had turned away from the city and gone through the sugar cane fields. The kids were disappointed; they wanted to experience a hurricane. It actually did come close to us - less than seventy miles away.

Richard Ward, a lovely man, who played one of the slaves collapsed on the ground one day. The heat was unbearable. There was no first-aid person on the set. Our unit manager had been too cheap to provide us with first aid. We didn't know what to do. We didn't know if Richard had had a heart attack or what. Kenny Norton began to pound on Richard's chest to revive him. We were all frightened and looked on, helpless. At last the ambulance showed up and the attendants took Richard to the hospital. We were all expecting the worst. Fortunately, he was suffering from dehydration. We made sure Richard drank lots of water from then on.

Our unit manager came on the set the next day and I blew up at him. "It's not fair to leave the crew without someone medically responsible for the set in case of an emergency. It's not our job to make decisions about how to help someone in trouble, when we obviously don't know what we're doing." Someone "medically responsible" was on the set from then on.

I was still low. The weather was too hot. The set was stinky. The subject of the film depressed me. All the foliage was overgrown and wet and I was always covered with mud.

There was one humorous thing that always tickled me. Frank, the caretaker for the estate, was really smelly. He lived in a little house on the property with seven dogs. I don't think he ever bathed; a stench hung around him like an aura. When he'd come up behind someone the person would begin to sniff and then slowly turn around to see Frank standing there. Quickly, they would find another place to stand, as far from Frank as possible. I'd get a kick watching this happen over and over.

Each morning, by habit, I'd climb on the bus and sit in the same seat each day. I had read that doing the same thing over and over puts you in a rut so I decided to see what happened if I sat in a different seat each day. I tried it and it did seem to help, but my frustrations and unhappiness were still with me and I started to question my way of life. Sure I needed to work, but did it have to take over my whole life? The summer working on *Fat Chance* had been so much fun I had no time to be lonely, but here in Baton Rouge I couldn't run away from my feelings. No matter what I did, there they were. I didn't know what to do. Did I want to continue being on one side of the earth with Patrick on the other? What kind of a life was that for my family?

In the meantime, Pat was having a wonderful time in Montana, not worrying about anything. I was still feeling sorry for myself and wanted him to understand, but he didn't seem to. James Mason talked with me about how, in the business, we sealed ourselves off in a plastic bubble at times so we wouldn't feel anything. He understood what I felt and I didn't feel quite so alone. I felt as though I was living in a void. I realized it was time to get clear about my goals, but this was hard for me. On the surface, my life appeared to be fun most of the time. What more did I want?

We finished the work in Baton Rouge and the weather began to break. It began to feel like fall. When I walked out of the hotel gate on the last day and climbed onto the bus headed for New Orleans, I never looked back. I was glad to leave Baton Rouge behind.

We stayed at the Bienvielle House Hotel in New Orleans, not quite the Royale Orleans where I'd stayed the last time, but we did have a nice, big room. It was nearer the Mississippi River, in a rougher part of town. The warehouse where we fitted the extras with hair and the wardrobe people would be outfitting extras with costumes was very close to our hotel. I began to feel more comfortable than I had in a long time. I could even walk to work.

The girls and I went out to eat a Mufeletta, a great New Orleans sandwich consisting of a large, round loaf of Italian bread with the top cut off, covered with all sorts of things like salami, peppers, olives, then doused with olive oil and covered in melted cheese. Yum! I also had a dozen raw oysters. Yum, yum!

Susan, our actress, was finished with her work on the film until we returned to Los Angeles and that gave me time to devote myself to our biggest scene. Alma, my hairdresser assistant, had arrived earlier and the area for the fittings was all set up right next to the wardrobe. Alma was a wonderful partner, no nonsense.

One day we did a scene of a slave sale at a marketplace. It was appalling. It really happened that way in the past. All the slaves were naked, men and women chained together. It was so difficult for the extras, standing there naked. Most of the crewmembers were men and I felt I should stay there since there were no other women on the set, but Fred wouldn't allow me to remain. He felt funny about me seeing all the naked men, but I only wanted to stay and support the women extras. I thought it would help them feel more comfortable, and the scene certainly didn't turn me on. I left, happy to get out of that awful scene.

On Sunday Alma, the kids, and I took a trip up the Mississippi River. It was such a different way of life on the river, barges transporting cargo up and down, inlets where I could see beautiful homes, and junky little shacks perched on the shore. It was peaceful, and I needed that after being so busy at work.

Our big scene was filmed at Beauregard House, the home of Francis Parkinson Keyes, the author of a great many books I'd read. I was impressed and utterly delighted to be in her home. It was on display for the public and we were going to work there for many nights, all night long.

While I was working there I discovered her library and office. I sat in her chair and meditated, hoping her talent would somehow penetrate me. It felt different from the other rooms. I felt blessed to be able to spend so much time there.

Our local producer was quite a womanizer and a real character. He'd find a pretty girl somewhere and, as producers have always done, promise her a part in the picture. But he was telling the girls the truth. Day after day a lovely woman who wasn't on the extra list would arrive to be outfitted. We had a hard time keeping up with him and his lovely ladies, and we were running out of hairpieces.

One day Tanya and Xochi decided they wanted to be extras, too. They were immediately sorry. They were outfitted in long dresses with flannel slips and all the trimmings. They had to stand out in the streets for hours in the uncomfortable shoes of that period. They could hardly wait for the day to end. They were miserable and didn't feel it was worth the fifteen dollars they earned. "Never again," they proclaimed.

One day an attractive woman stopped to watch us shoot. As guys do, our crew began to hang around, vying for her attention. She enjoyed it immensely and later we all had a great laugh when we found out that she wasn't a woman after all. The guys were so flustered and embarrassed, wondering why they hadn't known. They were so embarrassed in fact that they began to brag that they had known all along. Well, I don't think they did. The first night of work on the big scene, we began doing hair at 6:00 p.m. - head after head of hair, on and on and on. The scene was a party in a whorehouse. We filmed throughout the whole house. It was filled with extras. I have no idea how many hairdos I did that night. I didn't get to the set until well after midnight. They were still setting up the dolly track for the first shot where the camera moved through the whole house when I arrived. It was a complicated first shot.

The house was stifling, and we never did get an air conditioner; instead they hired a huge blower thing that blew air over chunks of ice, not sufficient at all.

The governor of Mississippi acted in the scene and so did his daughter who played one of the prostitutes standing on the porch. The governor was very handsome, yet his daughter was not attractive at all and I wondered how she felt to have a father more attractive than she was. Later on when we were doing her hair she mentioned how handsome her father was. It must have always been on her mind.

One of the last nights we worked at that house, we did all the hair and then I took the girls out for dinner before reporting to the set. They were twelve and fourteen and could stay alone in the hotel, but I wanted to spend some time with them. I'd had it with Creole food. My stomach had been in a constant uproar for weeks. We went to Victoria Station. It was heaven. That night a crisp, green salad, baked potato, and a rare prime rib were just what I needed. On Sunday we all went to the Royal Orleans Hotel for brunch - Eggs Florentine and Ramos Gin Fizzes, for the grownups at least.

Elizabeth Montgomery's agent called inquiring if I was available to go to Massachusetts for a week's location for *Lizzie Borden*, her next film. I told him I wasn't sure, but I hoped I could. We were working all night long and I was weary. At dawn we'd take off the extras' hair in the warehouse and then I'd shuffle home, barely able to put one foot in front of the other. It was getting cold, which felt good, but then I had to warm up before falling asleep. I was completely worn out.

The last night we worked, I went to Tres Jacques with the girls for dinner. It was very French and we sat down and ate whatever they served us. Later, at three in the morning someone brought in beignets and strong Morning Call Coffee, with chicory - my favorite. It was the first I'd had on this trip and it was the perfect ending to a difficult location.

We left New Orleans on October 5. Laurie picked us up at the airport and we stopped to see my mother in West Los Angeles on the way home. She had recovered and there was a little jauntiness in her step. It made me feel happy.

Our new house looked perfect. Laurie had fixed it all so beautifully everything looked great right down to the new plants she had bought. There were our dogs and cats galore; just the way I like it. My own bed had never felt so good.

We were working at Paramount Studio filming the interiors of the mansion we'd shot in Baton Rouge. The sets were rich and lovely. It smelled better too with no Frank lurking in the shadows. Yet when the stage door closed I felt encased in the darkness that appeared to be associated with this production.

Hal Lierly, the Makeup Department head at Paramount, gave me the script for *Lizzie Borden*. It was excellent and how I longed to escape *Mandingo*. It wasn't to be though. I planned to do a hair test with Lizzie while Hedy, a wonderful hairstylist who worked at Paramount, stood by with Susan on *Mandingo* for me. I did Susan's hair, but while I was gone there was a hat change. Hedy couldn't get it right and it turned into a disaster. I didn't realize Hedy had some small strokes. She's been such a top hairstylist, and I was sure I could trust her with Susan. But she fell apart and I got into trouble with the director. I had to come back to *Mandingo* and Hedy stood by with Lizzie. Lizzie, great gal that she was, was very patient with Hedy.

Kenny Norton, the one bright spot in my days, charmed and amused me. I'd be reading something and he'd take the book out of my hands and sit down and read it to me in a "Mammy" voice and I'd laugh till I cried. He had a hard time dealing with Susan, though. She was difficult. I did not like her much, either. She was mean to the costumer, if not to me. When she finished her part and said her goodbyes, I didn't say I'd like to work with her again. A few months later I saw her at CBS and she was quite sweet again. Perhaps *Mandingo* had gotten to her, too.

At lunchtime I began to do something I'd never done before. There was a little Armenian restaurant behind Paramount where I went to have a delicious lunch - a shish kabob along with a half carafe of wine. I never drank while working before, but at this point I just didn't care. At night too, I sat in my bath with a glass or two of wine. I was worried about my increased drinking. Here I'd been upset at Pat for his drinking habits and now I was acting just like him.

Gary, the second assistant, got rather nasty one day when he smirked, "Do you really think you are worth your salary?" I blew up at him; I knew I was worth it. "You have no idea what we have to go through in the dressing room behind closed doors. We have to deal with the actors before they come to the set. Do you realize we have the power to make your day work or not?" He only saw us sitting around the set all day. He had no idea how we had to baby the actors and the patience it took when they were troubled and needed consoling.

Kenny Norton was always accompanied by his friend, Bob. Bob would tell me how difficult relationships were for Kenny being a well-known athlete. Whom could he trust? Did the girls like him or just his persona? He'd been taken advantage of before. Bob said the surface of Kenny had just been scratched and there was gold beneath. I liked him so much. His parents came to visit on the set and we talked for a long time.

We were getting closer to the finish. Susan was gone and James Mason was next to wrap. I got a nice big goodbye kiss from him - nice lips: one of my most memorable kisses.

We wrapped on October 25 and it was the biggest relief I'd ever felt at the end of a film.

Chapter 36

LIZZIE BORDEN

My experience on *Mandingo* brought me to a turning point in my life. It forced me to question the direction my life was taking. Maybe it was the meditation I had begun, maybe it was loneliness. Up until now, Patrick and I had spent so much time together. Suddenly our lives were drifting in different directions. I'd been relatively content as long as I had my family and my love to come home to, but now my children were growing up and had lives of their own to live. Pat's work took him far away, or else mine did.

I realized that the changes in the movie business played a major role in my dissatisfaction. When I started out, not only had I been much younger, but the business had felt more loving, like a family. It satisfied any emotional needs that weren't being met at home. Now that the business was being run by accountants, its main concern was the bottom line. The art and soul of movie making seemed to have vanished. The hours had increased and it was all work, work, work, rush, rush, rush. There wasn't any time at the end of the day to relax and just do nothing. Still, the money I earned was more than I'd have been able to bring in elsewhere and there were still many wonderful people in the industry.

Elizabeth Montgomery was one of them. I loved working with her and I knew that *Lizzie Borden* was going to be a wonderful project. We decided to have her hair dyed a strawberry blonde. I sent her to Laurie Davis, a hair-tinting specialist, a wizard in my opinion. I didn't have the up-to-date knowledge in that area. The tint gave Lizzie's hair a great deal of body and made it much easier for me to work with. I styled her hair in the Victorian fashions and she looked lovely. Her costumes were made of beautiful materials and were enhanced with corsets that gave her a tiny waist. Her look filled the screen with such realism; you swore that she was the real *Lizzie Borden*. Lizzie loved that part

We worked hard on that film. The hours were long. It was only a three-week schedule and there was so much work to fit into each day. My work looked splendid, if I do say so myself.

The scene that stuck in everyone's mind was where Lizzie was supposed to eat the stew with the flies and maggots on it. It was an incredible feat. We nearly believed her. I never knew how she did it. It was so repulsive, but Lizzie pulled it off like the pro that she was.

Three young actresses were cast as Lizzie at younger ages. There were two redheads and a brunette. I couldn't understand why they had cast the brunette, especially this particular brunette. She was a permanent character on a series and I wasn't allowed to change the color of her hair. It was one of those times that I was tempted to walk away and quit. I couldn't do that to Lizzie.

I called Hal in the Makeup Department and explained the dilemma. "Come on up to the department and we'll search through all of the old wigs left there from days past." He said. Fortunately, I found something reasonably close to Lizzie's color. It had never dawned on me that we might need to order a wig for the kids, so I hadn't planned on it. I doubted the producers would have sprung for one anyway.

Lizzie was so happy with her love Robert Foxworth. They were living together and life was great. She seemed very content. At work she'd reach into her purse to find love notes or tiny presents tucked into her bag. Foxy was a special being.

Pat got a call from Bill Fraker to do *The Many Faces of Hong Kong*, a travel film, produced by Cathay Pacific Airlines. They would be gone for at least eight weeks. Bill told Pat that there were perks and that I'd be able to go along. It was quite unexpected. Cathay Pacific was going to give us a special deal on the tickets. The crew made a little less in salary, but the perks were great.

Pat left on November 9 for Hong Kong. I was still working on *Lizzie Borden*. Lizzie renamed me - no more Sugar, I now became Phoenix. I never knew why she came up with that, but perhaps I was being reborn without knowing it.

Lizzie Borden was finished. The three weeks went so quickly. I was in a better place mentally than I had been right after finishing *Mandingo,* yet I was very tired and needed some rest. I'd gone from one film to another. I was anxiously awaiting word from Pat about when I could leave for Hong Kong. I didn't want that opportunity to get away.

Pat was staying at the Hong Kong Hotel, in Kowloon. I kept picturing myself there too. I rested, napped and tried to regain some energy. I was impatient to leave. Everything was set at home. My mother would stay with the girls. I'd had my shots: cholera, typhoid and a second diphtheria, plus tetanus and gamma globulin. Dr. Pierce, our family doctor told me I needed to quit drinking alcohol. He believed my liver was bothering me. Here I thought that Pat had the alcohol problem.

I decided to buy my own ticket, rather than wait any longer. I was afraid the film would be finished before I got over there. I made my reservation for November 26. I called Lizzie to say goodbye and told her where she could reach me if she needed me.

The trip to Hong Kong took forever. Pat was so happy to see me and we had a wonderful time. I traveled with him for a few weeks, to locations. We saw the Gurkha Soldiers on the border of China, the oyster fields where people tried to escape by swimming from Mainland China. The temples, the factories, the oriental carpet making was fascinating. We took a ferry to Hong Kong Island and ate sumptuous meals. We shopped at the night market, buying so much, thinking we were saving lots of money. But it cost a great deal to ship home, so it might not have been such a bargain. I had clothes made and copied that never fit when I got them home.

It was such a wonderful, crazy opportunity and I loved being there. I flew back home the day before New Years.

Chapter 37

VISIONS

We began dining on traditional black-eyed peas for luck at New Year Day breakfast. It was difficult getting readjusted to California time. We'd been almost a day ahead for so long. The kids were fine and glad to have us back home. They had missed us at Christmas, the first time we ever had been apart, but enough family was around so they weren't too lonely. In truth I think I missed them more than they missed us.

We had plans to go to Vienna when suddenly the director who had hired Bill Fraker was fired and his replacement had his own cameraman. It wasn't too much of a disappointment to me - I was ready to stay home for a while, but Pat wasn't pleased about losing the $1200 a week he would have earned. I needed to diet and get back into shape. The past year had been so busy I hadn't paid much attention to my health.

We had plenty of spare time so we decided to catch up on the latest movies. We saw *Godfather II, but* didn't enjoy it as much as the first one. It was beautifully done, all it lacked, in my opinion, was a good script. It won an Oscar that year. What did I know? We went to see *Aloha Bobby and Rose*, a film Pat had worked on with Bill. It was surprisingly good and became a hit.

The movie business was quiet so I day checked on different shows. One of the shows I worked on was *Maude*, which I enjoyed. I loved Bea Arthur and her grand style of humor. I eventually had to apply for unemployment. During slow times like this I always managed to entertain myself. This time I browsed through country-style magazines, including *The Yankee*, which I subscribed to after discovering it in Montana. I also sent for catalogues offering cozy, country-style furniture. Looking at these magazines and going through catalogues I began to yearn for something I couldn't identify at the time.

I wasn't feeling very well. My gallbladder was bothering me and my hip hurt. Dr. Hovey told me that stress caused the gallbladder to react and there was certainly enough stress in my life. I was worried about not having work having spent so much money on the Hong Kong trip. I had expected to be able to work as soon as I got home, but it just wasn't happening. Toward the end of January I added up our income for the past year - $60,000 yet we had very little left. Where had it all gone?

Lizzie invited us to see the finished print of *Lizzie Borden*. So much was done to a film in post-production, we never knew what it would look like until it was entirely finished. I liked seeing the film on a large screen, but the public would only get to see it on television. Lizzie looked wonderful and her acting was superb. I loved the ending with the kids shouting and singing. I considered it a hit.

Finally I got some daily calls at CBS. I liked doing television shows with all the different talent. I worked around Dionne Warwick and Tennessee Ernie Ford on their shows. It was quite a treat to see and hear them live. I had my first experience working with Cloris Leachman on *The Cher Show*. She was difficult, always changing her mind about things and it was nearly impossible to get her finished on time for her appearance on the show. Working with Ethel Merman was a treat. She was full of vitality and could still belt out a song. Michelle Lee and Bobbie Morse appeared on the *Cher Show* too. I also worked on the *Dinah Shore Show* a few times. She was relaxed, charming, and lovely as ever.

I got a call from a makeup artist named Vern Langdon, whom I'd never met before, about some projects at the public television station KCET. They sounded interesting and different from what I normally did. It paid a little less than I was used to making, but there weren't any fabulous offers coming in so I took the job.

I was glad I did. The work was fun. Vern and his friend and assistant, Keith, were wacky and creative. Keith, who had been a circus clown, described his adventures of riding on the circus train from town to town and how things had changed after the trains went by the wayside. He was sad that the era had come to an end.

We worked in Hollywood on Sunset at a little, old brick studio. The project was called *Visions* and showcased many new artists. My favorite was Maya Angelou who came in to direct a play. Her warmth, graciousness, and talent were a gift. Vern and Keith bordered on crazy, but they were also great artists. They created a Death Machine that blew my mind. I believe they were the forerunners of today's fantastic makeup and special effects.

Pat was starting work on a film with a new cameraman, Matt Leonetti, who had been Fraker's camera operator. Pat enjoyed working with Matt because he gave him freedom to do the lighting.

Always searching for happiness in books, I read *Handbook to Higher Consciousness* by Ken Keyes. This book helped me to become aware that I was addicted to having things go my way rather than simply preferring things to go my way. I began to understand that my addiction to perfection would make me miserable whereas having preferences would make life more pleasant. I finally realized that I couldn't change anyone but myself. I wasn't able to control a situation, but I could control my reaction to it. I insisted that Pat read the book, too, as he often became upset and raged at things he couldn't change. It took a while, but finally he agreed to read it. It did help him change his outlook a bit, which made life easier for all of us.

While I was working at *Visions*, Pat became the wife. He cooked my dinner and had it ready when I got home. Something I seldom did for him. That was nice, but sometimes I felt compelled to eat so I wouldn't hurt his feelings even if I weren't hungry. One night we worked until 10:00 p.m. and the company brought in McDonald's burgers and fries. I ate because I was hungry so of course I wasn't hungry at all when I got home. All I wanted to do was take a bath and get into bed. But Pat had been saving dinner for me and he blew up when I couldn't eat. It was funny and not funny at the same time. He needed to be working again, too.

Meanwhile, I was reading about New England. I thought we might change our lives and move there to become innkeepers, something I had been attracted to for a while. I was even ready to sign up for at a hotel management school.

I began renting wigs and I formed a little rental company, Allspice Enterprises, to cover both of my names - Sugar and Ginger. The movie business was changing. One of the changes was the studio no longer had Makeup or Hair Departments so we had to bring all our own supplies with us and were paid rental for our cases. .

Toward the end of May, Hal Lierly, at Paramount, offered me a television series about Robin Hood called, *When Things Were Rotten*. Mel Brooks was producer, so I knew it would be hilarious. Even though I didn't usually do television I was ready to consider anything. I spent the rest of the month day checking while I considered doing the series. Finally I called Hal and said, "Yes."

Chapter 38

WHEN THINGS WERE ROTTEN

The phone rang; it was Natalie Wood calling to ask if I could bring her some curlers. She now lived in a wonderful new house on Canon Drive, in Beverly Hills. I'd never seen this house before so when I arrived she gave me the grand tour. Her house was lovely, just as I expected. She always had great taste. It was like a huge New England cottage - exactly the kind of home I wanted for myself.

Her daughters, Natasha and Courtney, had an adorable little suite filled with toys, a tiny fireplace, and a room for the nanny, all in shades of pink. It was delightful. Natalie's bedroom was in the process of being redecorated. A soft material was put on the walls first - sort of a soundproofing. Next they "papered" with flowered sheets that were quilted. It was an unusual treatment that looked lovely and muffled sound. Lace curtains hung in the windows making the room so very charming. As always, her home was comfortable and welcoming.

Natalie invited me to have a glass of wine. While Natalie and I were sipping wine she told me she had seen Dianne, the little girl who had visited her so many years before. She said she was a beautiful woman and often came to see her at the Sherry Netherlands Hotel when Natalie was in New York City. She seemed to always know when she was there. Dianne had told her to tell me hello.

Soon after, Dianne called my union, hoping to get in touch with me. She left her number, but I didn't call back for a while. Finally we contacted each other and talked on the phone every once in a while. After a few months, Dianne asked if we could meet. It seemed to be the least I could do so I agreed. We decided to meet at the Daisy, a restaurant in Beverly Hills.

I requested a table in the patio so I could see her approach. I sat there waiting and waiting. I ordered and waited some more. Finally after a couple of hours she hadn't shown up so, almost relieved, I paid my check and left.

When I got home, the phone rang. It was Dianne in tears. Her car had been broken into and the police had held her up. She still wanted to see me. I told her I wasn't willing to drive all the way back to Beverly Hills, but she was welcome to come to the house.

Dianne arrived an hour later. She was dressed in expensive clothes and was nervous. She kept opening her purse and fixing her makeup. She was gorgeous! Almost as pretty as Natalie.

We sat and talked. She told me that her father had died and her mother never spoke to her. She had been married three times. In any case, she was quite wealthy, but alone and very unhappy.

We talked until it was very late. I sensed the total unhappiness of her life and, though I wanted to be a friend, I didn't feel there was much I could do to help. Maybe just listening was enough. I had the feeling that at some time in the future she might choose to end her life - she had already tried a few times. Before she left, I gave her a hug and told her I'd be there for her if she ever needed me. I never heard from her again.

Pat was working in Baton Rouge. I was happy he was getting a taste of the heat, humidity, and discomfort I'd had to endure on *Mandingo*. Eventually he called and apologized for not having listened to my distress when he was in Montana and I was suffering down there. I felt a bit wicked, hoping he'd get a good taste of Baton Rouge before coming home.

Laurie had gone off to West Virginia to make her way, but nothing had worked out. I called her and told her to come home. She seemed so grown up, but she was still too young to be on her own and I was happy to have her back with us.

By June the industry began to come alive. I was scheduled to begin my series *When Things Were Rotten* toward the end of the month, but Hal assigned me to do a movie of the week called *Please Standby* first. It was about the famous Orson Welles radio show, *Invasion of the Earth*, which caused quite an uproar when it was broadcast on the radio in the Thirties. Many people had believed it was true and that Martians really were invading the Earth. It was a great project to work on with period clothes and hairdos, plenty to keep me busy. It was a relief to get back to work and know that I even had another job waiting after this one.

By the weekend I was exhausted. I hadn't worked a full week for so long and the hours were horrendous. But in spite of the hours, the crew was great and I was having a wonderful time working in Pasadena. It still looked like the Thirties in many parts of town. We had to film at night but the weather was balmy and warm, the crew friendly and relaxed.

During the second week, Hal told me I'd be taken off the film early to begin my series. I really wanted to finish, I preferred to do period work. In the meantime, Patrick was upset with me (again) about our finances and how much we'd spent on Laurie's plane trips, our van, the plumber, my bathtub, child support for his kids, my ex failing to pay child support, and me just being me put a lot of pressure on him.

The day we worked at Twentieth Century Ranch in the valley, I felt so happy that I sang all the way to Agoura. The location was beautiful, and later I had time to talk with June Sampson, our script girl, who was a favorite of mine. We talked about what I was reading at the time. Kurt Vonnegut wrote that we are each born into a carass - a group of people that we have a special relationship with. When we discover these people, we tune into them. That resonated with me as I often felt that way in the business. When I'd meet certain people, I'd feel as if it was meant to be, we just clicked as if we'd known each other forever. Sometimes I felt lonely and then I'd go to work and feel much better. Pat and I were having a difficult time in our relationship.

There was a Nobb Hill party scene in the film and my old hairdresser friend, Sherry Wilson now a successful realtor, came to work for a couple of days to help out - something she did each year to keep up her membership in the union. Seeing her was a real treat. We had a wonderful nonstop talk day. Although it had been years since I'd seen her, it was as though we'd never parted.

Our wrap party was held in the dingy radio station set. There was no wine served so I didn't drink. I'd had a wonderful time on the show and the director, Joe Sargent, was great to work with, but the party was rather grim. I guess we were all just too tired to enjoy it. The next day I wrapped my equipment, feeling like I'd been on a drunk the night before even though I hadn't had anything to drink. Somehow I could always conjure up the energy to cope with a project, but as soon as it was finished I'd collapse.

The following day I went in to prepare for the series, *When Things Were Rotten*. Tommy Miller, the makeup man, and I would work together. We had a room on the stage for our Makeup and Hair Department. Since this would be our home, I brought in plants, pictures, and other things to make it nice. I was happy to be doing a series. None of our stars were well known so they all reported to our place which was easier than having to run from trailer to trailer. The series had a huge cast of characters and we were always busy. I wasn't going to have to diet on this project - I was going to work my ass off. All our actors and actresses played two parts in the series. It was a real challenge. The stories were pure Mel Brooks, outrageous and full of spoofs. We had three stages full of sets. There was Sherwood Forest, the interior of the castle, and the places where Robin and his merry men lived. We only went on location for one day.

Pat was getting calls from a producer about a film called *Sorcerer* to be directed by William Freidkin. He and Bill Fraker had tested for it, but for some reason they decided to hire an English cameraman, Dick Bush. However, they still wanted Pat as gaffer. Finally David Salvin, the producer, made Patrick an offer he couldn't refuse. The film would go to Tel Aviv, Paris, New York, and Ecuador (which later became the Dominican Republic) and Mexico. It would be at least six months of work and he'd have to go scouting for weeks. I was so excited and happy for him. So was he and, for a while, our life at home began to improve.

I was having a great time doing the series. We were there to make laughs and it rubbed off on everyone - with the exception of Tommy, the makeup man I worked with. He had seemed so nice and kind before. Maybe he was going through a change of life or something. Anyway he was falling apart. He was angry and resentful all the time. It was awful. One day I sat him down and told him it was no fun working around someone who was always being so negative. That helped a little.

One day I was sitting beside the set when a lamp fell and hit me on the head, knocking me out. I opened my eyes and the whole crew was staring at me. I was stunned and had no idea what had happened. My glasses had been knocked off so I started to look for them. I was a bit goofy, but my head didn't hurt too much. When I felt blood dripping from my scalp, I decided I'd better go to the hospital to be checked out. Tommy drove me home that night and picked me up the next morning. The "kind" production company had immediately hired another hairdresser just in case I was unable to make it the next day. It made me realize how easily replaceable we all were.

Our one day of location shooting was at Lake Sherwood. I realized then how much I missed moving around and the changes of going to various locations. Perhaps security wasn't really what I wanted. A paycheck, yes - security, maybe not.

Norman Steinberg was our producer. He was nice and I liked him a lot. He was always proposing to me and I kept turning him down. Pat and I were still at odds and I jokingly wondered if I ought to consider his proposal. I had begun to question if Pat and I were really meant for each other. I loved him, but it seemed like it wasn't going to work. Maybe it was that seven-year itch. He didn't seem to realize that because we were apart so much I'd grown independent out of necessity. He felt left out, but I couldn't just change everything when he came home.

One weekend we drove up to Pismo Beach and camped with some friends. There was lots of drinking on Pat's part, some fun and companionship, and lots of wind and sand. By the end of the weekend I was sure we loved each other, but not sure that we needed each other. We seemed to be going separate ways.

Patrick and Dave Salvin had taken a liking to each other and spent hours in search of the "good life" in bars and restaurants. Some nights, Patrick would arrive home in a limo, arms laden with pizza from an expensive restaurant. I often laughed at the situation, but our relationship was falling apart.

It was mid-September and the series just went on and on. Sometimes it seemed that the actors' egos were like yeast. They were rising and filling our makeup room and smothering me. I was tired of doing the series. Only two more weeks to go and I was ready to quit, but I wouldn't let Norman, our producer, down so close to the end. Tommy was suffering under the delusion that he was a nice guy. He was driving me nuts.

Special guests like Dudley Moore, Sid Caesar, and the English actor Marty Feldman did provide some bright spots. It was a real treat when Marty directed a segment. He was hilarious and as homely as could be with his huge eyes. His jealous wife was always on the set. It was as though she had to fend off all the women waiting to seduce him.

Finally, it was September 30, and the series ended. In tears, I told Norman I wouldn't be back if it was renewed. I realized working on a series wasn't my thing. He said, "Don't cry, Sugar. If I had a choice, I'd do films, too."

Hal needed me for a few days on *Won Ton Ton*, a story about a dog starring many old stars. We worked at the Harold Lloyd Estate where I'd worked on *Peeper*. John Agar, who had been so beautiful when he was young, was one of the actors. Time had really taken its toll on him.

I was moving into my own spiritual world. I had discovered Seth, the first channeled writings I ever read (by Jane Roberts). They made sense to me. I also read a book about EST with instructions about visualizing a safe place that was just mine. I pictured a brown-shingled house hidden away on a hill surrounded by giant pines and other trees. It had a huge fireplace and was furnished with plump, soft couches, chairs, window seats and a big bed covered with comforters. The house was full of plants and flowers. At night, I'd take off in my imagination, open the door to my secret place, and glide inside.

Chapter 39

HELTER SKELTER
1975

The year 1975 was a tough time for me. I had little to no work, too many debts, and most important, my relationship with Pat had fallen apart. What I really wanted was for Pat and me to go back to feeling the way we had when we first fell in love.

As I write this more than twenty-five years later, everything is so clear. Communication and work were the only answers, but at the time I didn't have a clue about how to get help. I hadn't even thought of a marriage counselor. I did begin to change, though. I knew I had to stop being Pat's mother. It wasn't entirely his fault. I'd fallen into that pattern. It was what I did best at work with the actors. By taking responsibility for myself, I began to pay attention to myself and my feelings, a new dynamic that made it easier to make other changes.

A good friend who had always been generous with his hugs began to get closer. We were in similar situations - having troubles at home. I loved it. So much fun, so romantic. I acted like a kid, but in reality I had never gone through that phase when I was young. This was sort of like the young lovers in the movies, only we weren't so young.

We were an unlikely couple and no one ever suspected a thing. Our romance was mainly a flirtation, but I imagined I was falling in love. I needed someone to love and needed to feel loved in return. I knew we'd never end up as a couple, and I didn't feel guilty either. I just went with how I felt, not what was "right". I had always believed God wanted us to be happy and it was up to each of us to search for our happiness. Obviously it wasn't as simple as that, but for the time being, this worked.

Having lived through *Helter Skelter* I knew the terrifying, true stories about Charles Manson, his "family", the girls he controlled, and the ritualistic murders of Sharon Tate and the La Biancas. Warner Brothers was bringing it to the screen as a movie of the week with Tom Gries as director. Kenny Chase was the makeup artist. I called and told him I'd love to work on the film if he needed a hairstylist - my friend was going to be working on it, too, and I wanted to be near him if possible.

In the meantime, I was doing tests at Paramount for the part Marthe Keller eventually played in *Black Sunday*, directed by John Frankenheimer. Pat was still going through the turmoil of *Sorcerer*. First Universal owned the project, then it was sold to Warner Brothers, then everyone on the crew was fired, and finally they were rehired by Universal. What a deal. Friedkin's demands were causing difficulties at the studio. Eventually everything was all set. Pat called the production The Good Ship Lollipop Pact.

Kenny called me to do the test for *Helter Skelter*. The production company hadn't planned on using a hairstylist. Since Charles Manson looked so awful, they figured they wouldn't need anyone to do his hair all the time. How stupid! They had no idea what a hairstylist did.

The morning of the test I met Steven Railsback, who was playing the part of Charles Manson. His piercing eyes were just like Manson's, but his hair was too short. There was no way I could make him look like the wild Manson without extra hair. I rushed out and bought a couple of cheap wigs and tried one on Steven's head, placing it a little back from the forehead. I combed his own hair over the front. Then I sprayed brown Streaks and Tips on his hair to make it the same color as the wig. The spray made his hair dull and completely changed his look. He actually looked like Manson and I had a job for the next six weeks.

Kenny was delighted because he didn't have to deal with the hair. Steve was delighted at the way he looked. He fell right into his part. I was able to get a sense of the power Manson exuded thanks to Steven's portrayal.

We began shooting in Lone Pine. Even though we weren't supposed to drive ourselves to location, I decided to drive my own car. I stopped at the beauty supply to pick up the things I needed and set off on the three and a half hour drive. Lone Pine was the location I'd enjoyed so much on *How the West Was Won* years before. But this time we had a much smaller crew. I checked into the Dow Villa and had a delicious dinner at the Merry Go Round. Kenny arrived later that evening.

I had never been a smoker. Tobacco hadn't tasted good to me when I was young and I simply saw no reason to smoke. I had never smoked a joint either, mainly for the same reason. Kenny thought I should get high at least once in my life and I finally agreed. I wanted to know what it felt like. So the next night after work I went to Kenny's room and tried, but I only succeeded in coughing and having a great desire to brush my teeth.

The weather was cold and windy and we ate sand all day. My eyes got a wind burn even with my glasses on. The plane that was to bring the actors was late because an actor quit and there was a mix-up. But aside from that, our first day went well. We worked in Independence where they had actually caught up with Manson. Everyone there was amazed at how much Steve looked and acted like Manson. It was almost scary.

Kenny called and invited me to dinner the next night. By the time we went to dinner he had finally taught me to get high. I held my nose, inhaled, closed my mouth, and eventually succeeded. Success. It was a nice feeling, but I remember not being able to finish a sentence, or so it seemed. I felt weird, but nobody else noticed any difference. I didn't get much sleep that night. The next morning we had to pack and check out of the hotel before work because we would leave for home at the end of the day.

Our actresses looked awful. They had sores all over their faces done by the makeup man. They looked so real and I laughed as the crew looked the girls over and then looked away in disgust. I sat in the jail cell on the top bunk where the "family" had actually been held. Our crew began to pull closer that day. I think it was because it was so eerie filming where the events really happened.

The drive home was beautiful, but I was exhausted and had to stop for coffee, candy bars, and finally to meditate. I made it home only to discover that Pat had been gone away somewhere all the time I'd been on location.

It wasn't a very good week. Roselle, Natalie's stand-in, called to tell me our friend, Tom Collins who had been my neighbor and like a part of our family had been killed in a helicopter crash. There was a twenty-gun salute at his funeral. He was so young. We had been so close. I was devastated.

Pat was about to leave to scout locations in the Dominican Republic. In the evenings before he left, he cooked romantic dinners, complete with candles, then he'd get upset about one thing or another and ruin all his efforts. Other nights he'd get drunk while cooking dinner and by the time I got home from work he'd be angry or resentful about something. It was an impossible situation.

At the same time, work was very emotional. We went to Silverlake, where the La Bianca murders had taken place. The neighbors were angry because the movie company had been given permission to work there. I couldn't blame them. Who would want to be reminded of those horrors?

Kenny and I had a little trailer for our Makeup and Hair Department. He had a rubber belly made for the actress who would get stabbed that night. It was sickening to think of the reality - watching him put it on her, knowing that the scene we would be filming had actually happened.

When we filmed the Sharon Tate murders, we went to a "set" house, not the actual location of the murders. In real life, six little girls lived in the house where we were shooting. I don't think anyone could have handled another "real" location right then. We worked in the Lincoln Heights jail and other locations including the homicide office with its bloody garbage can, bloody clothes, and clues galore.

Our courtroom scenes were wild. Steve really got into the part. In fact the first time he did the scene he was so wild his wig fell off. The cameraman wasn't prepared for his antics either. After that I put the wig on so tight I used dozens of rubber bands. I didn't want it to fall off again. Luckily, Steve didn't mind all the bands and pins.

We were getting ready to do the scene where all the Manson girls shaved their heads. The actresses had agreed to really shave their hair when they signed their contracts, even though it was only for one scene. This was in the days of long, straight hair and I felt sorry for them.

Kenny offered to do a test to see if we could just cut their hair short and put bald caps on. It was better than shaving everything off. I was so depressed actually in tears as I gave them their haircuts. I got lots of hugs that day after people saw how upset I was. We really had a great crew and Tom Gries, the director, was perfect. He knew how to keep us all going and he helped us feel like a family, which we needed during this film. Usually it was "only a movie," but this time it was real life.

One day Charles Bronson came by to visit Tom Gries. I made a huge mistake. I should have known better. Years before when I'd worked with Charlie on *This Property is Condemned* we had talked about when he was young and living around the coal mines. At the time I hadn't known what that kind of life was like. But since then I had lived in Amigo, near the coal mines and now I felt I understood. Cautiously I went up to where he was sitting and introduced myself. Charlie hardly looked at me. I continued talking anyway and told him I now understood what he had been talking about so long ago. It was weird and I should have known better. He never even looked up at me or acknowledged me. I was so embarrassed. I walked away wondering how I could have been so stupid, or he so rude. I had heard how he behaved, but had chosen not to believe it. But the rumors were true. He had become just like the parts he played so well.

We worked at the house of Vincent Buglosi, the author of *Helter Skelter*. He lived in a sweetly decorated tract house on which he had taken out a million-dollar insurance policy just in case the movie company messed things up. Smart man.

I was being considered for a film with Jane Fonda. I'd been contacted earlier, but the project kept getting postponed. I had no job offers in my future, *Helter Skelter* was about to come to an end, and so I accepted.

The last day of work on *Helter Skelter* was hot and miserable, fitting for that film. It was an endless day. We worked from five in the morning until midnight. It was the most gut wrenching and emotional project I'd ever worked on.

During the filming I had to go to court one day because my dog had prevented the mailman from delivering the mail. The dog wasn't mean; he just scared the postman and the neighbor called the police to report the incident. I pleaded guilty, paid my fine of fifteen dollars and left the court. It was strange. Here I was in court because of a silly dog, while some of the Manson family was still out of jail and free.

Our last get-together was the crew party at Malibu on a beautiful day. We had been through a deep and gut - wrenching experience. It was time for closure.

Chapter 40

MARATHON MAN

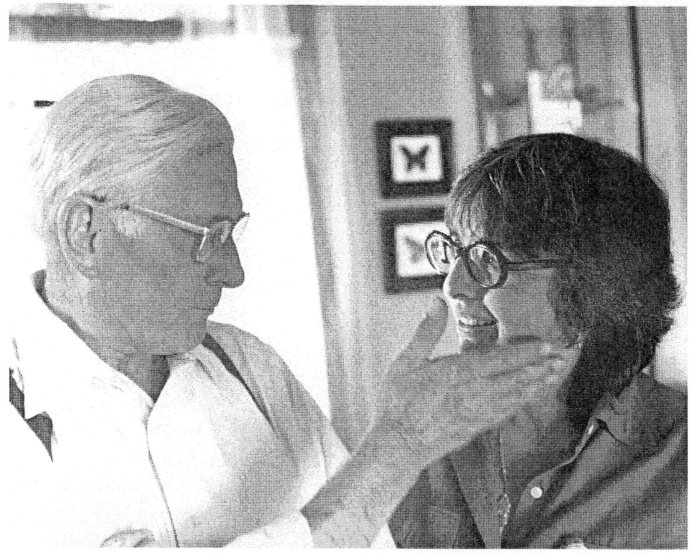

Ginger with Sir Laurence Olivier, *Marathon Man*

Reading had always provided me with a way to escape the "real world". At this point I wanted to escape my world with its traffic, smog, and, most of all, my unhappy relationship at home. I hungrily dived into books, losing myself in them whenever possible. I read Alan Watts who introduced me to a whole new spiritual world. I was getting an education about a life I never realized existed. Maybe this other world was where I belonged because, in my mind, the life I was presently living didn't seem to be working out so well.

Meanwhile I was still waiting to hear from Hal Polar, the unit manager on Jane Fonda's film. Finally he called and apologized. The studio now wanted another hairstylist for Jane. Hmm. Later I discovered that Sydney Guilleroff, who was designing her hair, had someone else in mind. I was disappointed, but knew that something better would come along.

It did. Ben Nye, Jr., the makeup artist on *Marathon Man*, being filmed at Paramount Studio, called in need of a hairstylist. Barbara Lorenz, who had started work on the film, had taken another project. He said it would be an eight-week job and I was happy to accept.

I encountered a couple of old friends from *This Property is Condemned* on this film - Howie Koch, Jr. now an assistant director and Bernie Pollack, a costumer. John Schlesinger was directing and Conrad Hall was the cameraman, both from *Day of the Locust*. Bernie and Howie had slimmed down since I'd last worked with them. They opened their coats to show me their flat bellies. I wasn't about to open mine and show them my rolls.

The fabulous thing about this job was that I was able to work with Sir Laurence Olivier! Just imagine. I'd admired him since I was fourteen and went to see him in *Hamlet* at the Stadium Theater on Pico Blvd. What a privilege it was to be in his company. Although he had been knighted, it didn't make him feel as though he was above anyone else. He was sweet, clever and so very charming. Before I was introduced to him, I was told not to shake his hand, as his skin was extremely delicate from some illness. Instead I gently patted his hand and he patted mine. His skin felt like satin.

The first day we worked in the Botanical Gardens in Pasadena. I had to put a wig on Olivier and it went just perfectly. On Christmas Eve we shot a scene where Olivier proceeds to cut his hair - actually his wig. He did it well, which was fortunate because I didn't have another wig. He was a real pro, but of course I already knew that. That scene only had to be shot only once.

The still photographer, Peter Sorel, wanted a haircut so he'd look nice for Christmas so he offered to take a photo of me with Sir Laurence in exchange. Later I received a beautiful picture of Sir Laurence reaching out to me. His writing on the photo has faded, but it said something like "What perfect molding." Wow!

Christmas came. I cooked and the whole family came over. It went well. Later that week Pat's friend, Timmy Griffith, came over for a few drinks. We got into a deep discussion about life and relationships. Timmy saw my relationship with Pat as one in which I had grown and Patrick hadn't. He told me I was trying to make Patrick change right along with me and it was throwing things out of balance. That sounded right to me, but I didn't know how to resolve it. I couldn't stop changing even if I wanted to. Perhaps Patrick had discovered me when I was in a period that appealed to him. But now I had changed. I was demanding more out of my relationships, and my life. No wonder he was upset. Taurus folks like things to remain the same and stable. Living with a Gemini made that impossible. It was helpful to see how an outsider viewed our relationship, but Pat didn't want anyone to know we were having troubles.

Work was thrilling. Just to be in Olivier's presence was enough, but we also had Dustin Hoffman with his own form of greatness. In one scene Dustin had to appear almost naked. He was uncomfortable about it so he used his humor to counter his discomfort. He proceeded to bring all sorts of surprises out of his jockey shorts, just like a magician.

Dustin had brought two women with him from New York - his hairstylist and makeup person. We called them the Salad Sisters. They were a couple of real characters. Being from New York, they weren't supposed to work on the set in California so I was their California standby. When I worked in New York, they had to pay a New Yorker to stand by for me, too. It was usually uncomfortable to be a standby because the actor really didn't want a stranger working on them.

Most memorable was the day of the scene everyone remembers from *Marathon Man*, where Olivier drilled Dustin's teeth and kept asking, "Is it safe?" Oh, it was awful. All day long we listened to the sound of the drill and it reminded us of what we feared most about the dentist. It was an intense, bizarre scene. Our director and cameraman were very intense folks, which added to our tension. At least I was aware that it was "only" a movie, not a true story like *Helter Skelter*. I could walk away at the end of the day and relax.

At the end of the film, Sir Laurence was supposed to fall down some mesh steps at the New York Water Department. The mesh steps were built on our set. They swayed back and forth when someone walked on them. My stomach got queasy and I hated going out there, but I had to touch up Olivier's hair. Olivier had a double that was a stunt man in the film named Len. I had bleached his hair white so he would look like Olivier. Actually he wasn't much younger than Olivier, but he was more fit and he also knew how to take a fall. Nevertheless, I was relieved when he finished the stunt safely.

One day Olivier saw me putting some gloss on my lips. "Oh, you're such a tart," he remarked. I bought him a bottle of wine and he was pleased. He told me how much he liked Natalie and Robert Wagner, who he called R.J. Whenever he came to town, they looked after him and always had him over to their home. Another day he describing what he loved to drink, he remarked, "A most comforting drink, Guinness Stout with a shot of good Irish Whiskey."

Toward the end of the film I asked Olivier what color he'd like to have his hair dyed when we finished. I wasn't there in the beginning so I didn't know his natural hair color. He surprised me by saying, "Make me look like Cary Grant. I'd like to be his color." I had no idea what color Cary Grant had been, but I thought maybe I could locate his makeup person and ask. No luck. Finally, using my own intuition, I picked a color and his hair turned out just fine. He was pleased. I couldn't understand why on earth someone like him would want to look like anybody else. I was sure he was just having fun with me and I was certainly having fun with him.

The last day arrived, the day when Olivier finished. I was very sad. Robert Evans came down to the stage to make a speech. I'd seen Robert Evans around the studio, but never had anything to do with him. He was a handsome man, a little over-tanned, his hair sort of greasy, and beautifully dressed. As Evans stood up and prepared to make his speech, the whole crew gathered around him. He called Sir Laurence up to where he was standing, praised him for his performance and a lifetime of work, and then he said, "Sir Laurence, in your country you are a knight, but in this country you are a king." I broke into tears. Bob Evans had touched my heart and I think he actually brought Olivier back to life, by putting him to work.

I wondered if Olivier would be able to make a film after *Marathon Man*. He was so weak that sometimes I worried about him. He had a scratch on the top of his head that just wouldn't heal. But he went on working for another ten years at least, traveling the whole world. I think it was because of the opportunity Robert Evans gave him to do *Marathon Man*. What a gift it was to be a part of that film.

Chapter 41

BLACK SUNDAY
1976

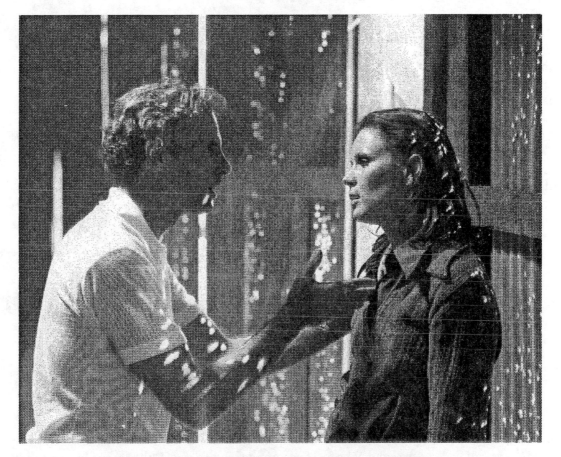

Bruce Dern and Marthe Keller, Black Sunday

February of 1976, I took off for Miami for a short location on *Black Sunday*. It was a film about terrorists with plans to blow up the Orange Bowl using a blimp as the weapon and starred Marthe Keller, Bruce Dern, Fritz Weaver, and Robert Shaw; it was directed by John Frankenheimer. John was a contrast to John Schlesinger, the short, round, dignified, English director of *Marathon Man*. Frankenheimer was all energy, tall and lanky, and always on the go. I liked them both. John Alonzo was our cameraman and my friend Don Merritt, the boom man, was working with us, too, which meant I'd have a pal to talk with on the set. Bob Dawn was the makeup man.

Marthe Keller, who had a small part in *Marathon Man*, was a lovely woman, very down to earth. She was from Switzerland and totally unimpressed with Hollywood. She liked acting, but just wasn't into the games that went on.

We reported to the Orange Bowl in Miami. The extras who were acting as CIA agents were supposed to arrive looking clean-cut, but they didn't, so I gave dozens of haircuts. Working in the stands, I went down line after line of men cutting hair. It was a short location, we wrapped by Saturday and I was home by Sunday. Production was set to start a few days later.

EST entered my life as I began reading a book on it. I was reminded that only one who controlled my life was me. I felt so heavy, that I decided to sign up for Schick to lose weight. They used a shock method that worked for smokers, so I thought it might help me with my eating. I was given instructions - bring all your favorite foods. So I brought all my favorite binge foods - Sees chocolates, Milky Way candy bars, those kinds of things to eat. My instructor told me to take a bite. Buzz. I'd get a slight shock. This was supposed to make my brain associate eating the candy with pain, rather than pleasure, making it easier to say "no". It worked for a while.

We resumed production and as soon as we went back to work I met Bruce Dern who appeared to be as strange as the parts he usually played. He wanted to change his image so asked me to watch his hair carefully. I wasn't sure what image he was changing to.

The Blimp base, south of Los Angeles was one of our locations. It was a long drive and took me an hour and a half to get home at night. I really loved the Blimp. I'd never seen one up close before. My friend Don jokingly said I had a crush on it. One day it was moving just behind me and I remarked, "It's following me. It likes me, too." One of the guys said it was the world's largest phallic symbol. Was that why I was so attracted?

One day Marthe and I were talking in her dressing room. She described what she felt made ordinary people artists at what they do. "It's their timing," she said. "Definitely their timing." She went on using Joe, Lizzie's limo driver who was working with us, as an example. "He knows when to talk and when to be silent. He is an artist."

Pat was still working on the *Sorcerer* project,

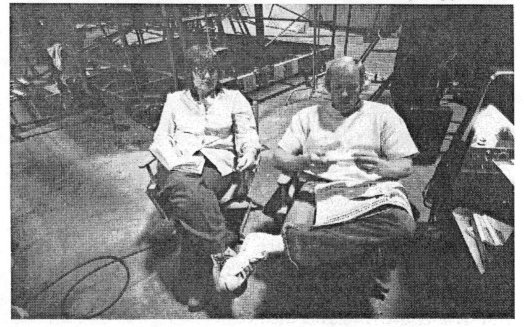

Ginger and Don Merritt on the set of *Black Sunday*

which seemed to go on and on. He was home often, working around the house, painting the front of our house white and Cape Cod blue. I was delighted with his artistic works.

When Marthe wasn't working, I didn't have much work, prompting Bob Dawn to remark that I was the highest-priced coffee maker around. I did make great coffee.

Trying to justify himself, Pat asked me if I'd ever had an affair and at first I denied it and denied it again. I felt uncomfortable telling a lie and I also felt sorry for him, so finally I admitted I'd had an affair. He went crazy. How could I do that to him? He himself had confessed that he had been untrue many times. Still, despite his numerous infidelities, he was unable to forgive me. He went on and on. I couldn't understand his double standard. He could have as many affairs as he wanted and it was okay. I had one and it was unforgivable?

Finally I said, "Go. When you leave for location in Israel, that's it, we're finished." He'd always imagined bedding a gorgeous Sabra, one of the Israeli girl soldiers. I told him, "You're free. I don't want to live the kind of life we're living now. I can't take it. Go find your Sabra."

He still wasn't ready to give up on me. He sent me two-dozen roses on the set, delivered to Marthe's room. I didn't even like roses that much. I might have felt differently about a spring bouquet. But the flowers became a hit in another way. Marthe loved them and when her ex, the father of her child, came to visit, he noticed the flowers and became quite jealous of Marthe's "admirer". She was thrilled and the roses did serve a purpose, if not what Patrick had intended.

He left for Israel and I was free. It was strange. For the first time in many years I could go where and when I pleased. The funny thing was I had no idea how to date and no real desire to either. Don and I would sit and discuss my situation. "Look, that young actor likes you a lot, Sugar. Why not him," he'd ask. "I don't really want to date. What would I say, how would I act? I prefer spending time with my friends and my kids." I replied. I wasn't in a hurry to make changes in my life. Being on my own was something I was enjoying.

We began to work in the harbor in San Pedro at night. It was very mysterious. We were taken in small boats to different places in the harbor. One foggy night I got a call that Frankenheimer wanted some of my good espresso coffee. I called back over the radio that I'd make it and they could pick it up in a few minutes. I was picked up in a boat and we putted somewhere in the fog. I got out of the boat and stepped onto a little pier. All of a sudden Frankenheimer appeared out of the fog, happily reaching for the thermos of coffee. Thanking me, he disappeared back into the fog. I must admit, it was an exciting adventure spending the night in the harbor. Each morning at daybreak I arrived home with cold feet; it took a long time to warm up before I could sleep.

One evening we worked on a huge freighter. Afterwards I had to climb a high wall with a ladder carrying my hair case. It was frightening and I was scared, but as I came to the top of the wall someone offered me a hand. What a relief! I made it. One evening Marthe got hurt on a speedboat so they sent us home early. They loaded us onto a boat and we all stood huddled together as if we were refugees sneaking over a border.

From time to time Dudley Moore would come by our set by for a haircut. He'd liked the cut I'd given him on *When Things Were Rotten*. Robert Shaw hadn't been particularly pleasant to me, or to anyone else for that matter. He was drinking pretty heavily. One day I was enjoying Dudley's company while giving him a haircut. Shaw walked up and asked Dudley why I was cutting his hair. Dudley explained that he liked the way I did it. Shaw was rather nice to me after that. I suppose that if another Englishman thought I was acceptable, I was okay.

One day Marthe was in disguise playing a nun. As I had nobody's hair to watch, I proceeded to give nearly the whole crew haircuts, nineteen in all. I kept the pile of hair I'd cut in a corner and by the end of the day it was huge.

With Patrick gone, my life at home was calm. I felt content and happy. On the weekends the girls and I would go to dinner at my favorite place, The French Cafe, at the corner of Sierra Highway and Soledad Canyon. They served delicious French food, home cooking, outstanding wine, and the prices were reasonable. I felt like I was in the French countryside when we ate there.

On the weekend I painted the kitchen light blue. Without all the tension, I found that I had plenty of energy to get all the things done around the house. I no longer felt tense and drained.

I decided to continue on my diet and of course told everyone. Frankenheimer picked up on it and watched me. Being a gourmet cook, he advised me to eat as he did. He was tall and thin, but his diet didn't seem to work for me and then I realized he never stopped moving. So I followed him around for a couple of days, moving my arms and legs like he did. Everyone on the set would laugh at us. As usual, I gave up. Frankenheimer lectured me and when I resisted he asked, "Well, why do you tell everyone if you don't want advice?" He was absolutely right.

Bruce Dern could be beastly at times. One day he totally embarrassed the second assistant's girlfriend. The assistant was leaving for the Philippines to work on *Apocalypse Now* and he was giving a goodbye speech. After he finished, Bruce walked up in front of the whole crew and presented the assistant's girlfriend with a dildo to use while her fellow was gone, totally embarrassing the woman. I was furious with Bruce and tried to stay as far from him as possible after that. I wondered how he could be so crude. In fact, not too long ago my youngest daughter, who is now a second assistant, met him and when he recognized her name, he mentioned that I had a very harsh mouth. Guess I made an impression on him. I'll also bet he never offered a woman a dildo in front of a crowd again.

At this time the newspapers were urging people to prepare for the coming earthquake - the big one. I bought into it and began to prepare. I bought plastic five gallon bottles for water, a transistor radio, and lots of canned goods, candles, flashlights, and batteries. I packed my favorite china pitcher so it wouldn't fall. I was as ready as I could be. That earthquake didn't happen until eighteen years later and fortunately I wasn't there.

Pat called from Israel. He said he missed me so much. He didn't really want a Sabra, but he wanted me. He asked if I would bring the girls and meet him in the Dominican Republic. I enthusiastically agreed. I hadn't really wanted to be apart from him, just away from the pain I was feeling about the failure of our relationship. I could forgive anything as long as we could grow together and move beyond the past.

Marthe was a great storyteller. She described a party she'd gone to in Hollywood where she met Warren Beatty. He had irked her and amused her at the same time, making a pass at her as though it was required of him. One weekend Marthe went to New York to meet Al Pacino who was thinking of casting her in a film. She had us in stitches. She is a tall woman and Al is a short man. She agreed to meet him at a restaurant figuring she could get there first and already be sitting when he arrived. And that way he wouldn't notice how tall she was. It worked for a while as they sat, talked and got to know a bit about each other. All of a sudden, Marthe spied Dustin Hoffman entering the restaurant. Dustin saw her immediately, but didn't see Al. Marthe (and many others) assumed Dustin and Al must be enemies. As gossip had it, they always were in competition for the same roles. Marthe tried to signal Dustin to go elsewhere, but he just headed straight for her table. As he reached the table, she realized that Dustin and Al had not actually met before so she introduced them. They sat down, happy to have the opportunity to get to know one another, amazed that they hadn't met before. Then trouble started. The phone next to Marthe rang. She picked it up and had to hand it to Al, but she didn't want to stand up all the way because then he'd see how tall she was. So she kept her knees bent, hoping he wouldn't notice. Seeing how awkwardly she was standing, Dustin asked her what the matter was. She laughed and finally stood straight up. She'd wanted to go to the bathroom for a long time. In fact, at the end of the meal she stood with her arms around both men, towering above them. She returned to Hollywood wondering if she'd get the part. She did. She even had a relationship with Al for a while. He didn't seem to care how tall she was after all.

We killed Marthe; it was so realistic I almost believed it was true. As she took leave for her home in Switzerland, she gave me her pet rabbit to take home and a beautiful antique tea set. I missed her.

They threw a fabulous wrap party on the set of the Israeli apartment. It felt like we were in a foreign country. At the party a wish of mine was granted. For years I'd passed by the window of a little storefront across from Paramount where someone had created a wonderful fantasy arrangement. There were dolls, unusual antiques, all sorts of fanciful things artfully arranged. Nothing was for sale; it was just a work of art. I was talking with an attractive young woman who introduced herself as Dora and after a while I discovered that she was the creator of the window. I told her how much I'd enjoyed her windows over the years and confessed I'd always wondered who created them. She told me the window displays were a labor of love.

That evening as I loaded all the books I had accumulated on the film into the car, John Frankenheimer came over and laughed when he noticed I had a copy of *Dr. Zhivago*. He told me that book was on a list of truly unreadable books. I felt relieved because I'd never been able to get very far into it no matter how hard I tried. As I hugged Frankenheimer, he said it wouldn't be fifteen years before we worked together again. It wasn't, more than twenty years have passed.

Chapter 42

SORCERER

With hope in my heart and understandably nervous, I agreed to take Pat up on his invitation to join him in the Dominican Republic. Would it work? I wasn't sure. Pat sounded sincere so Laurie, Tanya, Xochi, and Flump, our little Benji-like dog (who was too attached to me to be left at home) all decided we'd make the trip. All punctured with shots, I readied the garden for our absence. My banjo teacher offered to watch the house and tend to our other animals. Finally there was no turning back. We were on our way.

On May 19, we packed everything into the car (eleven bags plus carryon bags and Flump our little dog in her carrier) and drove to my mother's house in Los Angeles and left the car. From there we caught a bus to the airport. It was a night flight and I hoped to get some sleep on the flight to New York, but I was so nervous that sleep was impossible.

We arrived in New York at dawn and I took Flump for a walk before re-boarding her. Groggy, we sat around in the airport until 8:00 a.m. when we boarded the next flight that took us to the Dominican Republic. Full of babies and families of various sizes, the flight was noisy and fun.

Wild, colorful, noisy and hot, Santa Domingo slapped us in the face with heat and humidity. As we left the plane, sweat began to roll down my face and body. The luggage door got stuck and we had to wait and wait. I was worried about Flump, but she arrived seemingly unscathed.

As soon as we passed through customs, there was Patrick, looking terrific - tanned, healthy and seemingly cool despite the heat. He hugged and kissed me, then the girls got their hugs and kisses and he introduced us to Julio, his driver, who took care of our luggage. The crew was staying at the Jaragua, an older hotel. Pat in preparation for our arrival had stocked our rooms and the kitchen with everything we could possibly need. Exhausted, the kids and I fell asleep immediately.

After a couple of days in the crowded room, we realized we'd be much better off in an apartment. I was introduced to Toni who worked with the company and together we set off on an apartment hunt. I hadn't yet adjusted to being in the heat; if I was left alone for more than five minutes I fell asleep. It was embarrassing. I hoped that habit would pass quickly.

We searched, but it was very hot so we decided to take a day off and visit the beach as well as an unusual area called Tres Ojos (three eyes), a cool grotto with beautiful caves and pools of water. Later we swam in the hotel pool, had drinks with our friends, Punky and Flossie Grosso, and then went to Vesuvius for a delicious Italian dinner. A pitch-black hairpiece perched on the head of the little violinist who serenaded our table. His music was lovely, but I always found myself looking at his hair, doing my best not to laugh.

I had decided to wear higher shoes to give an illusion of slenderness, but Pat, who liked me short asked, "Why are you wearing those?" When I told him he said, "You could be a little less wide, but please no taller." So much for that idea.

One day I was out walking with another new friend, Jose, when he pointed out an apartment. Toni, my other friend, had mentioned that one, too. I looked at it and found that it was perfect - close to the hotel, furnished, lots of plants, and only a block away from Toni's place. Toni negotiated the price and soon we were happily ensconced in our own home. What a relief to have more than one room. We didn't have a television set, but since everyone on television spoke Spanish, it didn't matter. The girls diligently took up reading and have been avid readers ever since.

While living at the hotel, we learned from experience, to always carry a flashlight at all times because the electricity went out almost every night. Santa Domingo had been overbuilt and it was impossible to meet everyone's electricity needs. Luckily our new apartment was located in the same area as the president's home so we had no trouble. The president never went without lights. We had a veritable league of nations living in our building. One couple had come from the Simi Valley near where we lived. Others tenants were from Israel and Japan, there was even a belly dancer.

A woman gave ballet exercises at Toni's house twice a week and I signed up. I exercised until even the tops of my hands were sweaty; sure it was helping me lose weight. We needed to hire a housekeeper. Short, stocky Juanita arrived. We hired her and she did the cooking and washing and cleaning. She was happy to have a small room behind the kitchen that had been especially built for the maid.

I wasn't working, but I did give the crew haircuts from time to time. It helped me feel productive. I didn't have to feel too guilty, though, because the crew wasn't working that hard either. Shopping at the huge bustling downtown main market was quite an experience. It was filled with hundreds of people jostling about and we had to push our way to the counters to fill our bags. All the food was so fresh. One day I drank a delicious pineapple, fresh milk, ice, and sugar drink that was so good I bought a blender so we could make those at home.

Gulf and Western, who owned much of the country, had a very interesting arrangement with the film company. They paid soldiers to do whatever needed to be done and even had a General to manage things. It cost a lot of money to keep things going their way, but in a country where pay offs seem to be the custom, it all worked out. We were always aware of the armed military everywhere we went.

I developed a perfect routine for myself. Upon awakening in my air-conditioned room, I'd drink a couple of cups of strong Dominican coffee. I'd then sit in bed and read. Finally I'd get up and the kids and I would walk to the hotel to visit with friends and sit around the pool. While the kids swam and played, I sipped El Presidente beer, the best beer I'd ever tasted. Later I'd stroll home for a siesta and I'd be ready to go out for dinner when Patrick arrived home. As close to paradise as I'd ever been.

Patrick's routine was less relaxing. He'd arrive home, his shoes covered in pig shit, which was everywhere in the awful little village where they were working. It was supposed to be the pits, a kind of hell. It certainly looked and smelled that way. Roy Scheider, Amidou, and Bruno Cremer were the stars in *Sorcerer*, a remake of a suspenseful film called *The Wages of Fear* in which stranded men respond to a call to drive a truck full of nitroglycerin into the jungle to put out an oil well fire.

Early one morning we all went to the set leaving Flump home with the maid. We didn't want to take her to that smelly village. That night, Flump was missing. I was heartbroken and frightened for her too. How would we ever be able to find her in that huge city? Through the grapevine Juanita found out that Flump was at the ex-president's home. We called and sure enough, she was there. They gave her back, although they would have liked to keep her. Her bangs had been cut so she could see better, but I didn't care as long as she was safe.

The morning after Flump was found, I got ready for my exercise class and promptly walked right through the sliding glass door that led to the patio. Normally it was left open, but the night before I had closed it so Flump wouldn't run off again and then forgot I'd done that. The door wasn't made of safety glass so all the glass crashed to the floor. When I withdrew my leg, I could see that I'd cut it wide open. I could see the yellow fat around my knee. Scared wasn't the word for how I felt. I was terrified. I screamed so loud that I frightened the whole family. Pat came running down the stairs wrapped in a towel (he'd been sitting on the pot). Then Laurie arrived wrapped in a blanket, she'd been asleep. We were all frightened. Someone got a towel and wrapped it around my leg. Fortunately, there wasn't too much blood for such a dramatic wound. Laurie ran to get Toni who came right over with a woman whose husband ran a medical clinic. I was in shock at this point and didn't feel any pain yet. They rushed me to the hospital

Laurie, Toni, the lady, and I all took off in Toni's Volkswagen Bug. Patrick would have come, but I told him to go to work, I'd be okay. He was relieved. We hurried as best we could through the traffic to the clinic. Frightened, I was crying softly and didn't want to look at my leg. We pulled into the clinic and immediately I was loaded onto a gurney. Everyone was speaking Spanish, so I didn't understand much of what was being said. Soon I was rolling down the hall to the operating room looking up at the lights on the ceiling. I was reminded of the film *Seconds* in which Rock Hudson changed from an older man to Rock to escape his whole life. In one scene, the cameraman had made a shot from Rock Hudson's point of view while he was lying on the gurney looking at the ceiling as he was being rolled into the operating room. Funny how my mind turned to movies in the middle of such mayhem.

Lying on the operating table, scared and frightened, I kept crying and crying softly. Finally I was given a shot of Demerol so I could relax. Just as the doctor began to sew up my leg, the lights went out, and the electricity went off. Not unusual for Santa Domingo. The doctor was undeterred and kept stitching. Fortunately for me, the doctor was a plastic surgeon; he was taking tiny little stitches and it seemed to take forever. When he finished, I asked how many stitches I had. He answered, "Muchos." I had to laugh.

My leg was bandaged and a plaster cast was put on the back of it so I couldn't bend it. They were finished. I was given pain pills and sent home. I'd never experienced anything so traumatic. I was wiped out and immediately went to bed. I took the pain pills, afraid the pain might be too much, but it wasn't that bad. In a couple of days, I was able to walk to dinner with my family.

About two days after my accident, Ben Nye, Jr., the makeup artist, came by to see me. "Hi Crash - why didn't you get Polaroids for me?" "Sure, that's all I'd been thinking about at the time." Ben asked if he could at least take a photo. I agreed. Later we all went out for pizza and afterwards tried to find some ice cream, but the electricity had been out for quite a while, so there was none available.

A few days later Toni took me back to the doctor who was pleased with my progress. He was so gentle and wonderful that I imagined writing a story in which the patient falls in love with her doctor and remains in the distant country rather than return home with her husband. That's what was nice about considering myself a writer. I could embellish my own experiences.

I received a call through the production office from Bob Dawn, the makeup artist on *Black Sunday*. I tried to call him back, but his phone was out of order. When we finally connected, he asked me to come work in the British Virgin Islands. They weren't far from the Dominican Republic and the company could save money on my flight. I was to dye Robert Shaw's hair for the second unit of *The Deep*. It sounded perfect and by the time he needed me, my leg would be healed.

After the doctor took the stitches out, I noticed that I had inadvertently been given a "leg lift" - on one leg only. It looked odd, one young leg and one old leg. Pat announced that he'd pay for the surgery I'd had for my birthday present. What a generous man. The total bill was $250 plus the doctor's fee of $100, a real bargain for a plastic surgeon.

Walking home from Toni's house, I met a little man gathering plants someone had thrown out into the street. I began to talk with him, pleased to use my Spanish. He followed me home and planted the plants in my yard. Each morning, he'd show up and create a job he could do for me. Sometimes he'd come with a sad story like needing money to take the bus to visit a sick relative or some such problem that could be solved with a small amount of money. I always gave it to him. "Do you consider yourself the local social security office?" Pat asked. It was hard for me to turn down people in need when we had plenty.

Evenings were great fun. Pat usually came home early and we'd go here and there for drinks and dinner. One of my favorites was the New Santa Domingo Hotel that was decorated in a tropical theme. Huge ceiling fans circulated the air, the table linen was starched and white, drinks were decorated with tropical fruits, filmy curtains billowed in the breeze.

William Freidkin, *Sorcerer's* director, was sick and we took advantage of Pat's time off to walk around the city together. We looked at the Dominican rocking chairs wondering how we could import them to sell at home. One day while we were browsing in a jewelry store, a woman came up to me begging for money. Though I refused she wouldn't leave me alone, she followed me from store to store. Finally, in frustration I yelled, "Get away, leave me alone. I don't have enough to feed the whole world." In truth I felt bad. I would have loved to help everyone and I couldn't. She brought up my feelings of helplessness and I overreacted.

Toni became a great friend. She had worked with the whole crew and said she felt Pat was the only nice American there. He understood he was working in an undeveloped country and he dealt with the people from that perspective. She felt I had a Latin temperament because I was emotional. Most Dominicans felt that Americans had a harsh attitude.

A few days later Pat arrived home covered with bandages. He'd tried to save a little boy from being crushed by a falling sign and had taken the brunt of the blow himself. Now it was my turn to take care of him.

The biggest storms with lightening and thunder crashing right above us often happened at night. There was cement surrounding our apartment and the rain pounding on it echoed loudly. It was overwhelming and then in an instant the storm would be over.

I celebrated my forty-second birthday. Toni and some friends arrived with a birthday cake and they sang "Happy Birthday" in English and kissed me. Pat arrived home late and gave me my present, the $350 to pay the bill for my leg.

We had a long weekend so the crew and their families decided to get acquainted with the island and take a trip to the famous Porta Plata on the island's other coast. We all piled into the bus loaded with beer and food. It felt great getting away, escaping the city. The countryside was lush and green dotted with little shacks. Bananas and mangos hung ready for the picking from trees. Children played outside and the washing was hung from lines strung from tree to tree.

The people were friendly and waved as we passed by. People here were obviously poor, but I thought it must be less harsh being poor out in the country than in the city.

We had only one problem. Bathrooms were nonexistent and I had to go so bad it became impossible to enjoy the scenery. We stopped at one place and asked if they had a bathroom. They pointed to a door that, as it turned out, led out the back of the store. Eventually we realized we'd have to use the bushes.

The beach at Porta Plata was lovely, clean and inviting, much nicer than Santa Domingo. I wasn't ready to dip my leg in the ocean so I sat and watched the kids. Someone stepped on a sea urchin and got the spines stuck in their foot. It was very painful. We returned home that night around 9:00 p.m. thoroughly exhausted, but happy to have seen more of the island. Much of it was under development. Now I could understand why. It was so lush.

It was June 23, three weeks after I'd walked through the window. My leg was healing well. I massaged it twice a day with vitamin E, but I was still uneasy about exposing the cut. Even though it wasn't painful, it looked awful. That day I began taking KH3 or Gerivital, a vitamin B complex with procaine. I'd always wanted to try it, but it wasn't available in the States. It soon made a huge difference in my life. For years I'd been allergic to the sun, but KH3 eventually enabled me to enjoy the sun without the itchy after effects.

That day I went back to the exercise class that was now filled with wives from the film company. I carefully did my exercises, happy to be back. After class we all went to the hotel and I had a couple of my favorite El Presidente beers.

I received confirmation about work on *The Deep*. Bob Dawn was flying his own plane to Tortola. I called George Justin, the unit manager, to check in and ask about the project. He wanted me to make sure Bob had Nick Nolte's double's wig and also told me Jacqueline Bisset would be in the film and they had a diving double for her who was a very close match. Her name was Jackie also. She lived on Virgin Gorda, a nearby island. I was to take care of her hair on the second unit.

As it usually happened on location, Pat and I always attracted everyone to our home. People would drop by for dinner unannounced. Our maid had invited a cousin to visit and later asked if she could live there, too. I said it was fine, but there would be no extra pay. Now we had two maids. What luxury.

I got my British Visa and the reservations that would take me through Puerto Rico and on to Tortola in the British Virgin Islands. We'd be shooting and staying on Peter Island which was only accessible by boat. By this time, Laurie had enough of island life. She was ready to go home. We both left the same day; Laurie for home, me for location. She was such an orderly person; the chaos that surrounded our lives on the island had gotten to her. On June 30 we both took a taxi to the airport. I kissed her good bye at her gate, in tears and then I set off to find my plane to Puerto Rico.

Chapter 43
THE DEEP

Always worried that I might miss my plane, I rushed through customs in Puerto Rico. I hurried down the ramp looking for my gate to the British Virgin Islands. It wasn't well - marked and it wasn't a busy gate. I understood why when I saw our plane only held six passengers. I had to laugh as our pilot gave us the same spiel stewardesses give on big planes. He was very serious about it. Afterwards he climbed into the cockpit, closed his door, and we were in the air in no time. It was all in miniature.

The two passengers sitting in front of me were teenagers off to a summer class on a boat in Tortola. They were anxious and kept glancing back and forth at each other as we flew low over the water. The pilot explained that the things sticking out of the water below us were the tops of sunken mountains.

We circled Tortola, the capital of the largest British Virgin Island before landing. Bob Dawn and his family were already there having flown from California in his own plane. The production assistant came to meet me and a camp counselor met the teens.

My luggage was picked up and loaded into an open-air bus. We sped through the countryside past lush foliage, bright flowers, and pretty white cottages, the striped canvas roof of our bus flying in the breeze. Much classier than the Dominican Republic.

To catch the boat to Peter Island we pulled up to the pier where Bob was waiting for me with his wife Joan and his seventeen-year-old daughter Lisa, both of whom were very attractive. I asked him about his flight and he replied that it was exciting and quite an accomplishment for him in his little plane. I could sense the girls were glad to have landed.

The water taxi wasn't ready to leave so we wandered over to a local cafe and had a couple of rum punches. "Might as well enjoy" was my motto. This was one of the most beautiful islands I'd ever seen. I found the British - settled islands clean and lovely, the people so friendly and there was no language barrier.

We climbed onto the boat, stowed our luggage, and off we went bouncing over the waves. It took only half an hour to reach Peter Island - another piece of paradise. The resort, which was owned by a Scandinavian corporation, was the only hotel on the island. The main building, with its many windows, housed the office, the dining and gathering areas. The pool area was artfully landscaped with lush flowers, bright striped awnings, and bamboo chairs curved around the outdoor bar overlooking the ocean. Our rooms, for which the tariff was $400 a day, were set at different levels up the hill with a view from each window. I invited Lisa to share my rooms so Bob and Joan could have some privacy.

We always worked very hard on location when we were in production. I had learned to take full advantage of what was being offered during my free time. One day I took a run on the beach. By now my leg felt fine, although it was a bit disfigured. On the second day I took a speedboat ride to Tortola to do a bit of shopping. Bouncing over rough seas was fun. That day I met a native man who assured me that he liked Americans and was happy to have us there. This was at a time when anti-American sentiment was prevalent in the Caribbean Islands and it was nice to be accepted.

It felt good to be on my own again. I had escaped my problems and I had the freedom to be whoever I wanted to be. I didn't have to live up to Pat's expectations. I realized that I never would. Nobody is perfect, nor can we always please others. I think it's good, on occasion, for each of us to get away from everyone who knows us.

The hotel had a little beauty shop. No one ever used it so I decided to open the shop for myself. Some supplies were already there, but I had to go to Tortola for other things like rubber gloves for dying hair and wig blocks. By the time I returned, the employees had noticed that the shop was open and curiosity brought them in. Normally they had only been able to get a haircut when the traveling barber came by boat, once every two or three months. The first day I gave four haircuts. I was appreciated and my price was right. Free. Later, Lisa and I played tennis, showered, and joined Bob and Joan for dinner. Afterward we sat at the outside bar watching the dancers and listening to the music. I had a few tinges of guilt enjoying this luscious place alone.

The next day I actually did some work. We had a wig for Jackie, Jacqueline Bisset's double who lived on Virgin Gorda right near Peter Island. The doubles own hair looked pretty close to what Jacqueline Bisset's own hair looked like so I dyed her hair to match the double wig that had been sent. I figured it would be good not to have to use the double wig if possible. Seeing as the "real" Jackie hadn't arrived yet I figured it must be the color we needed to have. It matched perfectly which was fortunate. I was so very lucky to be able to find the right products to do my work. After all, here I was out in the middle of the ocean. It wasn't downtown Hollywood by any means.

My next project was unusual and a real challenge. All the underwater crew were great looking men. The divers, all in good shape, looked just fabulous in the little trunks they wore to work underwater. One fellow, named Jack, had been chosen as Nick Nolte's double. He looked very much like Nick with one exception. Jack had hair on his chest while Nick's chest was bare. I asked Jack if I could shave his chest and he said he'd rather not. "Okay, I'll try and bleach it and see what happens," Thinking to myself, I thought that maybe the camera wouldn't pick the hair up if it was bleached a light blonde.

Big, tall, handsome Jack strolled into the beauty shop, took off his shirt, and bared his chest. We giggled as I mixed the bleach, put a towel on his lap, and slathered the bleach all over his chest. We laughed some more and, Ron Talsky, the wardrobe man, poked his head in to see what was going on and he began to laugh, too.

I waited forty-five minutes then washed the bleach off. No change whatsoever. So I reapplied the bleach and we sat and waited another forty-five minutes. There was only a slight glint of gold to the hair. We decided to give up bleaching and wait to see what was really necessary. After all, Nick would be wearing a wet suit most of the time. If the hair really became a problem, we would shave Jack's chest on the spot.

The food on Peter Island was superb. Each night there were two entrees to choose from such as prime rib, fresh salmon, and lobster and numerous choices of everything else, including desserts. It was a welcome change from my Dominican diet, which included lots of rice and beans.

July 4, 1976 was the Bicentennial and here I was on English soil along with all the other Americans in the crew. Our company had planned to work, but the water was too rough so we had the day off instead. By this time Peter Yates, the director, had arrived and so had Jacqueline Bisset and Nick Nolte. They partied right along with us. Nick personified the ultimate beach boy and Jacqueline was the charming English woman. Our crew was now complete.

That holiday we all played instead of working, not that I'd been working much anyway. I went to the beach and swam and played in the surf with the chef's little son. Then I sat at the bar and drank rum punches with the crew and later took a siesta. After a shower I was ready at 6:00 p.m. for our Bicentennial celebration on the beach over the hill. I thought it was just great that the British were giving us a celebration for our independence from them. It turned out to be quite a party with fireworks shooting out over the ocean. For a desert they had made a huge cake decorated to look like an American flag.

Amidst all the commotion I heard someone calling, "Sugar, come to the bar." I jumped up and walked over to the bar. To my amazement, I was handed a phone. Who was calling me here in the middle of a beach party? I picked up the phone and there was Patrick on the other end wishing me a happy holiday. Great surprise! At 10:00 p.m. the party ended so we adjourned to the bar to dance and have a few more drinks. It was an amazing evening.

Each morning I awoke to the sound of a deep, native voice singing a lovely song. The man who cleaned the pool would be right below my room. His joyful sounds made me smile with pleasure, reminding me how fortunate I was to be here.

Jacqueline Bisset was amazing. I'd met her many years before when Pat was doing *Grasshopper* in Las Vegas. She remembered that we'd been planning to go to the farm and asked me how it was going. What a memory! One day while walking together she told me about her life in England when she was growing up. She always loved the outdoors and was very happy on the island. I don't think I'd ever met an actress with such warmth. I was surprised that she had remembered us. Most people in the film business are wrapped up in their own dramas. I was impressed.

Nick Nolte was a beauty. I'd seen him in the television show *Rich Man, Poor Man*. Upon meeting him, I saw a surfer, a happy-go-lucky kind of guy. He was sort of crazy too, in a nice way, Sometimes he'd stay up for days at a time. Years later I worked with him again on *Who'll Stop the Rain* and he was very different. Then I got it. He lived each part. *The Deep* called for him to be an attractive beach boy and he certainly was.

Robert Shaw was there, too, but not at the resort with the rest of us. The company had put him up in a hotel in Tortola. He had quit drinking by then, but the company wasn't taking any chances. They wanted to keep him away from the party atmosphere of our resort. Shaw's family was there. His new wife was trying to protect him from himself. He had changed since the *Black Sunday* days. I remembered I'd jokingly said to him, "Take me with you to the Caribbean when you do *The Deep*" and here I was. I cut and dyed his hair. He was charming and wonderful, so different from when he had been drinking. Location on *The Deep* was an interesting process, unlike any I'd ever experienced. Moby, who ran a tugboat out of Miami called *Moby II* (I don't know what happened to *Moby I*), captained our home base on the water. The *Moby II* was crewed by some young boys during the summer. I became immediate friends with them, especially James who was sixteen and Mike who was twenty-one. Pat was always sure I had a thing for younger men.

Our daily routine went like this: First Moby went out in the tugboat and anchored it above the wreck of the ship called the Rhone, just off Salt Island. When he was all set, he radioed us and we set out in a speedboat that transported us to the location. We pulled up right alongside *Moby II* and transferred ourselves and all our supplies for the day to the tugboat. It was very easy for all those long-legged guys to climb onto the deck of the tugboat, but for me it was a different story. It was scary and difficult. My legs were too short and not being the picture of grace, I'd take a leap as the boats came together. Inevitably as I stepped onto the tugboat my foot would hit one of the air tanks and it would start squealing, or I'd manage some equally embarrassing incident.

Finally, Moby noticed my predicament. He was about 5'5", 250 pounds and all muscle. He reached out his hand as I began to climb on the boat and once he had hold of my hand I knew I was safe. I was truly grateful for this.

Everyone's diving equipment was stowed on the boat and while all the divers were getting ready to dive I'd pin up Jackie's (the double) hair and put on her wig. They had decided to use the wig for some reason. I put it on very securely because no way was I going to stand by underwater.

Filming underwater was a unique operation. The script girl who wrote scene numbers on a slate with a wax pencil especially impressed me. Al Fleming, who headed the divers, directed the second unit for Peter. Guess Peter wasn't about to dive either. Al and Peter would discuss the upcoming day's work then Al would descend into the "deep" to direct it. A day or so later Peter would see the dailies and could make changes if necessary.

Off the end of the boat was a launching platform with a ladder leading into the water. That's where I sat while they filmed underwater. At night the crew surfaced slowly. They had to sit on a rope suspended beneath the boat for a while to decompress. We played music like "Thus Spake Zarasthustra" the theme from *2001*, while they perched on a long rope and waited to emerge from the sea. I couldn't really see the wreck of the Rhone, only its shadowy image. A replica was being built inside a huge tank in Bermuda where most of the shooting would take place.

Some days the ocean was quite rough. Luckily I never got seasick. I decided all the B vitamins I was taking helped and suggested the crew boys try it because many of them suffered from seasickness.

Around noon a boat would arrive with our lunch, catered by the hotel. One day we had spaghetti and I amused myself by throwing leftover spaghetti to the seagulls. They screamed and dived and it was comical as they tried to retrieve the spaghetti in the air before it fell into the water. Did they think it was alive?

After watching all the talented divers for a few days I finally decided to learn to snorkel. On my next day off I went into Tortola and bought fins, a mask, and a snorkel. I even ordered prescription lenses to go inside the mask. The next day, totally excited, I took my paraphernalia with me to the boat. After I put the wig on Jackie and everyone was below filming, I climbed down to the loading platform, put the fins on, and slipped on the mask. James coached me with the snorkel. Down the ladder I went, slipping into the ocean. I had no fear of sinking. It's difficult for round people to dive and they have to wear weights to stay down.

As I began to drift from the boat it occurred to me that I wasn't much of a swimmer. So I made my way back toward the platform where I could see the shadowy Rhone beneath the boat. I smiled and my mask immediately filled with water. James laughed and I soon learned not to express my emotions under the water. James pointed out a huge barracuda that was watching the shoot each day from beneath our boat. He mentioned they liked gold, shiny things like the necklace I was wearing. I quickly scrambled out of the water and took off my jewelry.

After that experience, I decided I'd better practice my snorkeling in the pool at the hotel. That night as we sat around the bar I put on my fins and began to walk toward the pool. It was difficult walking in the fins and the divers all laughed. "Walk backwards or put the fins on by the pool," they advised. I should have been able to figure that out for myself, but I had lots to learn. In the film business we often have experts working with us. They always make things look so easy. These divers were no exception.

Bob Dawn, the makeup man, was making me uncomfortable. I didn't know what had happened to him since working with him on *Black Sunday*. He was different. It almost seemed like he'd had a little stroke or something. He just wasn't on top of things like before. For example, he ordered Nick Nolte's double a wig, but hadn't thought to order a bit lighter color, which he should have because when hair gets wet it looks darker. After the first day's shooting the producers saw the dailies and didn't like the way the hair looked. It was synthetic hair and they felt didn't move right. Bob should have realized synthetic hair wouldn't work well in water. He was such a talented artist. Something was definitely wrong. I got on the phone and called Ziggy, our wig maker in Los Angeles, to explain our predicament. A few days later a wig made of real hair arrived and I relaxed.

I made another friend, Denny, who manned the boat that took us to Moby each morning. Every evening Denny entertained us with stories of his sea adventures. His family now lived in South Carolina because he wanted them to live in a nicer place than Miami. At the end of each job he went home to them. I also became good friends with the kids on the boat. One evening they invited me to the boat for a dinner of hamburgers and French fries. It sure tasted good; it had been months since I had eaten "real" American food. I invited Moby to come and stay with us in Santo Domingo on his way home after the shoot. They needed to stop in the Dominican Republic anyway. The kids could stay with us.

One day there was an emergency call at sea. We weren't shooting so Moby and his crew rushed out, found the boat, and saved the crew just before it sank.

My two weeks passed in a whirl and before I knew it the British hairstylist who was set to do the film arrived from England. She hadn't been able to finish her last film in time for the second unit, which is why I'd been called in. I had hoped I might be able to stay on the production, too, but it wasn't to be. I was lucky to have been in this paradise at all. Bermuda would have been nice, though.

My final workday was July 15, but I got a reprieve because there were no planes leaving for three days. So, although unpaid, I enjoyed three more days in paradise.

As I waited to board the boat that would take me to Tortola, I bid goodbye to my friends from the *Moby II*, nearly in tears, even though they would be visiting us on their way home. When the boat arrived to take us to Tortola, Nick Nolte, having been up for days, staggered off, dressed in a tee shirt on backwards and drawstring pants. He was so funny my tears just disappeared and I left in fine shape. Along with me part of the crew was also leaving, on their way to Bermuda to prepare for the rest of the crew to arrive. I felt better that I wasn't the only one leaving.

We arrived in Puerto Rico without a hitch, but they hadn't allowed time for US customs so I missed my plane to the Dominican Republic. The timing couldn't have been worse. It was Carnival in Santo Domingo and everyone was heading there. I sat anxiously in the waiting room, jumping up every time an announcement was made in Spanish. I drove the desk clerk crazy asking what had been said. Finally he told me, "Lady, just go back and sit down. We'll let you know when your plane is ready." But I was still paranoid about missing my flight. I was afraid I'd fall asleep and miss it again.

Finally I made the flight and took a taxi to our apartment. We now had three maids whom Pat called the three brooms. Only broom number one, Juanita, was there when I arrived. She told me Pat was upstairs in bed. I'd taken my pay, $2,000 in cash and I planned to sprinkle all over Pat to impress him. He'd been after me for spending so much money.

I went upstairs and there he was, lying in bed moaning and groaning in his dramatic way when he wanted sympathy. I laughed and kissed him. He was happy to see me. Then I took all the money out of my bag and threw it up in the air watching it all flutter down on Pat and the bed. He said, "Come here." Then he kissed me and we made love. He wasn't really that sick after all.

A few minutes later the doctor arrived to see Pat. He was very concerned when he took Pat's blood pressure. It was very high. Pat hadn't told him that we'd just made love. Before leaving, the doctor sat down with Pat and told him to take better care of himself and relax because high blood pressure could be serious.

Chapter 44

SANTA DOMINGO AND BIMINI

The Carnival was in full swing when I arrived in Santa Domingo. Crowds of people lined the downtown streets and music and food was available everywhere. Pat enjoyed himself immensely; he was never happier than when trying different kinds of food - all at once. I was standing on the street while he purchased his latest delicacy when a tall, dark, handsome stranger, with beautiful, deep brown eyes and an attractive mustache came up to me. He took my hand and kissed it. After all, this was Carnival. When I didn't reject him immediately, he gazed into my eyes and said softly, "I want your days and I want your nights." Wow! Hmm, I thought to myself, what a wonderful proposition! I told him "Thank you,", but I wasn't available. I've never forgotten his words. I'm sure they worked for him many times he was so charming. If Pat hadn't have been with me, who knows what I would have done.

There was so much excitement that Carnival week. My kids were in heaven, having fun on their own with new friends they had made. We all went out for dinner every night.

Pat began filming in Constanza, far inland, up in the mountains. Each morning he, William Freidkin, Dick Bush, and other department heads went to work by helicopter to Constanza and flew back home each night while the rest of the crew remained behind. On Friday night the whole crew returned to Santa Domingo, traveling back to Constanza late Sunday.

One Friday afternoon Pat surprised me by calling and asking us to join him in Constanza for the weekend. He said he'd send a driver for us and we could take the helicopter that brought the crew home for the weekend. The kids were at the beach and I had no way of reaching them. I called Toni who said not to worry; she'd look after the girls and make sure they got on the Saturday helicopter. This seemed like a good plan so I packed and took off as soon as the driver arrived to take me to the airport. The helicopter was a huge, 16 passenger Sycorsky. I'd ridden in a small one before while in New York on a publicity tour for Peter Gunn, but never one this big and I was the only passenger.

Saturday morning I awoke early, unable to sleep and walked out onto the balcony. The mist hung low in the valley and as the early morning sun began to shine through rays shone down from heaven. A neat patchwork of fields spread out before me with trees standing as boundaries, stretching out across the horizon. In the distance there were faint sounds of horses, cows, and donkeys. At 7:00 a.m. the church bells sounded and the little town began to come alive. First a motorcycle started up then a truck. Gradually the noise of the town took over. If the bed had been more comfortable, I might have missed it all.

The crew bus wasn't going to arrive with the kids until late Sunday evening so we decided to take a ride. The land reminded me of the bare mountains of Montana and other parts made me think of the lovely woods in West Virginia. I spotted a waterfall high up a mountain and suggested we drive up to it. I don't know why on earth I suggested it. I hate looking down from high places. Big mistake. The road was extremely narrow and the farther up we went the worse it got. Finally I got very nervous and suggested that we turn around. Unfortunately, that appeared to be impossible. While trying to turn around, we got stuck in the middle of road with no place to go except over the cliff. The front of the car was already heading that way. We needed to dig a niche into the mountain behind the car in order to turn around, but we didn't have a shovel.

With my command of the Spanish language, I figured that I could walk down the mountain to the houses we'd seen on the way up and borrow a shovel. Off I went down the hill. It was steep and I wondered how difficult the walk back up would be, but I trusted my energy would come to me as it usually did in an emergency. I knocked on the door of the first house I came to. The family was quite friendly and the young son offered to come with me to help us get the car out.

Luck was with us. As we started to climb back up the hill, I heard the sound of a truck engine and sure enough, there was Pat happily driving toward us. True to his luck, two men on their way down the mountain helped him move the truck. They had to assist him, in order to get by. They had maneuvered the truck back and forth, slowly and carefully while Pat looked on. What a relief.

We were emotionally exhausted after our escapade so we headed back to the hotel to wait for the kids and the rest of the crew. They didn't arrive until 9:00 p.m., but still had managed to have a good time. Flump, wiggling, and wagging was delighted to see me. We had dinner together and left the girls to play games with the crew in the lobby. Flump hopped up on the bed, happy to sleep with me again.

The next morning we were up at five o'clock. The bed was still terrible, but Flump hadn't minded. After a breakfast of filet mignon for Flump and pancakes for us, we packed up and drove out to the location. There our helicopter awaited us. This helicopter was small, like the one Pat rode in each morning. We got in - Tanya, Xochi, Flump and I - and Flump sat on the floor of the bubble looking down intently. I wondered what was going on in her furry little head. Would she ever be able to explain this to another dog?

Riding in the small helicopter was more pleasant than in the big one I'd taken on the way out. I felt like I was part of the sky like a bird. Most of the way home it was overcast, but I saw the most beautiful cloud formations with light blue reflections from the city.

A few days after our return from Constanza, Moby and the boys James and Danny called us. They had docked in Puerto Plata and were taking a bus to see us the next day. Moby needed a part for the boat and it was waiting for him in Santa Domingo. They arrived, hot and sweaty from their ride. After a shower we all went to Di Ciro's for dinner. On their last night we talked into the wee hours and I agreed to meet them in Miami over Labor Day weekend and to take a trip to Bimini with them. They always loaded up the *Moby II* with kids and food and headed to Bimini Island for the holiday.

Although it was now August 21, 1976, the American Embassy threw us a bicentennial party. We were excited about going to the embassy. It was a lovely place with beautiful, huge trees shading the backyard where the party was held. We had an all American barbecue - hot dogs, hamburgers, and fried chicken. Most of Santa Domingo was hot and humid that day, but in that yard it was shady, cool, and breezy.

One afternoon we bought a featherless parrot on a street corner. They said he was just a baby. We named him Jefe. I don't know if his baldness was due to age or what. His wings were clipped for his trip home with us and we had a cage made for him.

Pat was having difficulties at work. Freidkin didn't like Dick Bush, the English cameraman, who he described as "a fucking nut". For some reason Freidkin wanted Pat to say something to Dick, but Pat didn't feel it was his place. Freidkin had already replaced crewmember after crewmember. Pat talked with Mark Johnson, the production assistant, about his dilemma. Working on this film was great experience for Mark's future job as a producer. He had to deal with the toughest of problems.

They called a meeting that Pat had to attend with Dick Bush and Freidkin. At that meeting Dick decided to quit. Pat came home all stressed. He hated confrontations and avoided them whenever possible. He was relieved when things were finally settled and Dick was replaced.

Time drew near for my leaving. We got the bird's health certificate. We went to our favorite restaurants for the last time. I was both sad and relieved about leaving. I had to admit I was homesick, tired of the heat, the commotion, the beggars, and the constant noise. Downtown Santa Domingo was one of the world's noisiest places. Every store had the radio blasting out a different station and everyone sat on their car horns. By then I just wanted to go home. I didn't mind stopping in Miami or in West Virginia to see Mammy and Pappy, but I longed for my own bed and surroundings.

Our day of departure, September 2, was a stressful day. It started with the company car that was to take us to the airport being late. We made it to the airport barely in time, checked our baggage and the pets before going through immigration. Then the immigration officer stopped me saying the girls needed a visa extension that they didn't have. My heart nearly stopped. Before leaving I had checked this out with the production secretary who told me it was unnecessary. Now I didn't know what to do. Ordinarily someone accompanied folks on *Sorcerer* crew from the army who looked out for them. I wasn't a crewmember and there was nobody there to help me.

The officer was being a true son-of-a-bitch and there I was with soldiers standing all around with their guns. There wasn't time to go back to town and get the extensions and I was frightened the plane would take off without me leaving our pets to an uncertain fate. I began to cry. An American from the airline crew came up and asked me what was wrong. After I told him he took me aside and said that if I had a photo of the girls and $20.00 the officer would fix things and we could leave. Luckily I had their school photos in my wallet so I gave them to him plus the $20.00. It never occurred to me that the immigration officer just wanted some payola. Normally the movie company would have paved the way.

We boarded the plane at the last minute. What a relief! I couldn't wait to get out of there. I never wanted to see the Dominican Republic again. As fate would have it, that wasn't to be the case. We had a scary, bumpy landing in Haiti where I deplaned, bought some rum, got back on the plane, happy as we took off for the good old USA.

I had put some of my special Gerivital vitamins on top of the suitcase to see if customs would confiscate it, but they hardly looked at anything so taken were they by Flump and the parrot. Moby met us at the airport and took us out to his boatyard where we met his family. We went out to dinner and then headed home where we immediately fell asleep as soon as our heads hit the pillow.

The next morning we took the animals to the kennel to stay while we were on the boat. Moby took us to Hialeah Race Track to see the flamingos. It was a classy pink place, but it was raining so hard and thundering that the flamingos were all huddled together. Later that afternoon we boarded the tugboat. Lots of people were going on the trip with us, mostly kids. There were many staterooms so Tanya and I shared one and Xochi shared one with another woman. We took off down the canal at 11:15 p.m. in the evening. It was warm and we saw beautiful homes with gorgeous landscaped yards that came right down to the canals and docks with yachts tied up at them. We sat on the deck and I enjoyed the balmy evening.

By the time I awoke the next morning we were in Bimini. The kids had already eaten breakfast and were having a glorious time jumping into the ocean from the winch on the end of the boat. *Moby II* was quite a contrast to the elegant yachts docked beside us. But our passengers seemed to be enjoying themselves far more than the yacht occupants.

One fellow with us was a professional diver who worked all over the world. During one job he had worked for the Shah of Iran putting a guard fence in the ocean at his summer palace. He and Xochi and Tanya swam to the concrete boat that had sunk during the Second World War. He taught the girls to snorkel. They learned quickly, surpassing their mother in no time.

I was content to poke around on the surface of the water. When the current changed and the *Moby* began to drift toward the concrete ship, I clambered aboard; content to sit on deck and watch the girls dive.

Bimini was Hemingway country and that evening we all went to the Compleat Angler - a bar that Hemingway had frequented. It was dark and full of Hemingway memorabilia collected over the years. The bar looked exactly the way I imagined Hemingway's hangout should. I loved being in a place he had actually written about. I doubted the kids even knew who Hemingway was, but they had a great time anyway. They were doing a dance where they hit together at the hip. Most of them were quite bony so they invited me to join them. At least I was comfortable to bump up against.

The next day we had a feast. The guys went diving and brought back sixty-one lobsters. We gobbled down that meal, and then went in search of Moby. The rumor was he was dancing somewhere, but we never found him. It would have been a sight to behold.

I was so proud of my girls, joining in with everyone and learning how to snorkel. How lucky they were to have all these adventures. We left Bimini the next morning, towing three boats behind us. Moby always picked up a little extra cash that way. I watched Bimini fade into the distance, and then went up on the top deck to watch a little longer. Who knew when I'd return? I enjoyed the sun even more because fall was on its way.

We had the greatest dinner that night with Moby at a pizza joint that served knots of pizza dough dipped into a sauce of garlic, parsley, and butter. Scrumptious! We picked up Flump and Jefe so we could leave early. The next morning, after kissing Moby good-by, we boarded the plane to Charleston, West Virginia. On our arrival, I rented a big Pontiac station wagon, packed us all in and off we drove the sixty miles to Beckley and Mammy and Pappy's house.

Chapter 45
TURNING POINT

I was happy to be at Mammy and Pappy's house. The maple tree out front was already beginning to turn orange. The air was cool and crisp. One of the first things I did was go to Hills Department Store to buy a nicer cage for Jefe. Some of the kids who were staying on the farm came by and in the evenings we sat out front talking while my kids went off with the friends they'd made years before.

I drove to Amigo to see our farm. Nothing much had changed, but that's the way of things in Appalachia. I visited with the friends I'd made when I lived there. (As I said before, that's another whole book). I loved those folks and it was nice to be with them again. At that moment I felt such warmth, as if the Earth had wrapped its arms around me. Even though I now lived in the city out of necessity, I felt far happier in the country.

The trip back to Los Angeles was an ordeal and felt like forever. We loaded everything into the station wagon, headed to the airport then boarded a plane in Charleston. Our connections in Chicago were so close, and we barely made it. Finally we landed in Los Angeles where Laurie met us. She looked great and so did our house. I was ecstatic about being home. I got into my tub for a nice soak that night, before climbing into my own bed. To top it all off, it was cool and the rain was falling softly.

The next morning I took Xochi to enroll in Cow Pie High, as the kids called it. She walked in with me and appeared to grow smaller by the minute. She never did like starting at a new school, but after a couple of days she'd settled in and did just fine.

The union called wanting me to do a film out in our Newhall area called *Flush*. It was about a sanitary company and a man who drove the truck called the Brown Bumble Bee. It was truly a shitty story. A call to work on *Turning Point*, a story of ballerinas with Ann Bancroft, Shirley MacLaine, and Mikhail Baryshnikov and the American Ballet, saved me from that fate for a while.

At the Shrine auditorium, during rehearsals, I watched Mikhail Baryshnikov dancing and leaping across the stage. He was amazing and fantastic - flying through the air across the stage. Never having attended a ballet, I didn't realize that Misha was, at that time, the very best. I decided to make a point to begin going to the ballet until someone enlightened me to the fact that I was seeing the greatest ballet right there. It was unlikely I'd ever see better than what was happening right before my eyes. I spent a week working at the Shrine Auditorium watching scene after scene of beautiful people with gorgeous bodies dancing. I helped Misha with his hair a couple of times. He was arrogant, but with his talent I was ready to forgive him anything.

I had always admired Shirley MacLaine and was happy to work around her. I had the feeling she and I had lots in common. I told her how much I enjoyed her book about China.

I went to see the showing of *Marathon Man*. It was a great film, especially the dentist scene, which I figured would hit home with everyone. It did. I loved seeing my friend Sir Laurence Olivier again, if only on film. He didn't look so kind in the film. Nothing like the lovely person I knew he was. But his wig looked fine.

While I was still on *Turning Point*, John Rogers, head of production at Fox, called to see if I was interested in working on *The Other Side of Midnight*. It would star Susan Sarandon, Marie France Pisier and John Beck. I'd read the book already and was excited. Lee Harmon was doing the makeup. John gave me a time for an interview and I met Jack Bernstein, the unit manager, who knew Pat and obviously liked him. Jack took me into his office and asked what I expected for a salary. I wanted $800 for 60 hours and $1050 flat for location, which included Paris and Washington, D.C. plus $15.00 per day for my cases. I let him know that I'd love to work on this film. A couple hours after I returned to my job on *Turning Point* Jack called and said I was hired. Hurrah for me! Later Pat called saying that he was regretful about letting us go home. He was lonesome and now I had to tell him our paths might not cross for longer than he had envisioned.

Meanwhile I was working on the house getting it in good shape. There was one problem, though. Gene, the young fellow who had watched it while we were gone, had been growing a crop of pot in a small bedroom. He had quite a set up and each day he'd come over to water and talk to his plants. I told him the plants had to go. It was illegal and I was afraid our maid might just open the door, see the set up, and call the police. I didn't need that kind of trouble, especially since I never used the stuff. It was like telling him to sacrifice his children. He slowly took everything down. I felt like a murderer. He didn't have another place where he could grow them, but I didn't feel I had a choice.

On September 27 we did hair tests at Fox with Susan Sarandon for *The Other Side of Midnight*. It was a busy day. Susan had been working on location and I only had a short time to work on her hair. It was a Forty's film and lots of period hairstyles needed to be created. Susan rushed in and I tried working with the curling iron then with bobby pins, which were correct for that time period. She hadn't had time to wash her hair because she'd driven in from location for the test. This made her hair difficult to work with, but she was so great it didn't matter. I tried many hairdos on her. I threw hairstyles up and together quickly so I'd have time to fit them all in during the allotted time.

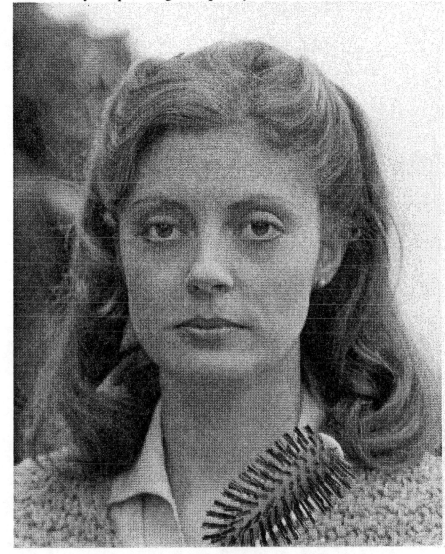

Susan Sarandon

That day I saw Howard Koch, Jr. who was now a producer on the film. When I first met Howie, he'd been a production assistant. His dad, Howard Koch, Sr., was the greatest producer at Paramount and a wonderful man. I hoped Howie had turned out like him.

The next day was the test with Marie France Pisier who had come all the way from Paris. She also had allotted a very short amount of time, too. I did at least fourteen hairstyles on her and everything looked quite good. When we saw the dailies of Susan's hair, I was pleased. The styles weren't picture perfect, but we had a look we could go with. The last test of the day was a riot. They were testing bats for a cave scene by throwing small, black pieces of material tied like bows in front of a fan and that was exactly what they looked like. Back to the drawing board.

I was all jazzed up thinking about my upcoming trip. There were wigs and supplies to order. I was going all over the world and I wanted to be prepared. Marie's character was going through many changes in the film and she needed a wig so I went to Ziggy the wig maker's home to measure her for it. I went to the set of *Audrey Rose* to meet John Beck, our male star whom I'd only seen on beer commercials. He was a handsome man with a full head of hair and a large mustache. I wondered if the '40s hairstyles would do him justice. It didn't in my opinion. His double needed a wig and a mustache, too.

Howie Koch and Charles Jarrot, the director, and I went through all the photos of hairdos to decide what would go best and where. An old time designer, Irene Sharaff, was designing the clothes in London.

In the Forties, they didn't have billboards with huge photos on them. Instead, they used paintings. I mentioned this to Howie because there was an important scene in the film where Noelle, played by Marie France, was pictured on a billboard. Howie asked me if he'd have to pay me more for that information. I said, "No," but as it turned out, he did in a way.

Part of the movie was to be filmed in Greece. I'd always wanted to go there - even without a salary I would have gone. One day while talking with Howie about the doubles who would be working in Greece I had a bright idea. "How on earth," I asked, "will anyone know how to fix the doubles' hair? Only I know what they are supposed to look like." Howie bought it. I was sent on the second unit to Greece. Thanks Howie.

The movie business never failed to amaze me and even with my frustrations it was fantastic how things changed so rapidly. Suddenly I had to go to London to do Marie France's hair so they could take a photo of her looking like Marie Antoinette for the billboard they were going to have to paint. Would wonders never cease?

Before I left for location we went to the little French Café in Newhall and I told the owners I was going to Paris. It was unusual to have such a wonderful place to eat in Newhall, but what was even more amazing was that the owner's brother had a restaurant in Paris right across from the Meridian Hotel where we would be staying. She insisted that I go there to meet her brother and gave me a note to give to him.

I went shopping to get things I'd need for location - comfortable shoes, warm clothes, etc. Paris would be chilly and on the way home we were stopping in Washington, D.C., which would be cold, too. I needed to pack for all kinds of weather.

I missed Patrick a lot especially because I was unable to contact him by phone, or even by mail. They were now behind schedule, which worried me, as I wanted to connect with him before I left for Europe. The location manager told me I could trade in my first class ticket for a $600 credit that Pat could use if he had time to visit me. I thought that was great, but later when I told Pat about the deal he responded, "I only travel first class."

On October 13 we celebrated Laurie's birthday at the French Café then went home to a Baskin and Robbins ice cream cake. We all ate too much and sat around complaining, rubbing our over-full bellies. I was supposed to leave for London on October 15, but suddenly they needed me there a day early. Pat was due home that Sunday, but I was leaving Saturday. What a crazy life. I took the girls to Laurie's apartment for the weekend. They would all pick Pat up while I was off on my next European adventure.

Chapter 46

THE OTHER SIDE OF MIDNIGHT

I arrived at the airport loaded down with baggage, including wigs, my usual hairdressing case, and clothes for all sorts of weather - many, many bags. No one from Fox Studios was there to see me off, but a man from British Airways came to my aid. My luggage costs came to more than $1400. Astounding! The studio had only given me a $250 luggage allowance. Did they think I was just taking a vacation? After a call to the studio, I got an okay for the additional charges and was off to London.

Since London is eight hours ahead of Los Angeles, I wasn't really awake, but I stirred when the stewardess put a tray beside me, my eyes all scratchy and dry, and managed to eat and then fall asleep again so that by the time I arrived in London I felt really rested. My luggage went through customs without a problem and it even fitted into the Volvo belonging to the location man.

Typically English, the Churchill Hotel was a lovely place. My room had a great bathtub, though not as large as the one I'd enjoyed at the Dorchester on my last trip, but nice enough. I was thrilled to find myself only two blocks from Marks and Spencer's Department Store because that's where I could always find large-bottomed pretty underpants. The value of the dollar was quite high at the time, but it only took me an hour to spend $200 for, among other things, a curling iron and a plug for my hair dryer. By this time I was drooping so I went back to the hotel and ordered room service including a half bottle of wine - for $70. After eating I fell right to sleep.

The next morning I got ready, packed the wig in a bag, grabbed my case, and went downstairs to wait for the driver. While I was looking through the magazine stand I left my bag with the wig out in the lobby, certain nobody would steal anything in this dignified hotel. Wrong! When I returned to the lobby, my bag was gone. I panicked - my wig! A man, who turned out to be the hotel detective, was watching me suspiciously. He came over and asked if I had left a bag in the lobby. "Yes," I answered. "Please come with me," he ordered. Walking me into the office, he explained that nobody should ever leave a bag anywhere in public, in London. It was too dangerous; it could possibly be a bomb. That had never occurred to me. After a short lecture he returned my bag to me. In the meantime he told me about some of the rich people who stayed at the hotel. He described an Arab man who forgot to take his change so the detective brought it to his room. In the room he saw jeweled daggers and other valuables just lying around. The detective suggested that they be put in the safe, as the hotel didn't want to be responsible if they were stolen. The Arab was unconcerned. Another guest had kept a whole suitcase of money just sitting in his room. What was a detective to do?

I was driven to Berman's costume house where I met Irene Sharaff for the first time. Old and very thin, she reminded me of the wicked witch in the Wizard of Oz. She was an icon of sorts and appeared to be supportive and kind, but I was wrong.

Jack Bernstein arrived with Marie France and we hurried to a portrait gallery to take pictures of Marie France. She was ill with the flu, so I tried to hurry. I hadn't had an opportunity to fit her wig nor had I seen her costume so I wasn't sure how I would do her hair. The brush rollers with which I'd set the wig snarled the hair. I should have remembered that whenever I tried to hurry things happened that ended up taking more time than if I'd gone at my normal pace. I should have been like the big wigs and demanded enough time, but instead I tried to please, especially as Marie was sick. Finally, I got the hair in acceptable shape and they were able to take the photo. Soon Marie was back on the plane to Paris and her bed.

The next morning I had to leave at 7:30 a.m. to catch a 9:30 a.m. flight to Athens. My alarm didn't go off, but luckily I'd left a wake-up call at the front desk. This time a woman from the airline had been alerted about my overweight luggage so it was all taken care of in advance.

I looked out the window as we descended for our landing in Athens; the countryside reminded me of Los Angeles, all brown and dry. Kate, a production assistant, was waiting for me at the gate, but customs made me open all my cases before I reached her. They thought I might be selling things. It took forever, but finally customs was finished and Kate found me. We took a taxi to the Caravel Hotel to drop my things, and then we went to the office to meet Robert Watts, our production manager. He was so very English with reddish hair, freckles, and a round face.

By the time I returned to the hotel my neck ached and I was hot and sweaty. Jet lag was rapidly catching up with me. After sinking into a hot tub, I was asleep by 8:30 p.m. Time changes were tough on me and I hadn't had a moment to adjust since leaving Los Angeles.

The next day I was to drive to location, a picturesque ruin in Point Sounion, with Robert Watts. When I woke up that morning, the clock said 6:30. I didn't think that could possibly be right. It felt more like noon, but I didn't feel rested. A call to the front desk confirmed that it was indeed 6:30 a.m. We weren't going to leave until later in the morning so I went for a walk and bought a dictionary before going back to the hotel to wash my hair and to wait for the headache that had developed to go away. All my belongings were downstairs by noon, and then I waited and waited. Around 2:30 p.m. Kate came by with the news that Robert, who I was to ride with, had forgotten me. We went back to the office to figure out how to get me to the location. There was a VW bus that needed to get there too, but had no driver. I offered to drive it as long as they gave me directions. It was impossible for me to read the signs.

A Greek driver led me out of town and as he departed, he told me that all I had to do was stay on the road by the sea and eventually I would end up at my destination. At first I was nervous, but after a while I realized I was fortunate to be able to take the trip on my own. It was the most beautiful drive I'd ever taken. The water was a fantastic turquoise blue and the Greek countryside spread out with stone walls, sunflowers, and olive trees. People were working in the fields, it was so lovely - just like I'd imagined. I had become the producer of my own movie in my mind. It was music for my soul. I arrived at the Sounion Beach Hotel without a hitch and I happily thanked Robert for forgetting me while he apologized profusely.

The hotel was charming with quaint, little cottages up and down the mountainside. I settled in my room then went to the lobby to meet the English camera crew. I knew some of their buddies from my trip to the Dominican Republic so we had something in common and soon became drinking buddies and fast friends. The first night we shared a great meal and bottles of wine then drank late into the night enjoying Rusty Nails, a combination of Scotch and Drambuie. It was wonderful going down, but what a disaster the next day.

I woke up with a queasy stomach, but it was a small price to pay for the camaraderie of the night before. We had breakfast together and they seemed to be holding up better than me. I met Micky, the costumer and the only other American besides our director. It was raining so I went back to my room to work on the doubles' wigs. Then I went through the script again and tried to nap, thinking it would help me feel better. No luck.

We worked at Point Sounion, the beautiful ruin of a temple where Lord Byron had scratched his name. The Greek extras were marvelous and I had great fun trying to communicate with them. But as they say, it was all Greek to me. That night we rode home in a 1937 Rolls Royce after watching a beautiful sunset.

Our doubles arrived from Athens. I cut a wig and also cut a double's hair. The next day I realized I had a real problem. Raf Vallone's double was totally bald while Raf had a full head of hair and I hadn't planned on a wig for him. I sprayed his baldhead black When they photographed him through the back window of the Rolls his head shone like a bowling ball. Back to the drawing board.

In our business one has to be innovative. I decided to glue crepe wool to his head. Crepe wool is actually for stuffing hair, to make it look fuller, but I figured I could make it look like hair from a distance. I painted his whole head with wig glue then combed the crepe wool as thin as I could. I glued it to his head and formed it into a sort of hairstyle. It worked well and to my surprise the man slept with it on and came in the next day looking just fine, too. I was delighted and the children who worked with us were entertained and laughed at me as I did my work. He was accommodating and as highly amused as we were.

My friends and I had a wonderful dinner and we discussed their lives. I got a kick out of them calling their wives Duchess. David said he collected rocks and had now limited himself to one from each location because his apartment was getting too crowded. Chris, my favorite, told me he had never been happy. I assured him that as he was only twenty-eight, life would most likely improve.

We returned to Athens. The next morning and filmed at the Parthenon where we spent most of the day waiting for the sun to come out. It never did. We moved to the harbor to take some shots and someone from the Greek government tried to confiscate our film because of a problem they'd had on a previous film shot there.

The next day we went to the Acropolis then down to the harbor for a lunch of calamari and good wine. Mickey was so repulsed by our choice of food he made me laugh. He had traveled the world over as Yul Brynner's wardrobe man, but never tried any unusual food. He had no clue what he was missing, nor did he want to know.

The end of that day we went back to the hotel to check out. We had to leave for Crete that evening at 8:30 p.m. By the time we boarded the plane, it was so dark we couldn't see a thing. The Englishmen stated, "We were really - 'knackered' " - a perfect description for how I felt.

After we landed on Crete, it took us an hour to get to the Elounda Beach Hotel in Elounda. It was another fantastic hotel with tiny, cozy cottages and I had a cottage to myself. Dinner was waiting for us, but we were so tired we just sat and stared at one another. Finally, at 2:00 a.m., I went to bed.

Crete was a place I'd only dreamed of visiting. I was not disappointed. My little, enchanted cottage had walls of rough white plaster and two beds with brightly colored covers. Candles were placed on the dresser in case the electricity went out and flowers in vases were placed throughout the cottage. There was a dressing room with a huge, inviting bathtub. It was heavenly. What more could I ask?

At breakfast, the next morning, we were notified that the production company had decided to call it a rest day so I went back to my room and slept until lunch at 2:00 then met my friends and the script supervisor, Nikki Clapp, an American living in Greece. Nikki suggested she give us a tour of the town. She had a car.

Driving through the countryside of fields and stone walls toward St. Nicklaus Village was extraordinary even though it was overcast and rainy. Alongside the walkway in town, the ocean was rough and dark waves marched on forever. We walked past a yarn and weaving shop where the brilliant colors vibrated in the gray of the day. The day was cold and damp, but the inside shop was warm; the shelves lined with yarn dyed the richest colors - deep reds, purples, and dark greens. I wanted to crawl under one of the blankets they were weaving and curl up.

We found a little outdoor café with a canopy to protect us from the rain and settled in for lunch and ouzo. I enjoyed pouring water in the ouzo, while watching it turn white. Nikki ordered us all local food - octopus, squid, etc. It was a great day and we arrived home a little tipsy that evening.

The phone was ringing. Surely it was too early to be awakened! "Where were you last night?" Pat asked in a loud voice. Trying to wake up I stammered, "In town drinking ouzo with the British crew and the script girl." "That doesn't make any difference. The British fuck, too." Oh my, I thought to myself and laughed. I hadn't misbehaved, but then again the British aren't pushy.

When I told my British friends about the call, they laughed saying, "He gave you a bollixing, but you got pissed (drunk) not laid." I realized that Pat assumed I operated just as he had in the past. Maybe I should have, I thought to myself, I might have had an even better time.

It was still raining so we had another day off. I wrote everyone post cards. The following day it continued to rain, so no shooting again. After lunch I put on my big Eddie Bauer jacket and walked into the town of Elounda and bought some T-shirts. I said good morning in Greek to a man who taught me to say good afternoon and good evening, too. Now I knew three Greek words.

That evening we all went to a real Greek café for dinner. The men danced to sensuous music, hands on each other's shoulders. After downing shots of ouzo, our glasses were thrown into the fireplace. The wine and octopus were great too.

We were able to work the next day. The shoot was on a mountainside. It was still cold and I was the only one dressed for the weather. I shared a meal with Rick, who was a hippie kid that was standing in for us. I gave him a haircut, which was badly needed. Later he bought me roses. At one point a three-wheeled car came up the road. We pulled our equipment out of the way to let it pass and a handsome Greek man leaned out and handed me a yellow flower. Greek men were so romantic.

We wrapped early that night. After the cold day, the nice hot bath I took so felt good. That night the production manager told me I'd be leaving for Paris in three days. I was ready to burst into tears. I wanted this to continue forever. I didn't want to leave my friends or Greece. I knew that in our business nothing lasts, good or bad, but I wanted to hold on to this very special time.

October 26 was a very interesting day. Early in the morning I began giving haircuts to thirty of the male villagers who were acting as extras. They were supposed to be playing soldiers in the 1940s and their hair needed to be very short. These fellows hadn't seen a barber in a very long time. I hadn't been able to charge my electric clippers so I ended up using a straight razor to clean the hair off their necks. I cut and shaved neck after neck and actually ended up changing the look of the whole town. When I finished, I was exhausted so somebody brought me a shot of very strong liquor that was supposed to make everything better. It burned my throat going down and I did feel very happy and relaxed.

Our location that day was on an island called Spinalonga. At one time it had been a leper colony, a place where people with leprosy were sent to live away from everyone. Once there, they never left the island. Even water had to be delivered. I imagined what it would have felt like to be a leper, suffering as I know they did. After a cure to the disease was found, the island had been abandoned. Now it looked just like a movie set. Little huts were falling to pieces, just like the people who had inhabited them long ago. The wind had blown some of the graves open revealing old bones. I considered taking a souvenir home, but thought better of it.

We worked around the countryside for a couple more days and then, all too soon, it was time for me to leave. The company threw a good-bye party for me and another fellow who was also leaving. We had a huge dinner with lots of Greek wine and partied late into the night.

I fell into bed after tearfully bidding my friends farewell. At three in the morning I woke up to get ready to leave and began to cry, in fact, I cried all the way to the airport. Finally I understood what Melina Mercouri meant when she said Americans were so cold and controlled. I'd begun to feel like a Greek. My emotions got the better of me, and I had such a feeling of loss. I couldn't hide the way I felt.

Before leaving I had made sure the Greek accountant gave me enough Drachmas to pay for my overweight luggage. It turned out that she gave me exactly the amount I needed - I was left without a cent of Greek money. At the airport in Herraclan I wanted a cup of coffee to settle my nerves and keep me awake, but I had no Greek money. Luckily a man saw my dilemma and bought me a cup. I gratefully accepted and sat with him, drinking my coffee. He worked for the airline, which turned out great for me. He upgraded my ticket to first class so we could continue to talk on the flight to Athens. I no longer felt so sorry for myself.

Nobody was at the Athens airport to meet me and all the directions were in Greek so I was completely confused and nervous. After bumbling around a bit, I found my way to the correct gate and got on the plane headed for Paris.

On my way to Paris, I sat next to a Japanese businessman who had traveled all over the world. He enjoyed telling me about his adventures, his business, and how he always brought wonderful gifts like jewelry and fur coats for his wife.

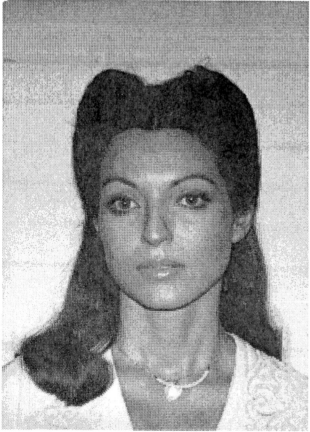

Marie-France Pisier,
The Other Side of Midnight

I was exhausted by the time I landed in Paris and overjoyed to see a card with "Sugar" written in huge letters. It was in the hands of a movie company driver. At this point I needed to be rescued. He took me to the Hotel Meridian, a huge place that didn't seem very French at all - except, of course, for the people working there. It was one of those hotel chains that exist all over the world. They all look alike and one can travel anywhere and everything is familiar, nothing changes.

I was in the lobby checking in when someone kissed me on the neck. What a nice way to be welcomed to Paris. It was Larry Jost, the sound mixer. I was hungry, so after I saw my luggage safely to my room, we found Clint Althouse, Larry's partner, the boom man, and we all went for a walk and a snack. That evening the makeup man, Lee Harmon, arrived. I was happy to see him again. I hadn't seen him in years. We had become friends while working together on the Batman television series.

Later I settled into my room, unpacking my things. I had so much stuff because of all the hair supplies I had brought. I was almost done when Fred Brost, the unit manager, called and asked me to go dye Marie France's hair. Great. It was the last thing I wanted to do after my late night and the flight from Greece. Nevertheless, I went taking her hairpieces along so I could match the color. Now, I wondered was it possible that I could find the right tint? I wandered around the stores a while before finding a drugstore that had exactly what I needed - and a clerk that understood my French. What luck! A gift from the angels. I hailed a taxi and hurried to Marie France's apartment. First I cut her hair then colored it. She was very gracious and fixed me a tasty green salad. I was hungry and appreciated her hospitality.

The next morning I woke up at 6:00 a.m. feeling more human. I still missed my English friends, but a good night's sleep always made me feel better about everything. The first thing I did was go to the Production Office to collect lots of francs for my per diem. Paris was very expensive. Then on to J.V. Studios to meet my helper, a French hairstylist named Danielle. I enjoyed using my high school French even if it wasn't perfect. I saw Mickey, the wardrobe man, at the studio and brought him up to date about my experiences in Greece.

Mid afternoon I reported to Charles Jarrot's house where our director was working with Marie France. Her hair appeared a little dark, but I felt that after it was washed it would lighten up a tad and be fine. We were still doing prep work for our shoot. Lee took off for Holland for the weekend; Larry, Clint and I went out for a Chinese dinner. We had a Cote du Rhone wine that my English friend Chris recommended. It was excellent.

The next day, Saturday, I made a huge blunder. Terry Lewis, our prop man, had asked me to send some large black and white photos of Marie France to his room; he needed them for a prop photo in a scene. He gave me his room number, 7051. I put the photos in an envelope enclosing a silly, provocative note all in jest, knowing Terry would laugh, but it wasn't Terry who received it. The phone rang and it was Lewis on the line, not Terry Lewis. This Lewis's apartment was 7015. I had mixed up the number. I began to laugh, realizing I had made a mistake, but Lewis kept talking as though I was Marie France. "No way," I said. "I look nothing like her. Believe me, but I'm much older. Perhaps wiser, but I definitely do not look like her." I'd made a big mistake. Lewis was disappointed and confused; He sent me a note, which I still have, that read, "I have two pictures of you. I am not confused (which was underlined). You are very beautiful. Call me." Finally I was able to convince him and we both had a good laugh. I know he was quite disappointed. Sorry about that Lewis.

The walls of my room were dark brown and it was dreary, especially after my bright cheery room in Crete. I went out and bought some brightly colored dahlias in a vase and also a poster of a little French girl in a park. The room felt brighter.

The Russian Ballet came to Paris and it was absolutely fantastic. My favorite part was where the dancers were dressed in long robes and appeared to glide across the stage. They squatted down and kicked their legs with such energy provoking excitement. I loved it.

My stomach began to rebel with too much rich food. I had found the restaurant belonging to my friend's brother. In fact it was right across from our hotel. It was also called Café de Paris. I told them of my indigestion and they doctored me with Fine Branchia, an aperitif that settles the stomach.

The next day, I couldn't resist going to dinner with Clint Althouse, one of the nicest people I've ever met. Larry was to go too, but he insisted on Chinese and who needs Chinese in Paris. We ditched Larry and went to the Lagoste Amorouse. The chef selected our meal - crab curry on artichoke hearts, turbot with a sauce, green salad, white wine, coffee and a fabulous chocolate dessert. Not bad for someone so miserable the day before.

The next morning was a day off and I did my washing, paid the hotel bill and took a long walk. I still longed to be with my friends in Greece. I was disappointed that our American crew was not like them. The French were nicer than I expected them to be and they would generally smile back at me if I smiled at them. Often though, they looked down their noses at us, but then again, our crew wasn't much better, especially the camera crew. Fred Konacamp, our cameraman and his gaffer and a few other men would sit in the hotel lobby saying they were bored. I wondered to myself, how anyone could be bored in Paris, unless they were boring themselves. I guess they wanted Paris to discover them. I realized that one must go out to taste, feel, hear and smell Paris. It can't be done from a hotel lobby.

We worked French hours, which were normally 8:00 a.m. to 4:00 p.m., no time out for lunch, but food was made available all day long. It was great for most of the crew, but not for Lee and me. We had to begin work two hours earlier than the rest of the crew to get our actors made up. It was quite a process. Production would locate a hotel near each location. We'd be picked up and taken to the hotel and an assistant would show up with mirrors and lights and (hopefully) croissants and coffee. After we finished our work we packed our kits and went to the nearby set.

We never stopped for lunch, but a little trailer with a small kitchen was always near the set and we could get our food whenever we had the time. I had ham and cheese sandwiches on French bread most of the time and was often wearing breadcrumbs on my chest that fell from my sandwiches. I envied the flat-chested ladies who could stay so neat. There was always beer, wine or coffee available.

The weather was very cold one morning while we were working at Montmartre It felt as if it was about to snow. Wrapped in layers of clothing, I felt too large for the small apartment where we were working. That night after we wrapped and hurried to dailies, to my surprise I found my friends from Greece were there. We hugged. They had missed me too. We went out to dinner and they told me about their dinners in Elounda where everyone danced and broke their plates. I was jealous. Paris wasn't the same as Greece and I bid them goodbye more easily that night.

The French crew liked me because I tried to speak French. Although I had studied only high school French, they appreciated my effort and I found myself able to communicate most of the time. Nobody else on our American crew even tried to speak French. I found the French were happiest when they were eating and drinking. The French must have a Taurus soul. Pleasures of the flesh occupy the happy sensual Frenchman, eating, drinking, and making love. When we all sat down to a meal together, the French crew became very happy.

Paris had a huge flea market and one Sunday I decided to go to it. I found my way through the winding streets. It was a damp, drizzly day and there were sad-looking Africans sitting on the sidewalks selling carvings. They were shivering and sitting all huddled up. I felt sorry for them, but consoled myself thinking at least they were here in Paris, not in some African mines where they wouldn't be treated like a human being. I found woolen stockings to keep me warm at work. I got lost for a while in the puzzling streets and eventually found the Metro and went home.

One rainy morning we left for work at 6:00 a.m. for our makeup hotel. The lobby of this hotel was filled with Japanese people on a tour. After we finished our work, we tried to get on the elevator. Lee, a husky, teddy bear of a guy and I towered over the people and every time we got on the elevator the buzzer screamed "Overload, Overload". We finally had to leave by the stairs going through the kitchen.

Patrick phoned me in the middle of the night to let me know he was arriving the next day. I was so excited, and I could hardly wait.

The next day I had to climb a one-story platform at work. The boards were laid out on the staging, but not nailed together. It was frightening, and I'm a big chicken when it comes to heights. Lee teased me and called me a tightrope walker. When Pat arrived on the set, I was immediately needed more than usual. Par for the course. By the time I got home that night Pat was asleep, so I soaked in a hot bath before waking him up. We had a great evening.

Things were difficult the next morning. We had another 6:00 a.m. call and I was exhausted. Marie France was late, so Lee and I just dozed. When Marie arrived, her hair was still wet. This was the first time as she had always arrived with it dry. I'd left my dryer in the prop truck and I was panicked and angry because I was so tired, but I should have been prepared.

Frank Yablans, our producer had arranged for the crew to see his newest film, *Silver Streak* about a train. They threw a buffet dinner for us. Later, Pat and I went out to an Italian place for dinner. I wondered just how we were able to eat so often.

The next morning he left for Los Angeles. I didn't go downstairs to tell him good-bye because I knew I would cry. After he left, I took a nap and I was still tired when I got up. Later I went to a little café for a home cooked steak and green beans. I took a walk, sorting out my feelings. We were still not where I wanted to be in our relationship. Here I was, in the most beautiful city in the world, feeling so miserable. Patrick wanted me to change, but I liked being comfortable with myself and others.

The Eiffel Tower was such a cold set and all I could think about was getting home for a hot bath. Lee and I met for dailies after work and for the first time he asked if I'd like to go to dinner. His buddy John Beck had left for home. We went to the Left Bank for dinner and I began to wish that I'd discovered this place before. I would have taken Patrick there. All kinds of exotic food were displayed in the windows: Greek, Vietnamese, you name it. We settled on a smoky place upstairs with high chairs, enjoying a delicious Armenian meal with lots and lots of wine. Normally Lee kept to himself, although we had been working together for weeks. That night I got to know him much better which was good. We'd be working together for the next few months.

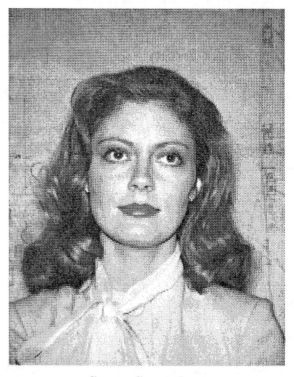

Susan Sarandon,
The Other Side of Midnight

Our last day of work in Paris was November 16. We finished at lunchtime with a champagne toast. The French crew gave me an orange trophy, which was for being the best-liked American on the crew. I was impressed. We hurried home to pack, which was a huge job for me. I had all my goodies from Greece, and what I'd bought in England and Paris.

Our parting dinner with Lee, Larry and Clint was at the same place Lee and I had eaten the night before. Later we met Severin, our French production assistant, and all of us piled into her car to go see the show at the Lido. We drank more champagne. I noticed that things had changed since I'd last been in Paris. Now the dancer's breasts were hardly bigger than those of petite Marie France Pisier, before they had been far more voluptuous. I didn't notice the guys being disappointed though. We got home at 3:00 a.m. rather woozy.

We flew off to Washington, D.C. the next day. I was extremely tired from too much booze, not enough sleep so I slept through most of the nine and a half hour flight. I arrived at customs with my own seven suitcases and Terry Lewis piled all his prop cases on my luggage. I think I frightened the agent. He just passed me right through, not wanting to open all of that. I do look trustworthy, which helped. Our crew stood by and laughed at me. We finished at customs, climbed into a bus and were off on a two-hour ride to Luray, Virginia where our location was shot in the caverns.

The Holiday Inn in Luray was a far cry from our top-of-the-line Meridian Hotel in Paris. It didn't matter. I was so very happy to be back in the USA. I'd had enough of Parisians. I checked into my room and felt right at home. What a difference in attitude. The politeness of the Southern people, their friendliness and smiles were appreciated.

Wiped out that next morning, thanks to the long flight along with the previous night's partying, I dragged myself to work. Production had called in extras and I needed to look at them and give instructions. The men's hair was much too long for the time period so I located a spare hotel room, turned it into a barbershop, and went to work cutting hair. I set the double wig.

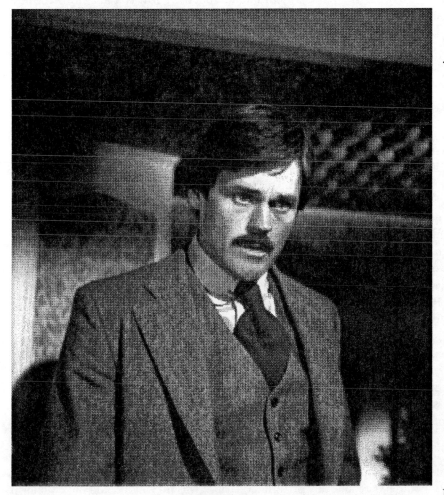

John Beck,
The Other Side of Midnight

Lee came in; we sat and talked while I cut his hair. It felt good to slow down. Bruce Barrenger, our publicist, joined the conversation and a little later John Beck arrived with the news that he was leaving his wife. I guess I wasn't the only one with problems.

In Paris we had filmed sequences with Marie France, in Virginia and Washington, D.C. we were doing the sequences with Susan Sarandon. Both women played parts with John, but in the film they never met.

The first morning we descended into the bowels of the Earth - Luray Caverns. The caves are more than 200,000,000 years old. Dripping subterranean water that added only one cubic inch to each formation every 120 years formed the outcroppings. Inside the cave it was warm, humid, and dark. My lungs felt heavy as I descended into the cave and it became harder to breathe. Astoundingly beautiful with all the huge stalagmites standing up so mightily, it was difficult for the crew, carrying all the equipment deep into the cavern.

We filmed a scene with Susan, who played John's wife. He had fallen for Marie France and he wanted to get rid of Susan. It appeared divorce didn't enter his mind because then the author, Sidney Sheldon, wouldn't have had such a great plot. In this scene, John leads Susan down into the cave with plans to leave her there. He doesn't kill her with his own hands, but it was still premeditated murder. When she realized she's been abandoned, she panics and hearing bats flying past her, she falls down an embankment. The screen is in total darkness as John disappears. At least, that was what was supposed to happen.

Thanks to all the humidity in the cave, Susan's hair began to frizz and it didn't match the shots we'd already done. I was anxious to finish the scene and get out of there. I couldn't fight the problems I had. We all had problems. Most of all the prop man had big problems. Before the scene was ready to shoot, Terry Lewis had brought the bats to show the director. They were made of rubber, but still looked phony so finally it was decided that real bat footage could be spliced in later.

The scene was supposed to be scary, but it just didn't feel frightening, there were too many lights and even with Susan's acting it just didn't appear to be realistic. Here she was screaming and yelling and groping around as though it was dark and it wasn't dark at all. It was hard to take the scene seriously and we had to cover our mouths tightly to stifle our laughter.

We finished and took off for Washington, D.C., riding in John's comfortable motor home for the two-hour drive. We stayed at the Key Bridge Marriott, a luxurious hotel. The weather was getting cold again and I relaxed knowing, no matter how cold it was or how tired I might, be there was a lovely room waiting for me at the end of a long day. If the bathtub was deep, all the better.

Settled into our rooms, Lee, John and I took off to see the dailies of the cave scene with Susan. When the film came on, we realized something was wrong. It looked exactly as it had in real life - Susan was still groping and screaming, but the film wasn't dark or scary - it was as bright as day. Sometimes a night scene looks bright when it's being filmed, but when it's developed it looks like it's dark. What on earth had happened? It was a disaster. Nobody wanted to go back and shoot in the cave again plus it would cost far too much.

Fred, the cameraman, wasn't my favorite person. He was seldom pleasant to Lee or me so the fact that the lighting was his blunder made it even funnier. No sympathy there within our black hearts. John, Lee, and I began to giggle. The harder we tried to stop, the worse it got. We just couldn't help ourselves. In hysterics, we sneaked out the back door and grabbed a taxi back to the hotel.

I talked with Pat. He was leaving for Mexico on Saturday. I was supposed to be home Friday night. Talk about ships passing in the night.

We filmed Susan by the reflecting pond. Lincoln stared down at us from the other end of the pond, which turned to ice before our very eyes. Susan was freezing and shivering and, to make matters worse, as we filmed, her hair kept alternately collapsing or curling up. I could hardly control it. Finally we had to quit shooting, it was just too cold. We went back to the hotel, ate lunch, and returned to work in the evening. Brrr.

The next day we left for Los Angeles. The ride to the airport through the wooded countryside was quite beautiful. We entered the airport in Washington, D.C. and I felt like I was on a different planet. It looked like outer space to me, after being around all the beautiful old buildings in Paris and then in Washington.

Pat met me at the airport, flowers in hand. We hadn't seen each other since Paris. We went by my mother's where the girls were waiting for us, and drove home and spent a wonderful afternoon catching up. Patrick was thankful we hadn't totally missed one another. I was sorry it was so short. The next morning I took him to the airport and saw him off to Mexico. We downed a couple of Ramos Gin Fizzes at the bar, which only enhanced my sadness as I kissed him good-bye. Knowing he'd be back in a few days didn't help. We hardly had a relationship anymore.

I called Fox and talked with Howard Koch, Jr. My daughter, Laurie, had finally gotten her Screen Extra's Guild card, which was a difficult process. Howie assured me she'd get to work on our show.

The kids had done well in my absence, they were quite independent now, but still they were happiest when I was home. I settled in and napped a lot to catch up on my sleep.

Saturday, November 27 was Tanya's sixteenth birthday. I rushed around doing wash and errands and gave the kid's friends haircuts. In the evening we went to "our" French Café to celebrate. The food was far better than it had been at the brother's Café de Paris in Paris and I told them so.

It took a few days for the filming to resume. In the meantime Howard Koch called me. Irene Sharaff, the designer, had called from England to tell him that she didn't approve of the way I did the hair tests. Nobody had told her how little time I had to do them, but I doubt it would have made any difference. There was no way I could have pleased Irene. She was of the old guard and didn't approve of my low-key work style. She wanted the producer, Frank Yablans, to hire Sydney Guilleroff, her old buddy from days past to design the hair. Howard didn't appreciate being in the middle and he wanted to know how I felt about the situation.

Truthfully, I was relived. Frank Yablans had done such weird casting choices for the film. I was worried about whether I was going to be able to make the women look as great as he expected. With Sydney designing the hair, I wouldn't have to worry about pleasing Frank. I'd always been grateful for the kindness Sydney had shown me when in my stockroom clerk days at MGM. Not expecting any problems, the change was fine with me. Howard was relieved and I was too, now that Irene would be off my back.

The first days back we reported to the studio at 10:00 a.m. with plans to put the makeup trailer together and to unload the truck that had arrived with our stuff from Washington. I tried to get everything put away to surprise Lee, but didn't quite finish before he arrived. I was glad to be there for him, though, because he was more upset than I'd ever seen him. Lee was married to a very attractive actress. Although she had made the rounds of most of the television shows that needed attractive women she never really made it "big".

She had made a few changes around the house while we had been in Paris. She bought a $1,700 antique chair. Lee was shocked. Although I wouldn't have called Lee cheap, you might say he was careful with his money and he could see no reason to spend that much on any chair. She had also had all the trees and bushes in their yard trimmed which he interpreted as an insult since Lee had been a green man (who supplies sets with greenery and flowers). He liked to take care of his own garden. To add insult to injury, she had the exterior wall at the back of the bathroom shingled. Lee got into a fit of anger when he thought about someone else working on his home and he yanked the shingles off and as he was having the tantrum a pipe burst and water had sprayed all over him - the carpenter had hammered a nail right through the pipe.

Now I could sympathize with her because Lee was never home, but I felt sorry for Lee, too. Still it was amusing to see him so worked up about inconsequential things. He was like a tomcat that had marked his territory only to have it invaded by another cat.

Sydney came to work and checked out our trailer. He had his own dressing room, his own chair, and a sit-down breakfast served to him on the set as part of his contract, which dumbfounded the Production Department. He worked in our trailer though when he did the actress's hair.

Work was exhausting and Sydney drove me crazy. He would tell Marie France that he didn't approve of nudity just as she was preparing for a nude scene in the bathtub. I was shocked at how hostile Sydney had become. He'd always been outspoken, but not angry. He had gotten very old. I felt sorry for him. He told me how his adopted children had caused him heartache and disappointment. Now I began to realize that perhaps his judgmental attitude was what caused him the most problems, not other people's actions. I tried to be patient, but felt I needed to put up mental barriers around him so as not to absorb his negativity. I was having enough problems at home. I didn't need more at work.

One day, while Sydney was doing Susan's hair, he looked at me and asked, "Where are the bobby pins?" I handed them to him explaining that they were right next to him. "I can't see that," he replied. How was he able to do hair if he couldn't see something that was so close?

We were all intimidated by Sydney. Susan hated the way he did her hair and Marie's head hurt from all the pins he used. He still did hair the way he had when he worked on Greta Garbo. The ultimate goof came when he turned Susan into a Barbie doll.

Sydney was upset because Lee and I allowed people to visit us in the trailer so we tried to stay as far away from him as possible. Sydney wanted a second hairstylist. We found him Kay Pownall, one of my favorite people whom I had known since I began in the business. Normally Kay worked with Faye Dunaway or Barbra Streisand. She had some time off and was willing. Her presence was calming, which we sorely needed.

We worked at Marineland in Palo Verdes. It resembled the Greek coastline. One morning we waited and waited in the trailer for Sydney to arrive and do the hair, but he didn't show up. He refused to work until he had his breakfast! Production finally got fed up; they didn't appreciate his behavior and demands. They fired him. What a relief! It wasn't that we were happy he was fired, but he had become such a bear to work with.

Even though Pat and I were back together, we didn't seem to have enough time to work out our relationship. There was still a lot of work to be done and at times it was tough for us both, but finally Patrick began to calm down a little and that made my life easier. He was leaving for Mexico on December 13. I figured he wanted to leave with me feeling good about him. We decided that Xochi and Tanya would spend Christmas with him in Mexico.

Shooting continued at Marineland. It was a long drive from home, but it was nice coming home to a clean house. Tanya having learned from Pat drew my bath and had rose petals floating in it, and love notes from them. The girls even did the dishes. I loved having their support and I felt good about them going to Mexico for Christmas. A major earthquake was predicted for Los Angeles at that time and while I had to be there for work, I wanted them safe.

It was a treat working with Kay Pownall, who had taken over doing Marie's hair while I did Susan. The two actresses never worked together so when Susan worked. Kay supervised the hairstylists who were doing the extras. When Marie France worked, I supervised the extras. I liked the variety and it took the stress off both of us.

I had lots of time to think while driving to work. Mostly I wondered about my relationship with Patrick. We were still going round and round in circles. I felt like I was treading water. In order for things to work out Patrick would have to let go of his jealousy.

While I was in France, I had invited Severin, the French assistant director, to come and visit telling her she could stay with me. One day she arrived on the set. Surprised, I asked her why she hadn't come to the house. She replied that she could not believe I meant what I'd said. I finally convinced her I had meant it and she came to stay with us. Severin was strange. She got upset at how friendly Californians were, saying it felt phony. She hated stoplights telling her when to walk or not. I thought it was funny since I had found the majority of the French quite unfriendly.

The girls left for Mexico and I knew I'd miss them a lot. I told them they'd probably see the earth opening in wide cracks beneath them as the plane took off. "Don't say that Mom," they protested.

The house was empty, but I didn't have much time to think about it. We worked such long hours due to the number of large extra calls. The day Laurie got her first call as an extra, I told her to come in with her hair all done up in pin curls, which she did. When she arrived at work the next day, her hair was amazing. With all the pin curls it was so thick that the hairstylist could hardly get a comb through it. By the time Laurie was made up with her hair done and in costume, I hardly recognized her. She had a great time.

I thought I wouldn't enjoy Christmas without Tanya and Xochi, but I was wrong. Severin and I went to my mother's for dinner and later to Fred Broast's home. His wife, the great cook who had made the soup during the hurricane in New Orleans, fed us again. We had a lovely evening with a second traditionally French Christmas dinner.

On New Year's Eve I picked Tanya and Xochi up at Mexican Airlines. They'd had a wonderful time, although not really a Mexican Christmas as I'd hoped. At least the predicted earthquake hadn't shaken Los Angeles.

Nineteen seventy-seven was finally here. I wondered what changes it would bring (many as it turned out). I was still working on *The Other Side of Midnight,* which was both fun and exhausting. There were some problems with Frank Yablans, our producer. He was a unique character and I liked him a lot. He loved to kid, sometimes very strongly. It appeared that he must have come right off the streets of New York, but his enthusiasm for and love of making movies won me over and his jokes relieved the tension that built up on the set at times.

Frank pushed and pushed us and although everyone did their best, it never seemed to be enough. We were all totally exhausted, especially Marie France. In her role she was supposed to be a lovely, rich woman. While they were shooting someone changed the schedule for the benefit of production. That meant she had to change back and forth between her younger character and the sophisticated woman she becomes. It wasn't so difficult for her acting skills, but it was a pain having to change her makeup all the time. Production refused to give Lee time to take off her makeup and begin fresh so it caked, which didn't look good. Lee was exhausted and depressed and others felt the same way. Frank's pushing made it impossible to do our jobs correctly.

He got wind of our dissatisfaction. Goodness knows that I'd told him often enough. Early one morning he called a meeting of the crew and announced that he wanted to hear any complaints. He said he was willing to listen. Seeing as I was standing right next to him I spoke up first explaining our problem with Marie France. She was being pushed too hard and on top of everything else she had to learn English. Frank remarked, "It must be that time of the month." I was angry. "That's not it at all," I retorted. "She's just exhausted."

With my complaints registered I waited for the others to speak up. Nobody else opened their mouth. I couldn't believe it. I was really annoyed at all the wimps who had complained behind Frank's back yet were afraid to speak up now. Later in the day the art director commended me for telling the truth and apologized for not speaking up himself. I learned something about men that day. They were too afraid of losing their jobs and would rather bitch and complain than confront the problem head on. I don't think Frank liked what I had to say, but I believe he respected me for saying it and I wasn't fired either.

Bruce, our publicist, was writing a book called, *The Making of "The Other Side of Midnight"*. He hung around with us in our trailer. He was getting frustrated because there was very little excitement among the stars, nothing of interest to write about.

Susan had a boyfriend who kept her off-balance. She'd come in with circles under her big eyes, looking sad. Lee would make her up as best he could, but he had to fight with the cameraman about how to light her so she would look her best.

Charles, our director, joked about Frank's casting saying here he had this wonderful story filled with romantic characters and Frank had given him Minnie Mouse (Marie France), Olive Oil (Susan), and Ichabod Crane (John) to work with. We tried very hard to make them look their best and then we begged the cameraman to do his magic. It seemed to me, Fred, our cameraman, didn't care about the overall product. He didn't seem very enthusiastic about his work, nor did his assistants. The only time I saw him excited was when we shot a scene with Susan where the rain poured down on her and Fred used the fireman's hose to aim the water at her. Maybe he should have been a fireman. He might have enjoyed his life more.

Marie France was so short and John was so tall they designed shoes with five inch platforms for her to wear. If you noticed the shoes, it looked terribly silly. We joked that whereas in the script she was to die at the firing squad, in reality she might die falling off her shoes.

John (who was still with his wife) complained that he had to take off his clothes for the bathtub scene with Marie France. In actuality he was worried about what his wife would say. I couldn't believe it. "Didn't you read the script?" I asked. "It's all in there." Soon after the bathtub scene we shot at Lincoln Heights Jail, which was in one of the sleazier parts of Los Angeles. At lunchtime John and the boys sneaked off to a girlie show. When they returned, I asked John, "Why is it okay for women to take off their clothes and you guys watch them, but it isn't right for a man?" He mumbled a reply.

Finally Bruce decided that his book would have to be written from the point of view of Lee and me in the makeup trailer. He felt we were more interesting to write about than anyone else.

The film went on and on. It was really a creative job for me doing all the period hair work and the changes back and forth. It amused me one day when my sister talked about the film not being "morally perfect". How righteous! I wasn't there to judge the film, but to do the best job I could. I was proud of what I accomplished.

The film wrapped in February. What a relief! Pat was back from location. Our relationship still needed a lot of work so I decided we needed to see a marriage counselor. Glen, the counselor, came to our house to talk with us and gave us each a questionnaire to fill out. After we filled out the questionnaires and Glen had a chance to look them over, we met again. Glen told us he felt we really loved one another. We just had to open the lines of communication, share our feelings, and listen to one another - which I was happy to do. Now that there was an unbiased third party, for the first time each of us was able to speak without interruptions. Then Glen asked us to repeat what we heard the other person say and then the other would say if that was what was really said.

What a relief to be able to communicate with Pat again. We began to come together again. The girls were happy, too. The tension had disappeared. The family was healing.

Life was on the upswing. I was glad we were doing our emotional work rather than going our separate ways. We both knew it wouldn't be easy, but then anything worthwhile takes work. As for me, I no longer wanted to use work to avoid my problems. I was learning how to deal with them instead.

Toward the end of the film, I'd started on a liquid protein diet, an incredible feat for me. I ate nothing, just drank sweet tasting protein and lots of water. Each day I went to lunch with Lee and Kay and inhaled the smells of their food, vicariously enjoying their meals. If they ordered cold food, I was disappointed because it had no smell. In my deprived state, sniffing foods became equated with eating it. Strangely enough, I didn't feel hungry and I lost thirty pounds, which pleased me no end, but I did wonder what it had done to my body in the process.

After finishing the film I went to do publicity with Susan who lived in Manderville Canyon, a lovely section of Los Angeles. I'd loved working with her. She was so genuine with an open sweet manner and always shared her life with us. I hoped I'd get an opportunity work with her again someday.

Chapter 47

WHO'LL STOP THE RAIN

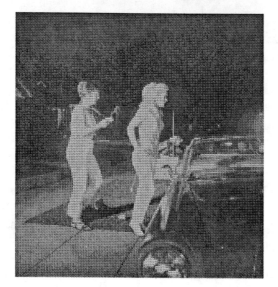

Sugar and Tuesday Weld, *Lord Love a Duck*

I got a call from Shel Schrager about doing a film called *Dog Soldiers,* later named *Who'll Stop the Rain*. It was a story about some Vietnam veteran smuggling drugs and then getting his wife involved with gangsters. It was directed by Karel Reisz and starred Nick Nolte, Michael Moriarty, and Tuesday Weld. My old friend Dick Kline was going to be the cameraman. It sounded okay, but after I read the script I realized the story was a real downer.

I met Karel Reisz and Michael Moriarty at the Chateau Marmont. I immediately loved Karel. He was a small, very gentle, sweet man. Michael was intense. He was sure I must be a New Yorker, something many people had said to me over the years. I asked him why and he replied that I had the enthusiasm of an easterner. Most Californians were so laid back. Now, at last I understood what people meant when they said that to me. It was true that I always felt very alive and energized when in the east.

Michael was balding and wanted to try a hairpiece so off we went to Ziggy, the wig maker, who designed a piece for him. But after trying it out in a screen test Michael decided he didn't like it.

It was fun to work with Tuesday again. I caught up on her life. She was married to Dudley Moore at the time. An unlikely choice for her, I thought. He was so funny and she seemed sort of negative, at least that's the way she acted. They had a baby daughter. Tuesday was just as attractive as ever. I ordered a wig for Tuesday also, but later we decided against it.

On April 10, 1977, we left for Stockton, staying at the Holiday Inn, the motel of choice for a movie crew. Pat said he always liked staying in it because when he woke up in the middle of the night he knew just what direction to head for the bathroom. Throughout our years in the film business we spent so much time in hotels that a Holiday Inn did begin to seem like home. I hadn't been to Stockton since I was a kid. I'd loved the long hot summers I'd spent there. On this trip we worked down by the river, an area I hadn't discovered in my teen years. It resembled Vietnam, which is why we were there.

We were shooting a scene from the Vietnam War with napalm bombs exploding. This particular scene would reveal the reasons for our characters' disorders later in the film. I was almost sick thinking that was what really went on during the war. For this scene they created the most terrifying explosion I'd ever seen. I couldn't have imagined it no matter how hard I tried. A 250-foot long pipe was set up to contain the area where the explosion would take place. We were all sent far away from the set because they didn't want anyone to be hurt, so we watched from the river.

We were told not to look, but when the director shouted, "Roll," it was impossible not to react to the explosion. It flashed brighter than anything I'd ever seen and the sound was incredible. I could feel it inside my heart where it vibrated and filled me with terror. This was not a fantasy to those who had endured the war.

After the explosion was filmed, they went in to shoot close-ups. We went back to the set. All of us were affected in one way or another. For the rest of the day they burned tires to simulate the smoke of the war. It smelled just awful and by the end of the day I was covered with the black film from the burning tires. That night it took five showers to get all the gunk off my skin. It had even seeped through my clothes.

The next day they set off several smaller explosions and there was mud everywhere and helicopters, too. What a mess we all were. I was glad when we finished that scene and left for Berkeley.

In Berkeley we filmed on a huge freighter that sailed out into San Francisco Bay. It was empty so it rocked from side to side like a little rowboat bobbing in the water. Sometimes when trying to walk up a staircase I would find myself walking horizontally instead of vertically. Shel, our unit manager, ever the manipulator, had loaded the ship with more crewmembers than he had permission to have. I was instructed to hide in a closet if we were boarded so he wouldn't get in trouble. Nice going, I thought to myself.

Our hotel in Berkeley was in a lousy part of town and barely adequate. Prostitutes roamed the streets. I felt sorry for these young, long-legged, short-skirted women out in the cold of the night. The funny thing was that nobody would stop for me when I wanted to cross the street. I guessed they thought I was out hawking my wares, too. No way. Well, then again somebody might have wanted a woman with a little meat on her bones. Who knows?

Many of our extras were Vietnamese immigrants. They were so nice and most of them allowed me to cut their hair. One man wouldn't allow it on the first night, but got his grandfather's permission and came the next night for a cut.

After seeing Nick Nolte's hair in the dailies, they decided it needed to be a bit lighter. During the war sequence it hadn't mattered because he had been filthy. But now it needed to be lightened. I went shopping and found the necessary products. Since we didn't have a real shop to work in, I took Nick to my bathroom. There I was standing on the toilet seat while Nick stood in the shower with me pouring water over his head, both of us laughing at the outrageous situation. It worked though.

Arnie Schmidt, our first assistant, was such a nice man, but Shel was different and not always easy to deal with. Shel was wise to put a person like Arnie on the set with the crew. One evening I went with them to San Francisco where I experienced another Hyatt Hotel. It was similar to the one in Atlanta only a bit more luxurious. All open inside with plants and glass everywhere. The construction of these places never failed to amaze me. We ate a sumptuous Italian dinner, took a tour of art galleries, and finished up with an Irish coffee.

We worked a few nights on the pier and were exhausted at five in the morning when we finally wrapped. After breakfast we'd fall into bed and sleep until our call the following afternoon.

We worked in a bookstore in Berkeley. What a treat for me, the book-a-holic. I could browse through the books and not have to buy all those that appealed to me. At lunch I went to an authentic Berkeley-style coffee house. People sat around the tables deep in conversation. It was one of those places I'd always wanted to go to or even run. I ordered cappuccino and drank in the atmosphere. I hadn't gone to college and that hadn't mattered to me, but if I had gone to places like this I might have changed my mind.

One evening we worked in a dark, smoky nightclub with topless dancers. I went home smelling terrible, my hair full of tobacco smoke and my lungs hurting.

Pat was writing lovely letters and calling. He missed me a lot. I could feel it had been good for me to go away for a while leaving him with the kids and his feelings. He needed the time alone to become aware of what he really wanted out of life and our relationship.

We had a wrap party in Berkeley. I drank too much wine and in the next morning it was difficult getting packed and off to Los Angeles. We were all exhausted, having been pushed to the limit working long hours that changed back and forth from day to night.

It felt great to return home to Pat and the kids who were all happy to have me back. Before the weekend, we worked a couple of days more in Los Angeles and when the weekend finally arrived I collapsed, tired to the end of my arms and the bottom of my feet. I had to lie in bed and just let the tiredness flow out of me.

We were working on the stage at MGM, it was dark and the feeling on the set was dark, too, thanks to the story.

Michael was very intense and sometimes it took more than twenty takes before he was satisfied. Nick would come in and have his Morning Thunder tea and get ready for the day. That tea was powerful stuff. Nick was always fun and delightful even if his character was intense. Tuesday said we were too happy for her.

At this point Shel told me that I wouldn't be working on the second half of the movie that would be shot in Mexico. I was both let down and relieved. The film wasn't a whole lot of fun. Tuesday wasn't pleased, she wanted me there for her, but they didn't want to take anyone who could possibly be left behind. Nick's makeup man, Eddie Enrique, was in his contract so he would be going. I gave him my hair stills so he could advise the Mexican hairstylist who would take my place.

Before they left for Mexico, we worked in San Diego, out in the desert, and at various airports around town. The film came to an end for me on May 26. I was relieved. I hadn't had any time for myself during the shooting. My relationship with Pat was improving, but I needed time to get to know myself and Pat. After all these years I was finally beginning to feel that there must be something more to life than work.

Before she left for Mexico I gave Tuesday lots of healthy suggestions for taking care of her baby while she was there. I enjoyed her even though she complained about my good humor. I don't really think it bothered her.

Chapter 48

HIGH ANXIETY

The production manager on *High Anxiety*, a Mel Brooks film, had called toward the end of *Who'll Stop the Rain* to ask if I'd be available for work. If so, when? The film was already in production. Linda Trainoff was the hairstylist on the film, but when she was hired she told them she was going on a Caribbean Cruise halfway through the film and they hired her anyway, knowing she would have to be replaced. They had given another hairstylist Mary Keats a try, but that hadn't worked out so now they were calling me, hoping number three would be the charm.

I thought about it for a few moments then realized I wanted to do a comedy after the black drama I'd been working on. I took the job and was immediately told to order a wig for Cloris Leachman, who was playing Nurse Diesel. What a character Cloris was. Still is. She was even more eccentric than when I worked with her on *The Cher Show* years before, full of talent and oddities and I liked her a lot.

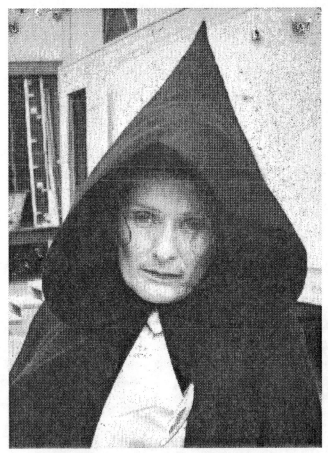

Cloris Leachman, *High Anxiety*

The first scene on the film was wild. A large group of people was sitting at a table eating an elegant dinner at the sanitarium where most of our action took place. All our stars were at the table, including Harvey Korman, Cloris Leachman, and Mel Brooks. The camera was on a boom outside of the set, while the action was going on inside. I watched as Mel shouted, "Action". The scene inside began, the camera began outside, but slowly it began moving toward the window as if it was coming in for a close-up. It kept coming and coming and then it just crashed right through the window. As it crashed through the window, the scene just went on as normal at the table, with the camera now inside the room.

Mount Saint Mary's on Sunset Boulevard was a beautiful spot, our hospital exterior. One of my favorite things about working on films was being able to work in the most marvelous places that ordinarily I would never be allowed into. This film was a spoof on Alfred Hitchcock's movies. We were filming a part of *Vertigo* in a bell tower there. The day was all foggy and felt very English.

One morning while doing her hair, I mentioned to Cloris about my wanting to have Juliette Prowse-like legs. "Oh how foolish! "She chided me. She had already been after me about my weight that morning. She got on her soapbox and said that I'd been acting like a cunt to myself (in her words) by not accepting my legs as they were. "When you are finished with my hair I want you to come to my dressing room," she demanded. When I got there, she closed the door and went into the bathroom. "Okay," she said, "now take off your slacks and look at your legs in the mirror. Just look at them. Tell them how much you appreciate them and thank them for carrying you around all this time." I laughed a little uneasily, but I slipped off my slacks and looked at my legs. Of course my legs were not Juliette Prouse-like, but they were sturdy and had never given me a bit of trouble. I talked to them and told them thanks and apologized for wanting them to be different.

From then on Cloris called me Legs.

Going from film to film plus all the emotional work with Pat had exhausted me, so when I had a day off I went to the doctor. He said I needed B12 shots. After picking up the hairpieces for Cloris I went home to relax.

This was a busy time in the film business and I got a call for *Going South* with Jack Nicholson. I wasn't finished with *High Anxiety* yet so had to turn it down.

June 17 was my forty-third birthday and Pat sent red roses to the set. The following day we saw the finished product of *The Other Side of Midnight*. I hadn't realized how much location there had been. All our interior sets had been matched up to the exteriors and it looked as though the whole film had been shot on location. I was proud of the work I had done. The period hair dos looked great.

The next day we went to Hollywood to the Grauman's Chinese Theater to see *Star Wars*. What a fabulous experience. The film was breaking all records. We stood way around the block to get in even at ten o'clock in the morning. Our seats were in the very first row.

Looking up at the giant screen as the credits rolled by, we were overwhelmed with the grandeur and the power of it all. The sound was incredible with the music surrounding us. I felt like I was right inside the whole adventure. It was truly impressive. Since we were in Hollywood, we went to see *Annie Hall* that same afternoon. Although it was a great film, it was tame compared with our morning's entertainment.

There were some great scenes during *High Anxiety*. In one scene Cloris, wore a severely pointed bra that looked like it was made of metal and had Harvey strung up on a rack above the bed which she let down little by little. I also loved it when she said, "I think I will let down my hair" because that morning I had put a five-foot long wig of black hair on her so she was really able let down her hair. She was evil and insane, a great nurse for the asylum.

Another time we did a scene in the mad house where a man was imagining himself to be a dog. He lifted his leg and peed on Mel Brooks, which broke us up. The strange thing was, when we saw the movie later none of these scenes seemed as funny as they had when we were filming them.

Cloris' call to be ready on the set was nine o'clock, but she always came in late. Terry Miles, the makeup man, a big strong man and I would literally throw her together. I'd be gluing on her hair lace wig as she was leaving the makeup trailer. Never letting her be late became a game with me, but it was stressful, because a hair lace wig is so delicate.

Mel Brooks would come in to get his makeup. Terry painted Mel's scalp with black stuff so his thinning hair wouldn't be noticed. Mel was very picky about the way this was done. If there was nothing going on in the trailer, he'd watch Terry work with an eagle eye, but when Mel talked with me he wouldn't pay as close attention. For the first time ever a makeup man asked me to talk to his actor while he was doing his makeup.

Mark Johnson, who is now a well-known producer, graduated to second assistant on this film. I first met him in Santa Domingo, when Pat was doing *Sorcerer*. He had been a gopher of sorts at that time. It was fun to see him again and we reminisced about old times in Santa Domingo.

I was reading a book called *Pilgrims Inn*. It was about a family who after the Second World War came to an inn in the forest to heal. There was a river nearby, a unicorn in the forest and many cozy things that made me want to move right into the story. I was having a fantasy of living in a thatched hut in the country.

One day on the set, I was reading *Yankee Magazine* and I noticed an ad from a realtor selling inns. Mark, who was looking over my shoulder, remarked, "You and Pat would be great innkeepers." I replied, "I've often thought about hotel management and all that stuff." "Give them a call," Mark encouraged. He then proceeded to tell me about all the great inns he had visited when he lived back East. He had even thought about running a bed and breakfast himself. I made the call, asking for information.

Phil Steckler, of Country Business Brokers in Brattleboro Vermont, returned my call a couple of days later. I asked him to send us a brochure and any information he had. I was imagining what it would be like to run an inn and live where the lilacs bloomed. I couldn't wait for the information to arrive.

Miltie, Elizabeth Montgomery's agent, called me. He said Lizzie was considering doing a seven-hour television show called *Awakening Land*. It sounded far better than the Jack Nicholson film I had been offered. Miltie told me to call Robin Clark, the unit manager, and talk with him about it. I did so, but was only offered the minimum salary, which outraged Miltie who felt Robin should know better - people who worked with Lizzie got top dollar. After Miltie was done with Robin, I did.

High Anxiety came to an end. I'd had so much fun working on it that at the end of the film I felt more peppy and enthusiastic than when I'd begun. Cloris thanked me and acknowledged that I had really done a lot for her by not allowing her to be late. That part had been rather stressful, but I enjoyed it nonetheless. Mel gave me a great compliment. "Sugar," he said, "you're good and you're smart and I'd like to work again with you."

My information package about the inns arrived and I could hardly wait to look it over. Pat and I sat down together to check it out. The price of the inns for sale was unbelievably low and the places seemed to be calling to us. Since the film with Lizzie wouldn't start until the beginning of September and Pat had some time off too, we just looked at each other and simultaneously said, "Let's do it." We had the time and the money and we both thought it would be great to go back to where we first met. So we did.

Chapter 49

A CHANGE OF LIFESTYLE

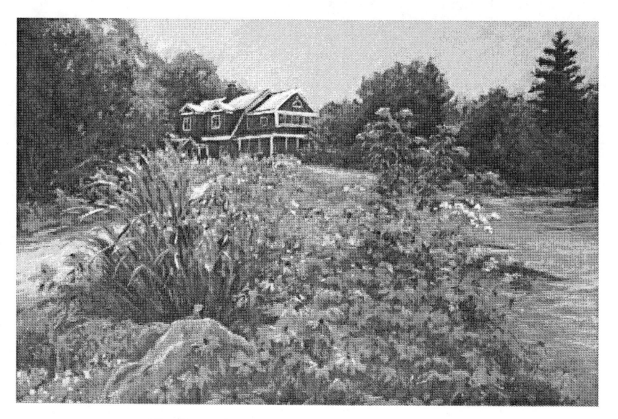

The Snowvillage Inn, painted by Gwen Nagel

July 23, 1977, we boarded a plane headed to Bradley Airport in Hartford, Connecticut. We were on our tour of inns for sale. I was so excited as we landed, that my eyes were watering. It was an hour later than expected and I was weary, but none of that mattered. My excitement carried me forward. We rented a car and headed north toward our first destination, Chester, Vermont and The Chester Inn.

Driving along the turnpike, I began to take in the scenery. There were lovely birches that grew on both sides of the road and sometimes even in the center of the road. These Birch trees were huge, unlike mine at home that had been growing for three years and still had trunks the width of a pencil. My excitement mounted as we drove along and I was beginning to feel that there just might be another way of life for me besides working in the movie industry. When we moved to our farm in Appalachia, I had learned that dreams could become reality. When I allowed myself the luxury of dreaming I knew my dreams could come true. Those beautiful birches became a symbol of a door that began to open that day.

I drove Pat crazy as we drove along. "Oh how beautiful, look at the trees, look at it all." He'd grown up in West Virginia amidst the mountains and forests took that all for granted, whereas I grew up in Los Angeles, which I considered to be a desert. I was absolutely enchanted. We arrived in Chester late that afternoon.

The Chester Inn looked immense when we pulled into the driveway. For some reason, I'd expected all inns to be cozy little places. This was picturesque, so was the town, with an inviting pond and flowers everywhere, in window boxes and along the paths - just what I'd imagined New England would be like. As we went inside to check in, an older woman at the desk greeted us with a friendly smile. We were shown to our room, which, though small, was quite nice. The wallpaper was flowering, fluffy, pillows adorned our bed, and the shower barely worked. But we were happy.

We made reservations for dinner and showered and dressed. That evening the experience in the dining room with all the candles lit and flowers on each table fed my desire to have an inn of our own. I began to make plans right then, forgetting we were only supposed to be looking.

Our friendly waitress recited the menu by heart. We made our selections and ordered a glass of wine. While we waited for our dinner, we chatted with our waitress who told us why she came to live in Vermont. With enthusiasm she described how she looked forward to the winters because she loved to ski cross-country. Being a California native, I had dreaded the thought of snow, but as I listened to her I began to understand how each season had its own special charm. Our meal was delicious, prepared with fresh vegetables and inventive deserts.

The next morning, after a breakfast that included blueberry muffins, we drove to Woodstock, Vermont. Wow! The only car dealership in town was the Mercedes Dealer, which impressed us. We found our way through that delightful village to check out the inn we had decided to stay in toward the end of our trip. It was different and much smaller than the Chester Inn. We loved Woodstock and thought it might just be "the place" for us.

That day we were supposed to meet Phil Steckler who was vacationing at Lake Winnipesauke in New Hampshire. He had wanted us to come at another time, but having two weeks off together was already a miracle so he arranged the trip for us and said to come by his family's vacation home while we were in the vicinity so we could meet.

His house was near Alton Bay. We followed the gravel driveway that led us right down to the lakeshore and found his lovely home situated among the trees. Phil came out and introduced himself and wife, kids, and dog. We liked him immediately. He offered us lunch, which we gratefully accepted. He told us we had to take a swim and since it was a warm day I donned my bathing suit and went in the water. We paddled around in a canoe for a bit, too. After dinner we went on our merry way to the next inn, Glen Gables.

Glen Gables was further west and south, but still on Lake Winnepausakee. Pat thought I was crazy because all the way there I kept sniffing myself. I smelled like pine trees and it was wonderful. I didn't want to take a shower and remove that wonderful scent.

Glen Gables was a disappointment. What a difference from the night before. It was more a bar and a restaurant than an inn. The innkeepers were a friendly Italian family, but the place had no atmosphere. Our room was unattractive and the beds were uncomfortable. Pat and I talked a lot that night. Was an inn really what we wanted? Of the two we had seen neither was close to my fantasy. Not a unicorn in sight. Perhaps we were just on a sightseeing trip after all. We were enjoying ourselves so we decided we might as well continue. It would be great vacation regardless of the outcome.

The next morning we ate breakfast in the main building which was really depressing. The whole family was sitting around a large table in the dining room trying to recover from the previous night's entertainment. I decided I wanted no bar atmosphere in my inn. We paid and the owner put the cash in his pocket. Mmm.

We set off driving around the lake marveling at the old homes. In Wolfeboro, N.H. we stopped at a cheese shop in a little red caboose and bought some cheese for snacks before continuing on our drive. We saw a sign that said, "Wolfeboro, America's oldest resort." It was such a beautiful place.

In Conway we located route 153 and drove south five miles, turned at Crystal Lake, went three quarters of a mile to a sign for the inn, and another three quarters of a mile up the hill. The day was overcast, but it was still beautiful driving through the woods. We went up and up. Suddenly a beautiful inn revealed itself.

It was perfect - a dark red, covered with shingles, surrounded by huge trees and bushes. Apple trees lined the driveway and we spied a clay tennis court beyond the stone walls, which just happened to be the widest stone walls we'd seen on our trip. We drove up the driveway and stopped at the front door. An older man greeted us. After introducing himself as Max Pluss, he asked for our bags and carried them to a room above the dining room. Then he told us when dinner would be ready.

We had earlier enjoyed a nice lunch with a glass of wine and were ready for a nap so after unpacking we crawled into bed. It was still overcast which added to the relaxed feeling and our need to take a snooze.

A couple of hours later I woke up and looked out the window. The view was absolutely incredible. We'd seen the brochure and it had shown a nice view, but there was no way a picture could do this view justice. The clouds were rolling away, revealing a green valley with a mountain range beyond. In the distance we could see Mount Washington for which the valley was named. It couldn't have been more beautiful. I'll swear I saw a unicorn for a moment. We were sold. I wanted to move right in.

At dinner that night Max was a little cool. Later we realized he didn't want anyone to know the inn was for sale. The meal was quite good, but not as fancy or creative as the night before. The dining room was un-crowded and very quiet so we tended to whisper. No alcohol was served. If people wanted something to drink, they brought it themselves.

After eating we wandered onto the porch, visited with a couple who were also guests, and went off to bed early. Max said we would get together to talk the next morning after all the guests left.

Our room was large with knotty pine walls. The bedspreads were something out of the 1940s, covered in huge flowers. The shower was good and we slept well.

The next morning Max was friendlier. He showed us all around the place and explained why he was selling. After his first wife died he had remarried. His new wife was from Switzerland, spoke only French, and was unhappy in Snowville. She wanted to go home and he wanted to please her.

The inn was an incredible place. There were eight rooms in the main house and a huge barn with eight more rooms most of which had their own private baths. I was already redecorating in my mind. Max had run it with only fifteen guests at the most and was closed in the winter. The inn needed new blood. I loved it! I was sure we belonged there. We still had more inns to visit before making a decision, plus Snow Village Lodge was the most expensive inn on our tour and we didn't know if we could even afford to buy it. Anyway we were just looking, or so we thought.

The next stop was Darby Field Inn also on a mountain, a little south of Conway. Our room wasn't going to be ready for us until late afternoon so we decided to take a drive to Portland, Maine, about an hour and fifteen minutes away. We roamed Exchange Street on the waterfront, thoroughly charmed, had lobster and oysters and white wine for lunch. We were pleased that Portland was so close to Conway.

Scott McKnight greeted us at the door of Darby Field Inn. It was different from Snow Village Lodge, but very attractive, too. Our room was small with slanted ceilings and had a musty smell. The shower was not great either, but the pub was attractive and the meal was one of the top five ever. The next morning at breakfast we enjoyed the view, but it couldn't compare to the view of the day before.

We took a tour and began to think that if we did buy an inn, this might have to be the one because of the price. Still the place seemed to be coming apart at the seams and I had a feeling it might be beyond our abilities to put it back into shape.

Our next stop was Sugar Hill Inn in Franconia. I thought this might be the one for us as it already had my name, but as we drove north we realized that we preferred the Conway area to Franconia.

By the time we finished the trip, we had decided upon Snow Village Lodge and I had fallen in love with New England.

Nothing should have surprised me. Under my calm demeanor changes had been brewing. My dissatisfaction with the movie business had been coming to a head once again. As I began to pay attention to my needs, I realized I wanted more time to myself. I was tired of work, work, work, all the time. We had a great house, and plenty of income, and our bills were all paid off. We were in demand at work. But still I didn't feel satisfied. I felt there must be more to life. Pat was on one side of the world, I was on the other, and the kids were at home. What kind of life was that?

So here we were driving toward Brattleboro, Vermont to see Phil, seriously considering buying an inn, which seemed unreasonable and unrealistic, but exactly what we wanted. We were ready to totally change our lives in an instant. We checked into the Colonial Inn in Brattleboro and made an appointment to see Phil. We told him that the only inn we really loved was Snow Village Lodge and asked how we could manage to buy it. After looking over our financial information he said, "If you sell everything, your home in Los Angeles and the farm in West Virginia, I think we can put this together for you." We were astonished and thrilled.

He gave us an SBA business plan to fill out, a complete plan for running a business and asked us to consider finances including back-up money, our family, our plans, our dreams, and our abilities - a perfect exercise. Had we done this before we bought the farm we might not have, but I was glad we'd had that experience, even though it had been overwhelming at times.

As we were filling out the forms, I remembered the visualizing I'd done when I read a book on EST. In my vision I lived in a huge, dark, red-shingled home where many of my friends, whom I never saw much of, because we were all so busy, could come and visit, and I was living in a never-ending forest. Well, New Hampshire was 85 per cent forest. I had also seen myself sitting on a window seat looking out the window and seeing people drive up the hill toward our home. All my random thoughts inspired, by a book, were becoming reality at Snow Village Lodge.

Phil took us back to the Conway area. We stayed at the Tamworth Inn this time while we contacted a banker. We met Randy Cooper, a lawyer who informed us of all we needed to know. Next, we all met with Max's lawyer and made the offer of $235,000, on the inn, with a $15,000 down payment. That was, all we had in the bank. It was accepted.

Max was pleased. His belief was that life has many Chapters. "When one Chapter comes to an end," he said, "we must close it, tie it up with a pretty silk ribbon, put it away and open a new Chapter of our life." He emphasized what a great life he had enjoyed for the past thirty years. He had lived in a most wonderful place like a rich man, which he never would have been able to do if he hadn't had the inn. I liked that.

Before we made the offer, I took Pat aside. I wanted him to be sure he was doing this because he wanted to do it, not just to please me. I didn't want to hear later that it was all for me, and he really hadn't wanted to do it. He assured me he had changed and wanted this as much as I did.

We gave Randy a $400 check for an appraisal and took one more walk through the inn. We had only been there twice and now we had a $15,000 deposit on the place and not one iota of inn - keeping experience. We had stayed at top hotels around the world. We knew what people wanted in a hotel and felt we could supply it. If all went as planned we would sell our home and our farm. We needed to come up with $105,000, including the down payment, and running expenses by May 1978.

We boarded the plane back at the Bradley Airport, hooked our seatbelts, sat back and looked at one another, and began to laugh. "We must be crazy. Nobody spends all that money on something they've only seen twice." Wrong! We made our decision without a second thought.

Chapter 50

AWAKENING LAND
Springfield, Illinois, Summer 1977

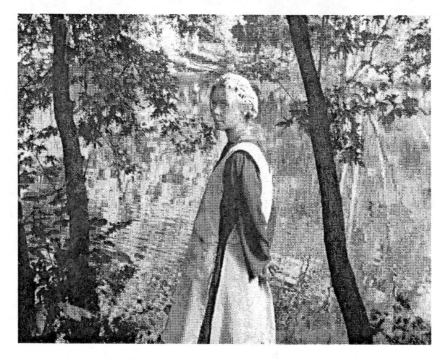

Elizabeth Montgomery, *Awakening Land*

The plane approached its descent into the Los Angeles Airport while we were still laughing at ourselves. We lived our lives differently from anyone we knew, but in truth I sensed we had made the right decision. Los Angeles's brown, smog-filled skyline only confirmed my feeling. Laurie met us at the airport and after piling all our stuff in the car we took off for home. The traffic was horrible and I missed those beautiful birches. Now that we had decided to really change our life, I saw Los Angeles through totally different eyes. I was very happy we had decided to make such a drastic change.

We transferred all our funds from our savings account to the checking account to cover the $15,000 deposit on the inn. We were down to zero savings again and it was quite scary. We still needed to raise at least $85,000 more.

The next day I went into to meet with Boris Segal, the director of *Awakening Land*, a multi-generational story of a pioneer family living in the late eighteenth to the early nineteenth centuries. We talked about how he saw the characters that comprised the film. In the story, the family first settled on barren land in the woods near a lake and then began to build a town, which grew throughout the film. It was a huge, challenging project.

Late in August we began to do tests with Elizabeth Montgomery. Her hair was to be very basic for most of the film, just tied back with a little leather thong. Sometimes she was wearing a mobcap, one of those cotton things that covered the whole head. All the characters had to look very simple, unkempt, and rather rough as they didn't have the time to spend trying to look beautiful, nor did they have a mirror in which to see themselves. It was all work and little play for these pioneers.

There were nearly a hundred characters in the film and almost every one of the males needed a wig. There also were Indians who needed strange, flat top haircuts that meant that I would have to buy wigs and cut them to fit the parts. I looked into renting wigs, but it was very expensive, so I decided to buy them myself and rent them to the company. It would be a risk for me and a large investment, but it would cost the company much less that way.

When the wigs arrived, I packed them up along with all of my other supplies. I had to buy many supplies; we wouldn't be close to any beauty suppliers and I wanted to be prepared for anything. We had a huge makeup trailer that left for location so I put everything I needed in there. Having prepared as much as possible, I relaxed a bit and went shopping for location clothes.

One of the actress's had quit and I suggested Susan Sarandon for the part, but she was already working on *Pretty Baby* which made her a star.

On September 2, we left for Springfield, Illinois. The Forum Hotel was a tall phallic-shaped building rising out of Springfield's downtown. What a dreadful design. The building was round; therefore, my room was pie-shaped - very narrow near the door and wider toward the windows. It felt weird and I didn't like it at all. Must have been bad Feng Shui. Our cameraman, Michele Hugo, was next door in a far bigger room with a kitchen. Each night I smelled wonderful food as he cooked his gourmet meals. My mouth watered and I happily accepted when one evening he invited me to dinner.

Pat came by for a visit on his way to State College, Pennsylvania where he was going to film inside a prison. He sensed my discomfort over my pie-shaped room and began to search the around for an apartment. As luck would have it, he found one that was perfect - within walking distance of the hotel and roomy, with two bedrooms. It had a kitchen and a living room. I was in heaven. I was going to be on location for a long time and needed a comfortable place to live. Pat went out and bought linens and kitchenware and I was set.

Lizzie didn't like the fact that I had moved out of the hotel. I wasn't sure why. All I could think of was that perhaps she might want me to visit her and she felt I was now too far away. I assured her I would be available whenever she needed me. I also explained that while she had a great suite at the top of the hotel the crew was housed in little, pie-shaped caves on the lower floors. For the same money I had a wonderful apartment with plenty of room. I don't think she really got it, but Joe, our Bluebird limo driver, understood. I was glad because he had known Lizzie much longer than I had.

I was very lucky to get a top hairstylist - Vivian MacAteer - to help me. She had been my teacher at my second hairdressing school and we were good friends. She was great to work with and happy to have had the opportunity to work with me. Her husband, Mickey, was head of Transportation on the film.

There was lots of work ahead of us. Getting the extras' and actors' wardrobes fitted for the film was a huge project. I told Robin, our Unit Manager that I was renting the wigs to the company, which would be a savings for them, and he agreed it was a good idea. I also told him that the wigs were not good enough to be shown close up without a cap. They weren't hair lace that would have cost thousands of dollars each. I told Boris, our director, that he mustn't ask the men to take off their hats. It seemed a weird request, but it wasn't a feature film and therefore didn't have a large budget so a few sacrifices were necessary.

The costumes were made of rough material and in simple designs. They actually looked as if they had been woven at home. The props impressed me. The bowls and kitchenware had been hand-carved and the spoons looked handmade.

It was a lot of work to get the wigs to look like real hair. Most of the wigs were too full of hair and had to be thoroughly thinned. I hoped we'd be ready for the first day of shooting. I really had no doubts, but there were times when I felt overwhelmed.

On the first day our call was 3:30 a.m. I went in and began dressing the extra's hair and later took a break to do Lizzie before continuing with the extras. Our assistant directors were not great, actually quite incompetent at times and by the end of the first hour I was furious and let them know. I got over it quickly, but it wasn't a good omen. With all the people we had to work on, we needed organization. Where did they get these guys?

Our meals were a problem, too, because we started work so early and were supposed to eat within six hours as per union rules. We had to eat breakfast by 9:30 a.m., but we were still putting on wigs. I argued with Robin over it. I felt that they should pay us a meal penalty (money added to our pay if we went longer than six hours without a break) and let us get our work done rather than holding up production to save a few dollars. But Production hated to pay the penalty even when it was necessary. They were absolutely unreasonable. We were working our rear ends off, but they didn't care. One morning after yet another argument over this, Boris asked me how I was and I burst into tears. I told him that we were trying to do our work yet were being hassled over the meal penalty. I never heard another word about it.

Sometimes Lizzie would tease me saying, "Sugar, thanks a lot. I get you on the film and then never see you." She was right. I wasn't spending much time with her. But in my defense I explained, "You asked me to do the whole film, not just you, to help Boris get it made. There's so much work and so little help and it's necessary that I always be on the set. I wish I could spend more time with you, but I can't." She knew that, of course. Anyway, she had Hal Holbrook, who played her husband, to talk with. They often played Backgammon together. Bob Foxworth came, too, which was great because Lizzie was happy when he was there and when she was happy so was I.

A new star arrived to play Lizzie's sister - a beautiful, young English actress named Jane Seymour. Jane had the most marvelous hair that reached below her waist. She brushed it with a special Mason & Pearson brush, and was very fussy about it. I didn't think I could handle her on top of everything else so I asked Vivian if she would mind doing Jane's hair. Vivian happily complied. She had such patience. As I watched her do Jane's hair, I was relieved it was she and not me.

When I gave Robin the bill for the hair rental, $1800 a week, he was shocked. He thought that was the bill for the whole shoot. I couldn't believe his naiveté. I reminded him that hair and makeup were not consulted when the budget was being put together. This wasn't unusual, but an accountant couldn't possibly know how much things like wigs, etc., would cost, especially when every man in the production needed one. I always wondered why department heads weren't consulted before the budget was made. In any case, I offered to write a letter to Warners explaining the expense. Robin said, "Please do, I would appreciate it." I did and there were no more questions. I received my wig rental on time each week.

One day there was an article in the paper with my picture doing someone's hair. I got a call from Kenny Norton's parents who lived in the area. They came to see me. We had a great visit. We had met on *Mandingo*.

We began shooting in an area outside of Springfield at a lake our company had created for the film. It was quite the mosquito pit on hot days. An old farmer taught me that Listerine Mouthwash was a good mosquito repellent so each

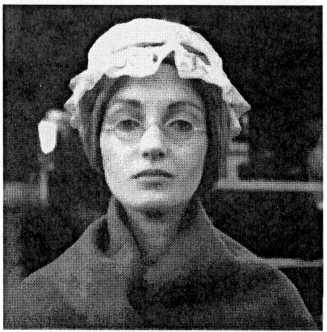

Jane Seymour, *Awakening Land*

morning after my shower I sprayed myself with it. During the day, the mosquitoes would fly toward me then suddenly hesitate and then turn away. Only when I washed my hands did they approach me and then only my hands.

It was exciting to see the log cabins being built in the forest. Everything came alive. It looked beautiful on film, because they kept a constant bonfire going in the center of the set. But I was happier when a few years (film time) had passed and we moved to Lincoln Land, a tourist attraction that was already a small village. It was closer to town and we didn't have to fight the mosquitoes plus there were many authentic buildings to work in.

One day all it did was rain. We all trudged through the mud and I held up better than most of the crew. It amused me that here I was heavier than most of the crew and yet my vitamins and attitude seemed to get me through in good shape. Maybe it was going to bed as early as possible that helped.

I missed Pat when he left, but it was okay. I knew that next year at that time we would be together in Snowville, keeping our inn. I pictured myself greeting our late guests, candle in hand. I even found a beautiful dark-green velvet robe to wear for the occasion. When I wasn't concentrating on work, I envisioned myself living at the inn. I couldn't wait for this new life to begin.

Before Pat left Springfield, the Small Business Bureau had approved our loan. Phil sent a business plan for Pat and me to fill out. Phil, our Realtor, was a slave driver, but he wanted the deal to go through as much as we did. After all, he stood to make about $25,000.

We spent Sunday writing up our plan. It was difficult, but we were full of enthusiasm and ideas. Just in case we needed extra money we had the movie business to go back to. Funny how that got us the loan, but later, when we wanted to borrow more for improvements, we couldn't use it as a source of income.

As I was filling in the forms, I pictured the living room of "my" inn filled with interesting people sitting in front of a roaring fire. Dinner was served in the dining room with the glorious view of Mount Washington and the valley. I could almost smell the muffins baking in the morning along with fresh ground coffee. What a wonderful future lay ahead.

In the meantime I was still working. Our sets were now located in a place called New Salem. It was now a town, no longer a little settlement. It was one of the first occasions that radios were used on the set. I don't know how we ever did without them. But there were still communication problems. Our nicest assistant, Al, was having a difficult time. He stuttered and when he spoke on the radio it was terrible. There we'd be waiting for an answer to some crucial question and poor Al was trying to tell us, but it just wouldn't come out. I wondered what had inspired him to take such a difficult and unlikely job. I was glad he was there because our first assistant, who will remain nameless, drove me crazy. I don't think he had a clue about how to make a film. It was important for the crew to work together and accommodate each other when things were difficult. This was especially true when operating on a tight budget. Cooperation was essential and somehow that first assistant just didn't get it.

One morning we had a call with all the extras in the first shot - meaning more than a hundred extras needed to be wigged. We were already coming to work before 4:00 a.m. as it was and Production had only allowed me one extra hairdresser. I put my foot down and insisted on another for these big shots. Luckily they listened, but even then the extras were sent to the set without a hairdresser standing by, which

ACADEMY

OF

TELEVISION ARTS & SCIENCES

Honors

SUGAR BLYMER
HAIRSTYLIST

THE AWAKENING LAND

PART III

FEBRUARY 21 1978   NBC

Nominated for

OUTSTANDING ACHIEVEMENT IN
ANY AREA OF CREATIVE TECHNICAL CRAFTS

1977-1978
TELEVISION ACADEMY AWARDS

Hank Rieger
President

Ginger's Television Academy Awards Nomination for
Awakening Land

was unheard of. The two makeup men, Tommy Tuttle and Mike Mochella were a little calmer, if not happier. They were old timers and it was normal for them to be grumpy at times. We were all worn out. Six - day weeks combined with long days added up. There was no time for anything except work. I was glad my life would soon be different.

The set kept changing as the years went by and rooms were added to buildings. The home where Lizzie and Hal and their family lived grew, room by room. I'd arrive on the set and the house would have a different shape. We filmed one scene in which the whole town got together for a barn raising. Another time they completed an unfinished church. It was interesting to see the town grow as the story progressed.

One day there was a scene in which about fifteen babies were on a bed in Lizzie's home. At first all the mothers were happy that their babies would be in the film - but not for long. This was another time our first assistant just didn't think. By rights the baby scene should have been shot early so the babies could go home. Wrong. He hadn't planned it that way and by afternoon the mothers were weary and the babies were hysterical. The scene was almost impossible to shoot.

In the meantime, Bob Foxworth and I had a wonderful time playing with the babies while Lizzie looked on disdainfully. She didn't like acting with children. She became impatient with them plus she felt they always seemed to steal the scene. Ironically, thanks to her series, *Bewitched*, she was doomed to have kids' attention everywhere she went. Kids just loved that show.

The Frazee family - Logan, Terry, and Logan, Jr. - was tops in their field and they did special effects for the film. They were each so different. The father was clever and funny, but quiet. Whenever I wore my huge moon boots, he'd ask, "Sugar, do you always have to drag your feet?" Terry was the star of the family. He was very attractive, loved racehorses, and also had a wonderful family. Logan, Jr. was the introvert - quiet like his father and as awkward as Terry was graceful. They were all good friends.

A few months before this, Logan's wife of seventeen years had left him and Terry decided it was time for Logan, his brother to begin to date. I thought it was a good idea too, but Logan was painfully shy so I offered to give him dating lessons. One Sunday afternoon there was a party and I decided it would be a great opportunity for a rehearsal date. Logan agreed so he and Terry picked me up at the appointed time and took me to the motel where most of the crew was staying and where the party was being held. Logan sat me down and bought me a beer then wandered over to talk with the boys. After a few minutes I went on over. "Logan," I said, "This is a date. You have to stay with me." We spent the day together and ended up having breakfast with Terry very early in the morning.

Later on, when we had returned to Los Angeles and had the Frazees over for dinner, Pat asked Logan why he was having such trouble dating. He replied, "When I was out with Sugar I was relaxed and had a good time. But when I go out with someone else my tongue turns to cement when I try to talk." So much for my coaching.

At this point in the shooting it was getting quite cold and we were all weary. There was a wood stove going in one of the back rooms of the house we were shooting in where we kept our hair things. One cold day as I sat in my chair near the stove, my Eddie Bauer jacket hood pulled up over my head, I fell fast asleep. I woke up abruptly when my name was called. I had been dreaming of more wonderful places.

Another day we had great fun learning how to hypnotize a chicken. This was very instructive. One of the stunt men picked up a chicken in the yard where we were shooting. He held it tight, put its beak down on the ground, and proceeded to draw a line. Then he set the chicken down and let it go. It didn't move. It seemed to be hypnotized. We laughed and laughed. I don't know how the chicken felt about it though. It wasn't hurt, but perhaps it didn't like being the butt of our entertainment that afternoon.

Around this time I got a call to do a film with Gary Busey, but it was scheduled to start before this film was finished so I turned it down. I got a call from Eddie Butterworth letting me know about Natalie, who hadn't done a film in a long time. She was going to do a film called *Meteor* and I was disappointed. It had been so long since we'd worked together so I asked if Eddie could find someone to take my place for the first week until my current film ended. Jan Brandow called to say she would be happy to do it. I was thrilled at the thought of working with Natalie again.

It began to snow. We were getting toward the end of the film and Lizzie's film family now moved into a grand home. At this point we had to film some pick-up shots at Riverside Park where our shooting had begun. The city had prepared the park for closing. The day of the shoot was cold, rainy, and messy. The wigs and costumes got so wet that they were still damp the next day when the extras had to put them on.

Every once in a while I'd join some of the crew at a local hotel or bar for a few drinks and some dancing, but I'd always regret it the next morning. When I'd been younger I could play more. Now I either was wiser or didn't want to suffer the consequences of too little sleep.

November 18 was our last day. Even Lizzie was happy to finish. I hadn't really spent much time with her and felt sorry about that, but I think she appreciated my work in making the film look great. The following year I was nominated for an Emmy for my work on that film.

I want to explain how you get nominated for an Emmy. You - the person who does the work - have to enter your own application to be nominated. Then, if accepted, your film is shown to the judges. This way even small, unpublicized films that usually fall by the wayside in feature film awards have a chance at an Emmy. One year I was invited to be a judge for the Emmy's hair and makeup awards. It was quite interesting. We went to a studio where we watched many different categories of film hour after hour. Then we voted.

Finally *Awakening Land* was finished. I didn't realize that it would be my last film with Lizzie. The morning we left for Los Angeles was freezing. Los Angeles was cold too, but still wonderful because I was home.

CHAPTER 51

METEOR

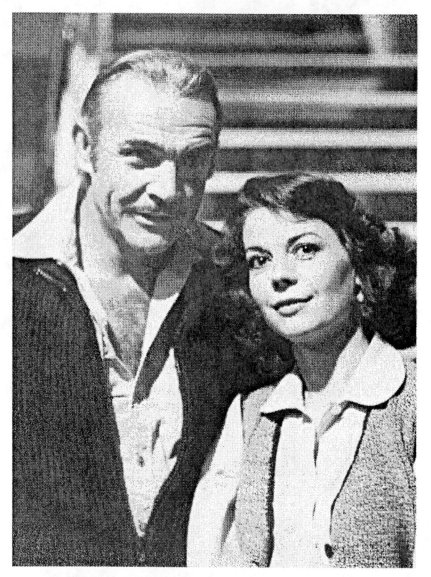

Sean Connery and Natalie Wood, *Meteor*

Ahh, home! My own bed. My children, my pets. Heaven.

As soon as I got home, I went into MGM to talk to Frank Bauer, the unit manager for *Meteor*. He agreed to my salary and case rental fee, no problem. I had learned that by not pushing I was more likely to get what I asked for.

The first morning back, Natalie hadn't arrived yet, but the rest of our entourage had. Ann Landers had retired. We all hugged, so happy to be together again. I missed Anne at times, but Peggy was nice, too.

Meteor was a disaster film, so popular at the time, about a group of scientists waiting for a meteor, which was going to crash in New York City. Their lab was deep underground and hopefully safe. In addition to Natalie, it starred Sean Connery, Brian Keith, Karl Malden, among others and was directed by Ronald Neame. Natalie played a Russian scientist. She actually spoke Russian, having learned it from her mother, but still needed to spend time with a dialogue coach to brush up. I tried to learn a few words, but soon gave up. My tongue just couldn't make it around those sounds.

This film had a different production schedule than normal. Natalie would come in and wait and wait and then there were days where she didn't have to come in at all. We'd come in just in case, but since the only person we took care of was Natalie we had plenty of free time.

Paul Lohman, the cameraman, kept his motor home right on the lot beside the stage. He loved hanging out there cooking gourmet meals. I loved Paul, but sometimes I felt he only made movies so he could afford to cook and enjoy making cappuccino for everyone. (But then, what's wrong with that?) Unfortunately, his photography left something to be desired. He didn't light Natalie very well and Natalie wasn't getting any younger. She was still beautiful, of course, but she needed help in the lighting department, which Paul didn't appear to care about. He'd have the lights too high which wasn't flattering. I always kept a huge mirror on the set so she could see how she was lit. If she didn't look good either Eddie or she would call Paul over and ask him to change the light. Pat came on the set one day and he could see Paul wasn't lighting her well. He didn't say anything feeling it wasn't his place, just joked about the high lights hoping Paul would get the hint. Nowadays a big star would get rid of a cameraman for this, but Natalie wasn't about to have Paul fired. That sort of thing hadn't happened yet in our industry. She just wanted him to make her look her best. Later on our industry changed and nobody was safe. People are fired so easily now.

Once the meteor fell the sets took a long time to get ready. During the scene they were filled with mud that then had to be cleaned up at the end of the scene. We were using Stage 30 at MGM, a huge place full of chutes with mud in them that were opened during the scenes. What a mess. The chutes went right up to the ceiling so that the mud, which was supposed to be pouring in through the subway corridors while people ran wildly trying to escape its fury, would have enough force to go where it was needed. Once in a while it just didn't work and mud exploded outside the set causing a major delay while it was cleaned up.

Before the mud began to slide, we were shooting in the lab and silicone dust sprayed down upon us from above, signifying that the meteor had struck. Then the set began to shake and down poured the dust. After all these years I think I still have some of that dust in my lungs.

The highlight of my day was when Sean Connery came to see Natalie. He was full of fun, flirting and laughing. One day he asked if I'd like to run off with him and take a bus downtown. Of course I would have loved to do that, but darn, he wasn't serious. He was a great storyteller and one day he told us about how he didn't trust film lawyers. "Trust the Mafia more," he said. It got so that each time he began a picture he'd start litigation immediately just knowing he was going to be jerked around in the end. He described a meeting with the lawyers where they all sat around a huge table, pens in hand. When the time came to sign something, nobody signed until all the others signed at the very same moment, so careful were they about not being first. Sean is a Scotsman, yes, but more than that he is an intelligent businessman.

Sometimes at the end of the day we'd sit in Natalie's trailer and chat while having a glass of wine. Natalie was frustrated with the director - actually all the actors were. He was critical, put them all down, and did nothing to encourage them. One evening he appeared at Natalie's door and joined us. He criticized Natalie for her makeup and hair people, saying it was old fashioned for us to be there with the mirror, watching her at every take. She responded by bringing up Paul's inability to light her well. Then she said, "I won't bother with my makeup people when Brian Keith takes off his hairpiece and Karl doesn't have the bald part of his head sprayed black." Touché! Ronald backed off after that. I remembered the wise director, Arthur Hiller, and although he may not have been the greatest director, he was smart enough to encourage the actors to do their best and then he picked the best they had done for the final cut. They made him successful. Ronald didn't have a clue about that.

Danielle, our craft service woman, who did clean up and supplied coffee on the set, was something to behold. Her bust measurement must have been at least forty-four inches. There was no hiding it, so instead of trying to do so she wore the most bizarre T-shirts with crude or funny sayings on them. Of course, she was always cleaning up the mud and needed to wear something that didn't matter. She was tough and we loved her.

At one point we all got bronchitis. Sean was the first down and by the end of the film it had gotten each of us. Maybe it was because it was dark and damp or because of the dust, who knows. But once it got hold of us it took forever to go away.

Natalie had turned off by the end of the film - the first time I'd ever seen her do that. She decided to do just what was necessary and no more. It wasn't a very good film so it didn't matter, but I was sad to see her so troubled. If it had been me, I could have quit, but a star, once committed and contracted, couldn't just walk away.

We celebrated New Year's Eve with the Frazee's at Terry's house. Pat rented a tux and looked absolutely wonderful. At the stroke of midnight I rejoiced, knowing that huge changes were coming in my life during the New Year.

At the finish of *Meteor*, we had our wrap party at the Rivera Country Club. Dressing up was required and we all arrived looking our best. We especially appreciated the opportunity after we had worked in our "mud clothes" during most of the film. We wanted to show off a bit. But the most wonderful looking one was Danielle of the bizarre T-shirts. She came wearing a long, strapless, black dress with a chiffon stole thrown over her shoulders. Her hair was up and she was looking gorgeous.

When Sean Connery arrived he was alone; his wife must have been in Spain. He came straight toward our table and sat down. We were impressed and pleased. During the evening he asked each of us women to dance. I loved being in his arms, dancing with my favorite star ever. He danced over and over again with Danielle. I'm sure he realized the pleasure he gave all of us that night. He was very generous with himself.

Normally at a wrap party the executives come with their wives, the stars hang out with the executives, and the crew sticks together. Not that night. I giggled silently as Sean danced by with Danielle while the executives' wives looked on longingly. We were all curious how Sean's

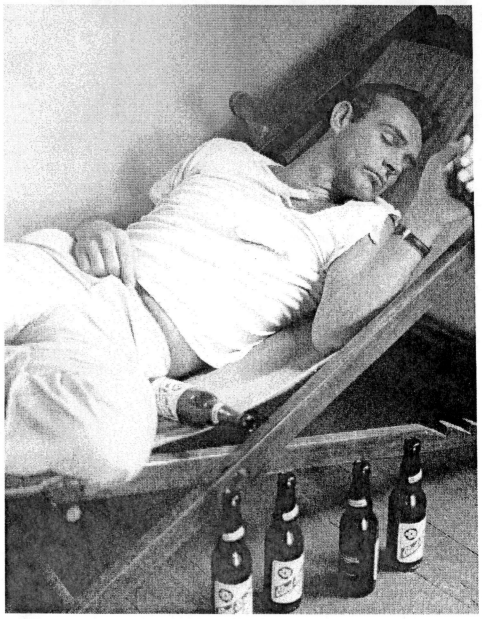

A Young Sean Connery

evening had ended and had great fantasies about him and Danielle. The next day at work Sean came to visit. He talked about the party and in a very nice way, made sure we knew he hadn't ended up with Danielle. A lovely man - and true to his wife.

When the picture ended, we were all relieved. Shortly after, Eddie and I went to Natalie's home in Beverly Hills to visit. Her new place was a beautiful Cape Cod style house. It was decorated in a comfortable style, just like all her homes, with tables of pictures everywhere. We drank wine together and she bid me well and wished me good luck at the inn. I hugged her and told her I loved her and thanked her for everything. Then I burst into tears.

CHAPTER 52

QUITTING THE BUSINESS

My mind was in Snowville, New Hampshire, but there was still a lot to do before we could actually move there. First we needed to get all the money by March. We were doing pretty well, but we hadn't sold our house so we had to refinance it. It became an ordeal because the bank wanted us to build a carport first. The garage had been turned into a playroom before we bought the house.

I called a contractor to make the necessary arrangements and Pat left for Georgia to work on a film called *The Double McGuffin*, starring George Kennedy, Ernest Borgnine, and Lisa Whelchel who later starred in the television comedy *Facts of Life*. Pat was delighted because Too Tall Jones and Lyle Azador,both pro football players, were also working on the film. Pat had always wanted Too Tall as an electrician. He didn't need a ladder to set scrims in front of the lights. Lyle and Too Tall signed baseball hats for us, which we later hung at the inn. I stayed home to recover from my busy year and to get things organized.

I was too fat and too tired from the previous year's work. I made a visit to my chiropractor, Dr. Hovey who looked burned out himself. He suggested that I might want to go a little deeper into my back trouble saying it might be emotional. He suggested I try Rolfing. I went for five treatments. I'm not sure if it helped, but now I know that emotions cause most back pain. The Rolfing did hurt and sometimes I ended up with bruises. The teacher was great though. At my last treatment he told me he should have sent me to a bigger practitioner, but he liked me so he did the treatments himself. Then he suggested I go to EST. He thought it would be helpful and I might even get quicker results. I'd wanted to take an EST course and so I signed up right away. I didn't tell Pat until afterwards because I knew he'd feel threatened and would also worry that I'd change too much.

Before Pat left for South Carolina, we took classes to learn about running a restaurant. The teacher's restaurant was called The Inn of The Seventh Ray in Topanga Canyon. It was a wonderful place that served all sorts of innovative vegetarian food. One thing we learned from our class was that people want to eat within three minutes of sitting down. Not the whole meal, mind you, but at least something. I found that to be true.

I took the EST course at the Convention Center in Los Angeles. It was exciting and I learned a lot about myself - mainly that I had an act, everyone does, but if you are unaware that it runs your life, it can cause you a great deal of trouble. My act was to be happy. Not a bad act, but an act nevertheless. I learned that it was all right to appear less than happy. What a relief. I was also reminded that no matter the situation, it is how we react that's important - in other words, we couldn't control anything that happened to us, but we could learn to control how we responded. I realized that as a child I had seen my mother thin and crying when she and my father came closer to their divorce. Somehow my five-year-old mind had told me that to be thin was to be unhappy. Oh these weird things we do to ourselves. We see them as true at the time and don't investigate further even as we grow older. I came away from EST a happier person, able to give myself permission to do and create and be. If someone became upset, well, that was their decision no matter what I did.

As I had assumed, when Pat found out about the EST he was worried I'd change, but I assured him on the phone that now there was just more of me to love him. After doing more wrapping up at home I left for the East Coast and for the inn where I needed to sign some papers with Phil and Randy, our lawyer. After landing in Boston, I rented a car and proceeded to drive for - the first time - in the winter snow. During the winter of '78, the snow was so deep that it reached almost to the first story of many homes. I saw snow banks so high I couldn't see over them, thanks to the recent blizzard. I got lost going east when I was supposed to head north, but eventually found my way and spent the night at the Darby Field Inn. I went by Snow Village Lodge and marveled at how perfect it still felt. I was anxious to move in, but we had to wait until May. I signed the papers and left to join Pat in Charleston, South Carolina and then Savannah.

It was great fun being a location housewife for Patrick. I had very little responsibility other than having some snacks ready for him when he came home and doing the wash. I would walk around town, do some shopping, stop by the set for a visit, give a few haircuts to the crew, and go home and take a nap.

I became good friends with the film's director, Joe Camp - famous as the director and creator of *Benji*. I met Benji one day, but felt our dog, Flump, was actually cuter and more loveable although perhaps not as smart and definitely not as well trained.

Every once in a while Joe and I discussed Lisa Whelchel who was there with her grandmother. Lisa was a great person and so responsible for a child. Joe felt sorry for her because her mother was a perfectionist and it seemed nothing Lisa did was good enough. Her grandmother loved her a lot, and was glad to be there with her. One day the mother showed up on the set. She was an attractive woman, but cold. I wasn't sorry when she left.

It was a close crew and we did lots of things together. Judy, the script supervisor, had a crush on Pat. Before I arrived on location, I'd told him that women on location sometimes get lonely. Yet it seemed that the only way they could get any men to show interest in them was if they wanted to sleep with a guy. I told Pat it was time for the guys on location to be nice - just friends with the women, but Judy didn't want to be just a friend to Pat. When I arrived, her first question for me was, "Are you really as great as he says you are?" "Of course not," was my reply. We became friends, but I think she was hoping I'd disappoint Pat so he'd come to her.

Back at home it was taking forever to get the carport completed. Was it going to be finished in time? I worried that Pat and I might end up with a lot of money, but no inn. I began to fret. For a while I forgot how I had been able to create things. Then Phil called to tell us that during the title search he discovered that Max's first wife had left a third of her ownership of the inn to the state of Israel. Max had never settled it, so it would take a while to get it all taken care of. What a relief. Now I knew we'd have our money ready at the time of the signing.

I was really proud of us; by April 1 we had $45,000 in the bank, $44,000 from the refinancing of our house, and we were looking forward to receiving $25,000 for our farm. A whopping $114,000 total and just a few short years before we had nothing at all and less than a year before we had emptied our savings of $15,000, not sure we could get it all together. But we did. I know visualizing helped make it all happen because everything just fell into place. I had even made $20,000 renting wigs on *Awakening Land* - a potentially risky investment of $3,500 that had paid off. We had worked hard, but now we were ready to begin a new life. In my mind I was finished, ready to give up the movie business completely, forever. I was sure that we'd be innkeepers for the rest of our lives and pass the inn onto our kids and grand kids. Still I wasn't silly enough to burn bridges so I kept my union card paid up and so did Pat.

We had so many adventures running the inn that like our farm experience, it would take a book of its own, so I'll only include a few stories here. Yes, it was very much like the Bob Newhart Show. The handy people and workers were all unusual with unique personalities. We were strange innkeepers and successful in many ways except in making a profit. But what the heck, life should be more about enjoyment than about making money. At least that's what we thought at first.

I now lived in the countryside where lilacs bloomed in the spring. I could really smell them. There were lakes everywhere with people of all shapes and sizes swimming in them and I was one of them. There were festivals, country fairs with animals and luscious foods. We pictured our inn full of guests with everyone sitting around the fireplace in the evenings, the dogs at our feet. My dream had come true.

Pat and I began to realize that the movie business had equipped us for the job of running our inn. We knew how to plan, order supplies, think on our feet, work with people, make things attractive, and feed people great food. What we didn't know, at first, was how to get people to come to the inn. Max had run it with the very minimum of people and his guests were folks who came from Europe to be with him. We soon found out that his clientele wasn't necessarily ours. We had to rebuild the business essentially from scratch. Toward this end, when a man named Igor came along and offered to open a ski touring school - he'd even build the trails - we agreed. Unlike Max, who had closed during the winter, we wanted to have year-round business.

Despite the lack of guests at first, I was in heaven. We had renamed the inn Snowvillage Inn (from Snow Village Lodge). No matter how often I looked at our inn, I couldn't get over how perfectly wonderful it was. The inn sat on thirty acres of land, mostly forested with a huge barn down below. I could imagine Teddy Roosevelt and guests of his time period vacationing at this summer home, sitting on the porch, watching the sunset, and drinking their cocktails. The main room of the inn was huge and warm with hand-hewn beams that spanned the whole room and windows that looked out on the most gorgeous view of the Mount Washington Valley. Huge pine trees were everywhere and I planted flowers along the circular driveway and everywhere else. In fact, the next year we won first prize for our landscaping.

The inn grew more beautiful each year.

We had loads of photos from our movie adventures, but I was reluctant to put them out and feature them. I wanted to have a new life. Like Max said, I was ready to tie up the movie Chapter. We finally decided to hang the pictures on the wall going up the stairs to the rooms in the main house. Yes, people were aware we had been in "the business" and they'd ask how it was to be around ordinary people now. I told them our guests were just as interesting as the stars, which made them feel good. It was true, too, at least most of the time.

Here I was living in my never-ending forest with my big house where people came to visit and stay for a while. I even had a window seat to sit in and watch people come up the hill. My dream had come true and yet inside I was a bit worried because it seemed all my wishes had been granted and that made me nervous. Everything I ever asked for had been granted to me, what more could I ask? In July I got a call from the EST people telling me there was going to be a big get-together in New York City and I must come. It seemed impossible, but I made it. In the middle of the night, I drove to Boston, hopped a bus to the Felt Forum and got to New York City just in time. It was a good thing because Werner Erhard said something that day I needed to hear. He explained that when one of our dreams comes true it is important to move on - to have other ideas, other dreams. It seemed he was speaking directly to me alone. I was so happy at the inn that a part of me had wondered if it might be time to die. Not literally, of course, but I guess I needed to hear there was life even after realizing one's dreams. I returned to the inn in a far better frame of mind.

I went to a lady's circle meeting and met Libby Edge, a fellow innkeeper from Rockhouse Mountain Farm. For the rest of the summer she sent us the overflow guests that she could not accommodate at their busy inn. When she asked if I liked inn keeping, I told her I loved it. She replied that during her many years of inn keeping, since 1946, she had been tired, but not tired of inn keeping. It was reassuring.

People were finding out about the inn slowly but surely. When they discovered our inn and stayed with us, they liked us and we liked having them. I was the accountant, secretary, bartender, and hostess. Pat was the cook, groundskeeper, and general handy man. He turned into a great cook. I set up the menu and did the shopping and he cooked. At first he wasn't very sure of himself, and often when I was taking an afternoon bath in the bathroom under the staircase next to the kitchen, he'd come in, sit on the edge of the tub, and ask me to explain this or that about a recipe I had chosen.

Tanya arrived after her graduation from high school and became a fabulous baker of breads and desserts. In fact, at seventeen she was written up in a book on inns describing her wonderful desserts. She also waited on tables with Judy our housekeeper that we had inherited with the inn. Xochi, who was fifteen, was settling in at her new high school and getting used to her new way of life. She joined the cross-country ski team even though she had never skied before. I went to her school and watched her in special events, which was so different from when I was in the movie business. I'd missed out on so much of my girls' lives.

I wrote to Natalie and Lizzie, inviting them to come for a visit. In fact, I wrote to everyone I could think of. I was in heaven and I wanted to share it. Bob Norin, a makeup man and friend was our first Hollywood visitor. He visited while he was working on a series in Boston. Judy, one of the Frazee's relatives, came and helped us clean out the cellar. She worked so hard she had to go home to rest. We offered her a real vacation the next time she came, but she never returned. Verne Caruso, a hairstylist from New York, also came up to see us.

One morning I awoke feeling panicky, but soon realized it was only a dream. I had dreamed that Natalie Wood and Howie Koch were coming to stay at the inn. We were rushing around trying to get the inn in the best shape possible, but there was so much to do. I was relieved it was only a dream.

On June 17, my forty-fourth birthday, I wrote in my diary, "I am happier, more satisfied, and fulfilled than I have ever been in my life." Pat didn't feel quite the same way. He tried to love the place like I did, but he'd never worked so hard in his life. He was used to carrying around a little meter and telling his men where to place the lights on the set. Here he was responsible for everything. It was too much at times.

He got a call from David Quaid, a cameraman who also lived in New Hampshire, to go on a show to Trinidad. We discussed it. It was true; our money was all going out and very little was coming back in, so we both agreed that he should go. It was only for five or six weeks yet I cried like a baby the day he left. Once again our happy home was breaking up. And thinking about running the place alone was scary. As it happened, in the end it all worked out and I was more secure in my ability to take care of things.

The Theater Guild approached me about wigs for their productions. Pat lit the haunted house for Halloween while I did the makeup and put wigs on people who were doing the haunting.

In November, Eddie called to ask if I was available to do a film with Natalie. I was putting down tender, delicate roots and wanted them to take hold. I didn't want to leave so soon, so I turned the film down. Kay Pownall began to do Natalie's hair. I was pleased to have her as a replacement.

Pat's folks came for our first Thanksgiving and it snowed. We had many people for dinner and it was like having a huge family. It was perfect. We opened a ski touring center and advertised everywhere, but still business was slow. Our savings were getting low - only $12,000 and falling. I wanted to open the restaurant to the public, but Pat said he'd quit if I did.

Pat hated the cold weather. He'd go around the inn muttering, "Only nineteen and a half years more." We still had that many more payments to make. I could feel his discomfort and it made me sad because I was so happy. I felt the friends I'd made would be here for years to come. I loved the changing seasons. I felt more secure than I ever had. In Los Angeles life was so transient. Everyone moved, things always changed. Here I had tradition and a steadiness in my life that I obviously needed.

My daughters were happy, too. Xochi was settled into her school and Tanya was now an accomplished cook and baker. Laurie, now twenty-one, was coming early in the next year. In fact, the change had been wonderful for everyone except Pat who was resisting all of it.

At the end of the first year we had lost $49,000. It was very wise of the SBA to demand that we have our running expenses in the bank. When we got a call to do a film the next spring, we left Laurie in charge and went to Madison, and Atlanta Georgia to do *Little Darlings*.

Chapter 53

LITTLE DARLINGS
Georgia, 1979

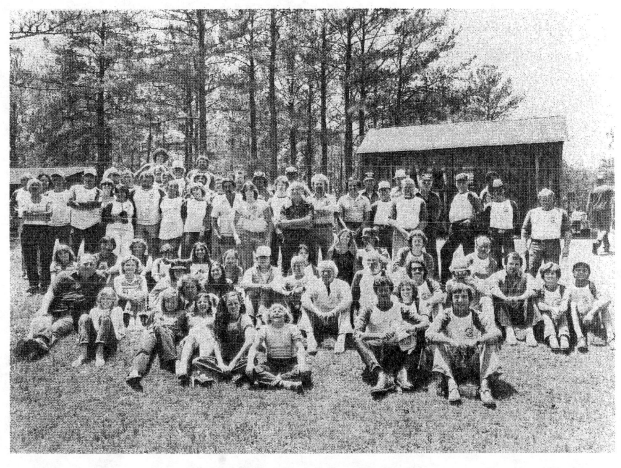

The Cast and Crew of *Little Darlings*

When the call came for Pat asking if he would go to Atlanta to do *Little Darlings*, I answered the phone. I talked with the production secretary and she remembered working with me in the past. Later, after Pat had accepted the job, she called back and asked if I would also be interested in working on the film. What a dilemma. I didn't want to go back to the film business, but we really needed the money. Our bank account was low and spring was a really slow season. If anyone did come, Laurie would be capable of dealing with it. Then I remembered we needed an ice machine. All last summer I made runs to the liquor store in town fifteen minutes away then rushed home to get it into the freezer before it melted. I decided to go. I can't say I was overjoyed, but as always I was ready to make the most of the situation. I wondered if I'd really escaped the movie business at all.

Off we went leaving the girls in charge. Luckily my ability to focus on the present kicked in and once we landed in Atlanta I was fine. In addition, this film was going to be fun. It was about a group of little girls at girls' camp and starred Tatum O'Neil, Kristy McNichol, and Matt Dillon along with lots of lively, young girls playing the parts of the campers. Ron Maxwell was directing and Beta Batka was the cameraman.

We began shooting in the Atlanta projects where Kristy's character lived. It was a depressing part of Atlanta. During the first scene, a boy came up to Kristy, who looked very appealing, although she was dressed in shabby jeans. Slyly, he said, "Come on Honey, you know you want me. Why don't you slide me something nice?" We heard that dialogue so many times that day, and it is forever etched in my mind.

We filmed in the parking lot of the Omni where we worked for a couple of days. It was hot and because of the reflection from the ground, my lips became covered in cold sores. I was a mess, but Pat seemed happy. He had drinking buddies, including the two makeup men I worked with, Tom Ellingwood of Burt Reynolds fame and Bill Turner. At the end of the day I'd fall into bed exhausted and they'd join each other for a "few".

We moved onto Madison a picturesque town full of old Victorian homes that had escaped the burning of the Civil War. We stayed in a Holiday Inn on the outskirts of town. It was comfortable and had a huge open area where we could hang out together on the weekends. The bar was awful, no windows, it stank of cigarettes and booze. I couldn't bear to go in there.

Our set was at a summer camp outside of town. The camp's surroundings were pure country and lovely. For the most part the kids we worked with were great.

I had been prepared for Tatum to be difficult and Kristy to be wonderful, but it was just the opposite. Tatum was great. She was a lot of fun and fit right in. Kristy, on the other hand, was a problem. She had hired a non-union fellow to do her hair, which wasn't legal at the time so she had him do it in the motel, and then she'd come to the set with it already done.

In reality, Kristy was an unhappy girl. I felt for her. She had a girl friend with her all

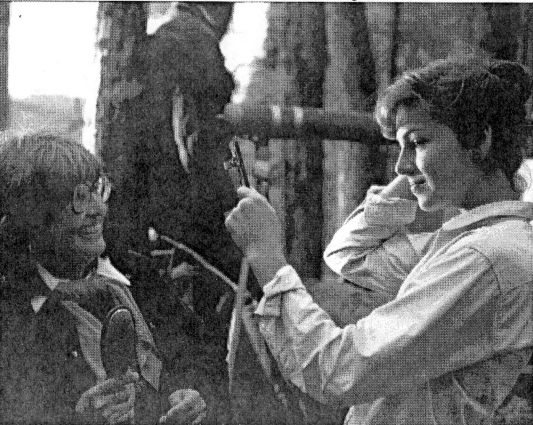

Sugar with Tatum O'Neal, *Little Darlings*

the time, a guardian and companion in one. Later, I realized her situation was similar to that of Lisa from *Double McGuffin*. Like Lisa, Kristy could never please her mother. She was a tomboy while her mother was glamorous. It wasn't a good situation and later when Kristy had troubles in her life I could understand. Actually she was quite lovable, but very good at manipulating us to get her way. Tatum was classy. She was fun and liked by the other girls. I ended up being sort of a mother to all the young girls. Most of them didn't have their own parents there and often needed some extra attention.

This was Matt Dillon's second film and I sensed he was a star in the making, so handsome with smooth white skin and nice as could be. I remember his white skin because of a love scene he had with Kristy in the woods. The Art Department had mistakenly chosen a site full of poison ivy for the scene, which nobody realized until the scene was shot and poor Matt's back was covered with poison ivy. What a catastrophe, the poor kid was in agony. His mother tried to make him comfortable, but it was near impossible.

Matt's mother was a wonderful person, happy to be there with him. There were many kids in his family and this was sort of a vacation for her, at least until the poison ivy attack. We would talk and she told me that Matt had been on the verge of getting into trouble when he was chosen for his first film. It had changed his life. At home they had a big house full of things the kids had collected, street signs and all. I remember her saying that the kitchen ceiling needed to be repaired because there was a hole and a raccoon used to sneak in through the ceiling at night and leave handprints on the fridge. I was sure that Matt was able to repair that ceiling and much more for his family.

Even though the cameraman Beta Batka was driving Pat crazy, in many ways he was having the time of his life. Pat was used to using small lights, but Beta Batka insisted on using huge brutes, the largest ones possible, at every chance. The lights gave off such heat that the actors were tortured with all that light in those tiny cabins. There was no changing Beta and at times Pat was frustrated. In his own way Pat took revenge, organizing a kazoo band that played in the van on the way home from location to torture Beta. It was a terrible sound, I hated it too, but it helped them get out their frustration. Nobody cared for Beta.

Someone else came up with another idea to torture Beta. One day he returned to his hotel room to find it filled with chickens, all cackling and messing about. He just didn't get it. All the little girls had it with him also. They were tired of enduring the heat of the lights, so on the last day of the film, as he stood at the end of a pier by the lake, with all his meters hanging around his neck, the girls pushed him into the water. Bill Turner's wife Keori did the body makeup and she became my friend. Bill met her while doing *Sand Pebbles* with Steve McQueen, in Hong Kong. Keori was Chinese and one of the loveliest women I've ever met. She taught me to eat an orange in the bathtub. First you peel it and then let the orange peel fall in the hot water. The hot water draws the oil from the orange and the skin absorbs it.

Keori was having trouble with Bill and his drinking, as I was with Patrick. One evening she decided to go to the bar on her own. She had a wonderful time dancing and got home around 1:00 a.m. The next day I was shocked by how mean Bill was to her. He couldn't forgive her for doing what he did every night. Keori came in so unhappy. She put her arms around me and it made me feel like crying. When I talked to Bill, he said, "Stay out of it. I know how she needs to be treated. You just don't understand." I certainly did not.

Pat's forty-first birthday, on May 20, was unforgettable. All the guys on the film loved him and wanted to do something special. At first they considered a helicopter ride, but then they decided to get him a slave for the day instead. One of the black waiters, at our hotel, said he'd take the part of the slave. He was paid well, but I could hardly believe that he'd do that.

Our makeup group always arrived at work earlier than most of the crew. We took the early van. On his birthday, we were munching our breakfast when the big bus arrived with the rest of the crew, including Pat. When the bus halted the crew got off the bus and stood in two lines waiting for Pat to disembark. Down the steps he came, followed by his slave for the day. It was not to be believed. Here was this guy all dressed up with a towel over his arm and a tray with a drink on it for Pat. He took Pat's breakfast order then took Pat's set bag over to his chair and stood by waiting for further instructions. Pat ate his breakfast, did the first set-up, and had a drink. Normally, he would never drink on the set, but this was his birthday and he took full advantage. It was funny and awful at the same time.

By lunch Pat was thoroughly sloshed and couldn't stop laughing. After his lunch was delivered, he gave his slave time off so he could play volleyball with the rest of the crew. After lunch, Pat passed out. His slave left around 4:00 p.m. It was some day. The nurse had been concerned that Pat might have a heart attack as he was laughing so much. I worried he might get in trouble for drinking, but nobody seemed to care. They thought he should celebrate and, believe me, he did.

Hurricane warnings were posted. On location, the wind blew and blew, the hurricanes power increasing by the hour. We were nervous, but the Production Department insisted on shooting. Telling them scary stories, we were able to convince the young actresses they shouldn't be there. They got upset and insisted we all go home early. We wrapped and returned to the motel. As luck would have it, not long after we returned to the hotel, the hurricane changed course and we had beautiful weather for the rest of the day. Production was upset, but unable to call us back to work once we had been dismissed.

We spent nearly two months on location. Our bank account grew. On our return to the inn, we ordered a big commercial icemaker. It was worth the time away and the new icemaker made our lives much easier.

CHAPTER 54
MY LAST FILM WITH NATALIE

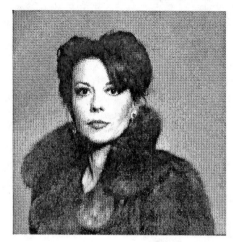 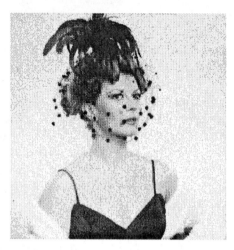

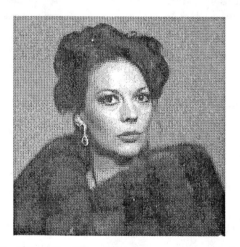

Natalie Wood stills, *Memory of Eva Ryker*

Our second year was more relaxing. We had a little experience, a little money, Pat had more confidence and our clientele was growing. At the end of foliage, late October, Pat left for Los Angeles to work on a film. He was out there when I got a call to do *Memory of Eva Ryker*, a Movie of the Week, with Natalie Wood. The production manager said it wasn't going to be a long shoot and seeing as it was our slow season and our income was still way below our output, I thought it over. Pat was already out there and I'd have a place to stay. I agreed to do the film.

During our first year of inn-keeping Natalie had gone to Russia for a television special. She later described her trip telling me that it was both interesting and awful. She had been chosen to host the show because she spoke Russian and also they really wanted her to host it. Before she signed the contract, she made many demands, basically simple things, like being able to speak with her children by phone each day. When she arrived in Russia, nothing worked like she hoped it would. None of the promises were kept. She couldn't get in touch with her children and in the end all she could think about was getting out of there and returning home. Kay Pownall, her hairstylist, went with her. I was glad I hadn't gone. Moscow had never been on my "need to visit" list.

Our living arrangements worked out well. Pat was watching a friend's place in Malibu so I had a place to stay. Roselle wasn't available so I asked Natalie if Laurie, my daughter, who was staying nearby with Gary Busey's family, could be her stand-in; I offered to get Laurie a dark wig if necessary. Natalie agreed. That was great; Laurie and I rode to work together so I didn't need to think about a car.

We filmed at Warner Brothers, which brought back wonderful memories of my times on *The Great Race* and *Inside Daisy Clover*. Irwin Allen, master of disaster films, was our producer. I knew this would be a classy television show. He didn't know how to do things any other way.

There were lots of flashbacks in the story so I suggested that Natalie should have a white streak in her hair for the present time seeing as she was older and normal brown hair for the past. Irwin Allen disagreed. "People often leave the room during a television show," he said. "It would confuse them to see her looking that different." He was right and he did agree to a different hairstyle, but not a different color.

Natalie's new house was beautiful. Since I'd been there last, she had done a lot more work on it. It was still so charming and I felt comfortable. Natasha and Courtney were older now and had their own suite. Willie Mae was still with the family keeping things in order.

One day we went to Natalie's house to do her makeup ahead of time. Her daughters were going to be in a presentation at school and she wanted to be there to see them. After Natalie was ready, we went by the school to see them perform with their classes. Natalie was a good mom.

The film also starred Robert Foxworth, Elizabeth Montgomery's intimate partner. We were old friends and he was as happy to see me, as I was to see him. Coincidentally, Lizzie was doing a film on the same lot so I went to her trailer and surprised her. She was glad to see me and gave me a huge hug. We talked for a while before she had to go to the set. I went to see her one other time and she seemed rather cool. It dawned on me it might have been because I came out for Natalie when she called and I hadn't for Lizzie. In my defense when Lizzie called I hadn't been able to leave the inn. It had been a busy time. Natalie's call came at a slow time at the inn. I never did see Lizzie again although she continued to send me lovely Christmas cards for a while. To this day, every time I light a green Rigaud candle I think of her. I knew she had grown up in the east and I kept inviting Bob to bring her to the inn, but she seemed to prefer staying at home.

Natalie's part in the film was rather strange. She played a woman frightened by the ocean, who almost drowns. It was really eerie, seeing what was to happen to her later. She never was comfortable working in the ocean.

I was having a rough time. Pat was drinking way too much. I didn't know what to do. Suddenly he got a call;

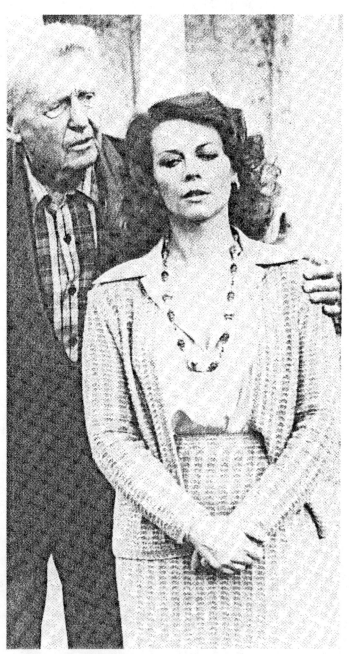

Natalie Wood with Ralph Bellamy
The Memory of Eva Ryker

Pappy, his father, was dying. He left immediately for West Virginia. I was heart-broken. Pappy wasn't supposed to die. I had pictured Mammy and Pappy coming to live with us at the inn at some point. On their first visit Pappy had been such a help. He did little things like dusting in corners - details nobody took the time to do. The day Pappy died, Tanya had to take our old dog Timber, who was in a terrible shape, to be put to sleep. I was in tears all day at work. I tried to make myself feel better by thinking that both Pappy and Timber were up there somewhere, free and happy to have shrugged off their painful, old bodies. It helped, but not much.

During the shoot I became friends with an electrician on the set who finally admitted to me he was a Hell's Angel. He was Mexican, huge, and very strong. We got along well and talked a lot on the set. His arms were covered with tattoos and he had a huge scar on his left arm that looked as if it had almost been torn off. He even showed me his special Hell's Angels belt buckle. He didn't let everyone know about his affiliation.

He described his home in Berkeley. He said he watched television over and over and when he saw something he liked on a show he built it into his own home. For instance he built a library with a rounded door that looked like one on some television show. He built a house for his cat, all in miniature of course. He even peeled a picture of a cat off a can of food and put it above the fireplace in the little house. I'd always thought Hell's Angels were tough, but he seemed very sweet. His friend who had introduced me to him warned, "Yes, he is sweet, but there is a really tough side to him you never want to meet." I never saw that side of him though. When we moved to the inn, he sent us videos and kept in touch for years.

That film with Natalie ended so quickly. It was a Movie of the Week and the schedule was short. I was anxious to get home, but happy to have done the film. If I had known what the future would bring, I wouldn't have been in such a hurry to leave.

Chapter 55

NATALIE'S DEATH
NOVEMBER 1981

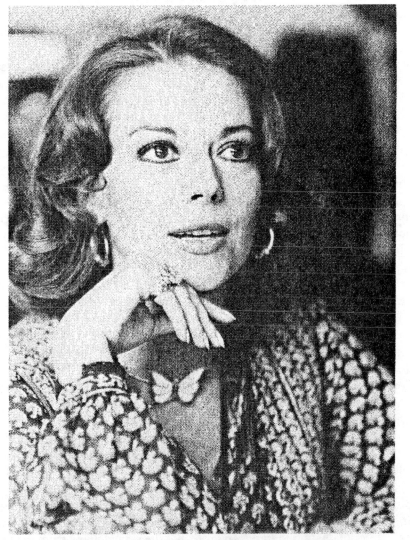

The way I remember Natalie Wood

I was alone at the inn on Sunday, November 29, 1981 when the phone rang. It was Liz, one of my inn guests. "Oh Ginger, I'm so sorry about Natalie." Anxiously I asked, "What happened? What do you mean?" Softly she replied, "Didn't you know? Natalie drowned last night. I'm so sorry." Stunned, I couldn't believe it. Later, after I had recovered a little from the news, I wrote in my diary:

Natalie is dead. She drowned in the ocean at Catalina. My God. I was stunned and still am five days later. What could have happened to that beautiful, little woman? How could it be her time when she has two small children she loved so much? R.J. Oh how badly I feel for you. She was your backbone.

I let myself feel my sadness and I've cried. I've been alone and pretty low all week. Natalie was a friend. She added so much to my life and to my career. She brought great value to my life and I ache inside knowing that her children will miss so much of what she gave me and so many others.

I cried when I read they performed an autopsy on that perfect, petite body. I cry when I think of R.J. having to identify her body. I think of all the wonderful photos that still must remain around their home reminding everyone of their loss. My eyelids are so swollen, and I can hardly see.

Dear Nat, bless you and may you find peace wherever you are.

Somehow, it never really did sink in that Natalie was gone. I knew it was true of course, but it didn't seem possible. When I'd go to Los Angeles, I'd still expect to get a call from her.

I wrote to Elizabeth Montgomery right away, I wanted to be in touch with her, and tell her I loved her. I didn't want her to slip away like Natalie had. Lizzie sent me a card and it was very sweet. She told me she was just fine and not to worry. Strangely enough, in 1995 Lizzie died at a young age, too. Before her death, there were rumors about her illness. Still, I was shocked when it happened. The day after I found out Lizzie had died, I went upstairs to my office and strangely enough found the card she sent me after Natalie's death on my desk. I reread it: "Don't worry," it said, "I'm fine." I was sure it was a message from her, not just a coincidence.

It was quiet at the inn after Thanksgiving, giving me plenty of time to think about Natalie and our lives together. I was thankful she and I had worked together the year before on *Memory of Eva Ryker*. I had felt so close to her then as we talked about our lives and our distress at both our husband's drinking. We talked about getting older and about things changing. She truly loved and enjoyed her family, her girls, and she realized that now she had to be more careful about her looks. We discussed face-lifts, but she said she really wasn't interested. "Perhaps just around the eyes if it comes to that," she said. She told me how she enjoyed my ease with people and wished it was easier for her. She was still very shy in many ways.

We had some interesting conversations. She spoke about Mart Crowley who had been such a close friend. During this film, he was drinking so much that she had told him to stay away until he got a grip on his problem. That hurt him, but Natalie had learned not to be an enabler. She was always supportive of her friends and I believe that finally, with all her therapy, she had learned that sometimes to "put up" with certain things was just not helpful.

After her death when her sister's book came out it was negative, putting Natalie down for not being there all the time for her. Lana felt sorry for herself, but didn't seem to remember all the things Natalie had done for her. I could remember when Lana was very small and we stopped by Natalie's mother's home, a ranch house in Sherman Oaks. Natalie was so sweet and kind with Lana. She was generous, too. I always felt Natalie went out of her way to make Lana feel good. She seemed to understand how difficult it was to be the little sister of a star. Sometimes I wondered how it must have felt to Lana, wishing she could be Natalie.

Natalie bailed Lana out time after time. In those days they didn't call that enabling, but it was. Perhaps she felt guilty for having so much, but regardless of the reason, Natalie was wonderful to her family and friends. Sometimes I wondered how she could put up with all the problems her mother caused and why on earth she didn't disown the whole bunch. She always seemed closer to her father than her mother or at least more comfortable with him. He was quiet and settled, whereas her mother seemed to always be conjuring things up.

I remembered how Natalie could set out to learn anything and she would master it. She may not have been the most outstanding actress, but she was capable of learning anything having to do with her parts and she gave so much pleasure to so many people.

One of our last conversations was about the drug culture. Even though I was four years older than she was, we both came along before drugs really hit the business. I was happy about that and so was she. Natalie enjoyed a glass of wine if she wasn't shooting, but drugs were out of the picture for her. She preferred to stay away from any Hollywood parties that included drugs. After her death, the *Inquirer* wrote that she stayed away from those parties because she was aging and jealous and didn't want R.J. to be around the younger crowd. I knew that wasn't true.

I remember working on *Penelope* when Natalie was so unhappy. At that time she was seeing her shrink, as she referred to him. She was going with David Lang, Hope Lang's brother, and it wasn't much of a romance. I remember wishing so much that she would find someone to love, who loved her for herself. It occurred to me then how difficult it must be for someone in her shoes to know if people wanted her for her, or the money, or because she was a star.

She wasn't herself on that film. I remember Roddy McDowall was in the doghouse for something with her at the time. I don't know why, they had been friends forever. He came to me, pleading that I try to help him get her friendship back. I never did find out why she was angry, but I knew she could be moody. Maybe it was because all her friends were having children around that time and she felt left out. But then I gave her the worst haircut ever on the film and she never said anything. Later we laughed over it and I told her she was too nice. She should feel free to show her displeasure when she felt it.

I thought of Natalie's friend, Norma Crane, who, during her last role in *Fiddler on the Roof*, refused to have a mastectomy because she didn't want to lose the part. Norma died before Fiddler was released. Natalie supported Norma throughout her career and this was her best part. I cried when I saw the film, knowing that Norma was gone. I remember Sir Laurence Olivier saying how Natalie always made sure he was welcome in their home when he came to Los Angeles. He felt her graciousness. And someone else told me about the time Natalie went shopping at an antique store and changed the price tags on things, putting high prices on inexpensive items and low prices on the high priced items. It amused me when she was naughty like that.

I thought of all the wonderful places Natalie had taken me, all over the world, and how my reputation had been built, thanks to her. I couldn't recall any really bad times. She spent her life

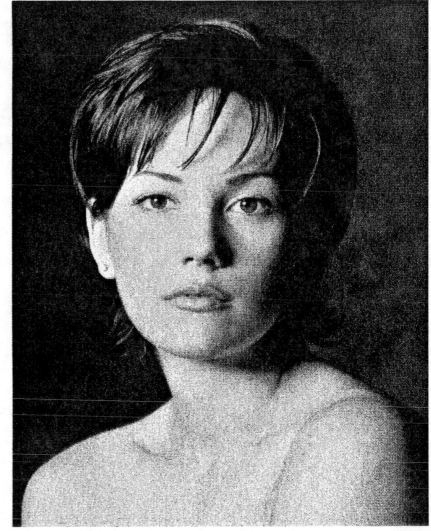

Natalie Wood's daughter, Natasha

supporting all of us, her family, her friends, and coworkers in so many ways. Sometimes I felt she needed to be more selfish, though. When I read in Lana's book that she was angry because Natalie didn't stay in contact with her, it made me angry at Lana. Actually I think it was better for Natalie not to be with her family. They manipulated her in so many different ways. The only way she could escape was by staying out of reach.

I saw a photo of Natalie taken not long before she died. I was stunned. She had circles under her eyes and the sparkle just wasn't there. I wondered what was wrong. I heard rumors of a romance with Christopher Walken, which seemed strange to me, but then it wasn't unusual for her costars to fall in love with her. She was so open and they just couldn't resist her loveliness. But screen romances were hardly ever consummated, just enjoyed. During a film it was easy to get carried away for a while, and then when the film ends it was over with it. Later I heard she was drinking during the production, which sounded so strange to me as that wasn't something she ever did. I couldn't help but wonder whether I could have helped her by being there. It wasn't meant to be though.

Perhaps she wanted to remain in the spotlight, but I had the feeling she was ready to relax and settle down in her later years, just do a play or a film now and then. Maybe it was too early for that, though. For myself I no longer needed the excitement. During Natalie's career we made the biggest, the best, and the most exciting films possible. Those experiences can never be repeated. So many people in the film industry today have no idea what it was like then.

I wrote R.J. a note and told him I was there for him if he ever needed anything. I didn't expect to hear from him, and I never did. I always wondered how it was for him. Natalie had really run their home, along with Willie Mae, of course. R.J. was a good person and seemed to keep the rest of the family together after her death.

A couple of years ago, my daughter Xochi worked on a show called *Models Inc*. Natalie's daughter, Natasha, was working on it, too. Xochi sent me her photo. She's so lovely. Natasha told Xochi she remembered me coming to her house and playing with her. She is very nice, just like her mother.

It has been so many years since Natalie died. She was born in 1938 and she died in 1981. Her life was too short. But perhaps a saying I'd heard and loved was true for Natalie: God takes you before something you can't handle comes up. Maybe that was it. I'll never know.

Chapter 56

MEETING WILLIAM HURT

When Pat worked on *Altered States* in Los Angeles, the previous summer, he became friends with William Hurt. This spring Pat was working on another film with Bill and also Sigourney Weaver in New York City. The film was called *The Janitor Doesn't Dance* then later it was changed to *Eyewitness*.

Pat and Bill had become close friends. At the finish of some scenes Bill, who was always sensitive, would ask Pat how he liked the scene, actually meaning his performance. Pat would reply, "It was great. You hit your marks." That seemed to work for Bill. Pat didn't know anything about acting and he knew better than to critique Bill's acting.

Peter Yates, the director, had been nominated for an Academy award for his film *Breaking Away*. He went back to Hollywood one weekend to attend the awards ceremony, giving the crew four days off. Pat had told everyone about our place in New Hampshire so Bill and Sigourney decided to come visit during this mini-vacation. It was off-season and quiet at the inn.

I cleaned and polished the inn to get it ready for our visitors. It was off-season so a bit dusty - not too bad. It had to be kept in order because we never knew when someone might come along and want to look around. Bill and Pat traveled up together. Sigourney was due to arrive the next day. It was exciting. For the first time, real, live actors were coming to our inn. I didn't act any different. I was used to being around well-known people.

The girls, went to pick Sigourney up at the airport, and were delighted when Pat gave them a photo of her. "Wow," they exclaimed, "She's the star of *Alien*." Neither Pat nor I had seen it, but the girls were very aware of her. They found her without any problems at the little Portland, Maine airport and brought her home. It was a quiet weekend. Everyone relaxed and hung out together. Sigourney hiked up Foss Mountain that has an amazing 360-degree view and she spent a lot of time being quiet up there.

Bill was taken with the area and began to think it would be nice to have a home here. He loved the outdoors and especially fishing. We made an appointment with a realtor to look at some houses. The realtor took us to Conway Lake which was a big lake and relatively undeveloped. Most of the homes on it were private and very expensive. We drove up to a strange-looking, small, brick house on the water. I wondered, why anyone would build a home with a flat roof in snow country, but Bill didn't seem to mind the design. There was an oriental decoration on the front door. When I suggested that it could be taken off Bill said, "Not at all, I like it that way." To each his own.

We went inside. Weird little place, I thought. The realtor explained that an architecture student had it built and it was paid for by his grandparents. Over indulgence was my opinion. It just didn't seem livable, the living room was a rectangle, very long and narrow and to the rear was the bedroom. Nothing about the interior appealed to me, but it did to Bill. However, I saw the possibilities when I walked out through the sliding glass doors and looked out onto the lake. The perennial gardens were just beginning to appear, and a canoe was tied up at the water's edge. With a little remodeling it had potential. The flower garden sold me.

Bill thought so, too. He bought the house and moved up after his film was done. We became close friends. At the time he was living with Sandra, a ballerina from the New York City Ballet. They seemed to be happy and enjoyed themselves when they came up. Pat and I would go to their place for dinner and they'd come to our house, too. Bill eventually remodeled the kitchen with lovely, dark red Mexican tile. After he put in a huge bathroom, the house began to grow on me.

Sandy became pregnant and later came with their son, Alexander, to spend time up there. Bill was always a little crazy. Aren't all actors? Sandy used to say that he was like a rushing river while she was a placid lake.

Bill loved fly-fishing and found a local man who tied flies for him and they became friends. He thought town was great because everyone treated him like an ordinary person. He also liked living on the edge. On a long weekend he decided to go camping far north. He packed a tent and some food into his four-wheel drive and took off toward the north, where exactly we didn't know. That night there was a dreadful storm with lots of wind, thunder, and lightening. We worried about him, but a couple of days later he showed up and told us about his frightening experience.

He had huddled in his little tent while the storm raged around him. He could hear tree limbs breaking and crashing to the ground. He thought of trying to make it to his vehicle, but was sure the road was impassable. Even though he'd been scared at the time, I had the feeling he'd been thrilled to have the experience.

Bill was reckless at times. One winter morning he decided to go cross-country skiing up Foss Mountain with his two dogs. He could have used our maintained trails, but that wasn't adventurous enough for him. He parked his car in our parking lot, checked in with me and took off with the dogs. I forgot about him until hours later a woman called from quite a distance from us saying Bill needed to speak with me. I couldn't believe where he had managed to end up. I got directions to the woman's house and went to pick him up. He was exhausted and so were the dogs. I gave him a piece of my mind, upset that he'd just taken off into the wilderness having no idea where he was going. What if he'd gotten hurt? But he survived, none the worse for wear.

Somehow our friendship survived. We just had to love him. I try not to judge, but to accept people for what they are. Occasionally when Bill came to visit the inn, he drove the help crazy. Once, he asked India, our cook Susie's ten-year-old daughter, a question and then berated her for not knowing answers to what he asked. Then he asked Xochi something about her complexion in a sarcastic way, embarrassing her. I was furious. "How could you do that to a young girl?" I shouted. He tried to apologize by saying he understood because he had pimples on his butt and it embarrassed him when he had to take his clothes off in a scene. "Not the same," I snapped.

Bill loved to hear himself talk, but the Yankees were not impressed. Our cook, Charlene, became bored with his dialogue and hated to see him coming. For my part, I'd stand behind the bar in the back listening to him for hours. Sometimes there was no point to anything he said. I've seen that part of him on the screen and it's funny. People think he is acting, but he's not. It's the real thing.

One spring he called and asked to stay at the inn even though we were closed. It was mud season and his place became impossible to get to that time of year. I guess he'd forgotten. He'd gotten stuck in the mud and a policeman had to pull him out. I said "Sure" and he moved into the inn, our only guest. We were in and out a lot during the day and he'd trail after me like a little kid after his mommy. There were many sides to Bill.

One weekend after he had filmed *Children of a Lesser God* he came to stay at the inn. We began getting these weird telephone calls. I couldn't understand the person on the other end. It happened repeatedly. Finally one evening he was standing by the bar when I answered the phone. He immediately realized what it was and said, "Hold on." He had just finished filming *Children of a Lesser God* and was going out with Marlee Matlin, who had a hearing problem. He rushed to his room for his brief case, opened it, and began to type in his conversation. It was a telephone for calling the hearing impaired. I was relieved to have those mysterious calls finally explained.

One weekend Marlee and Bill called and asked if they could enlist the services of our male cat to impregnate their female. Permission was granted. The next weekend we invited them to dinner and they brought the cat. The wedded pair romped in the basement for a couple of days and the honeymoon was a success.

It was amusing to see Bill and Marlee together. Usually Bill monopolized the conversation, but he couldn't with Marlee. He had to speak slowly and carefully so she could understand. He also had to listen more. It was one of the nicest evenings we ever spent with him.

Later, when she won the Academy award he was not happy. He felt she won it because of her condition even though she had done a beautiful acting job. I couldn't understand his attitude, but he could have been right, I suppose. Sometimes it seems they give awards for all the wrong reasons or just because an actor has been nominated so many times and never won.

Bill's reaction was very strange when he was nominated for an award for *Kiss of the Spider Woman*. He didn't want to go to the award ceremony, so Pat told him he could make a wonderful pitch for our inn if he won. Bill didn't take him up on the idea.

Chapter 57

FIRST MEETING WITH TOM CRUISE

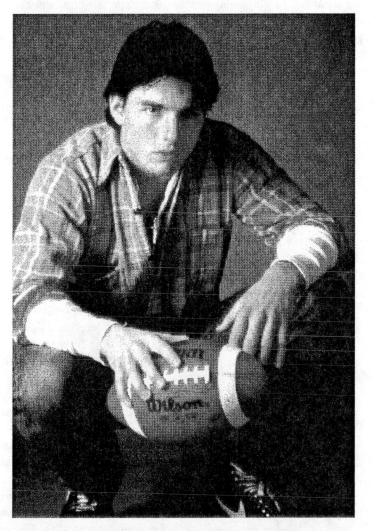

Tom Cruise, *All the Right Moves*

Spring 1981 rolled round and it was time for me to put in eight hours of work in the industry to retain my union card. I took off for California. Pat and Laurie were working on *Poltergeist*. Laurie was working as a stand-in on the set.

The apartment where we had lived in Lennox, before we went to the farm, was now just a shell of a building due to a fire. It was used as a flophouse for the guys, who lived out of town, when they were working. It had charred rafters and girlie pictures on the ceiling, quite awful to behold. Pat was living there and seeing as there were no other guys staying at the time, it also became my abode. A few days later Pat went on location and I was left there alone. Lying there alone at night, I could hear helicopters thunking against the night sky. There were sirens, shouts and even sounds of gunshots. I'd awaken in the night and find myself gazing at the girlie pictures, thinking what a far cry this was from our inn. I also knew that I had the inn to go home to.

On the set of *Poltergeist*, Steven Spielberg was having a wonderful time, setting off the lightning machines. Spielberg was planning for *E.T.* next. Pat was delighted to be working with him. With his brilliant mind, he challenged many of the old timers by demanding they do things differently. They grumbled to themselves complaining "We've always done it that way." They resented changes. Little did they know what was in store for the movie industry.

I did get my eight hours working on the set of *Pennies from Heaven* during a big call. Many of my old friends were there including Jack Stone. I'd known him since I was a kid. He questioned me, asking why I was so happy with my life. He had always prepared for disasters. His glass was always half empty. A few months later I got a letter from him, asking if there was some land nearby that he could buy for his kids. I never heard from him again and he died soon after that.

I worked on extras and spent most of the time on the stage talking to my old friends. I loved the opportunity to catch up and get reacquainted. I went on the stage and watched Bernadette Peters dancing and belting out a song. She was even more appealing in person, than on film.

I was ready to leave for home when I got a rush call from the union. They desperately needed a hairstylist in Johnstown, Pennsylvania. Could I take the job? It would only be for two weeks. I agreed, but had to fly home first to settle some business at the inn and gather my hairdressing supplies. I flew home, paid bills, gathered my things and off I flew to Johnstown.

I was replacing a hairstylist who was being fired. I had called him before I left to make sure he was okay with my taking his place. I wasn't about to repeat my experience on *Mandingo*. He was thrilled that I was coming. Getting fired is an awful experience. As I was later to understand, once it happens, you just want to disappear.

Johnstown was a depressed town and had been torn apart countless times by a rampaging river and floods. The closing of the steel plants had caused massive unemployment. The film *All the Right Moves* addressed many of the problems the town was experiencing. It was towards the end of the film and I arrived after most of the "bad boys" had gone home. They had left a bad taste in the mouths of the town's folk, due to their wild antics and tearing up the hotel. Everyone on the crew was depressed and weary after working in the freezing rain and mud.

I waltzed in, all happy, after my vacation in California. Instead of being resentful toward me, the crew was so nice, I was welcomed and I cheered people up. I had two main stars to work with - Tom Cruise and Lea Thompson.

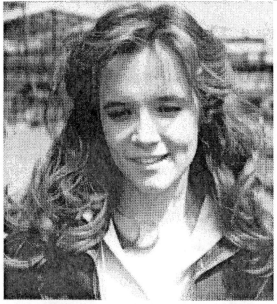

Lea Thompson, *All the Right Moves*

Craig T. Nelson of *Coach* fame was playing a coach. Tom was rather unknown at this point, *Cocktail* hadn't been released yet. He was handsome, kind, fun and cooperative. His part was that of a young fellow ready to graduate from high school that wanted to become a college football star. That's how many kids in those depressed areas escaped the hopeless towns. Tom threw himself completely into his role.

The first day the hairstylist took me into the makeup trailer and introduced me to Tom and showed me how he slicked down his hair. Sometimes replacing someone can cause problems, but Tom was great. He shook my hand, welcomed me and made me feel quite comfortable. Lea Thompson too, was very appealing, but frustrated and hurt because she couldn't figure out how to communicate with the director, Michael Chapman. He didn't seem interested in giving her any direction and he didn't seem to be comfortable with the actress. He seemed to do well enough with the men. After this film he went back to being a cameraman.

One morning we reported to a giant steel mill for filming. It had been deserted, but our special effects crew had built fires and along with props made the place look like it had never been shut down. In the film Tom's character had been told that he wouldn't make the team. He was condemned to failure, stuck in a life at the factory. But to his surprise, as he leaves the mill, the coach approaches him and tells him he has had a change of heart. He will make the team, after all. Tom was stunned and so happy he could hardly believe it. As Tom was acting, he threw himself into the part to completely that he actually hyperventilated and fell on the ground in a faint. I rushed over and sat beside him until the nurse arrived. He was just fine, just too highly motivated. We wrapped and he went home to recuperate that evening.

Despite its depression, Johnstown appealed to me. There were many nice things about the town, especially the friendly inhabitants, and the wonderful bronze statues in the park. They were sculptures of people sitting on benches, one standing outside the newspaper building. At first glance they all seemed real.

In the mornings I went to the local café for breakfast. It was close to the hotel and open twenty-four hours a day. Often some of the extras would be in there and they would come over and talk, which made me feel at home. I wondered why they hadn't left town to find work, but soon understood that they were very close with their families and didn't want to break them up.

We made a strange parade down the main street one night as we filmed a rain sequence. The camera was placed in the car, focusing on the two actors. Following the car was a water truck and a man sat on top of the water truck with a hose spouting water over the car in which they were shooting. It looked like rain from the inside the car, I guess. We all followed in a line of cars. First the set car, then the man with the hose, then the rest of our cars. Hilarious, strange parade.

I only worked for two weeks and it was fun. It was time to go back to the inn, do the spring-cleaning and get ready to open for the next season. I said my goodbyes and invited everyone to visit me at the inn.

Chapter 58

HURRAH, I'M A GRANDMA!

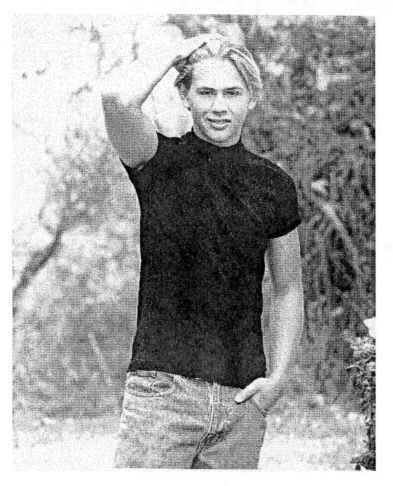

Sugar's Grandson, Patrick Blymyer at age 19

After *All the Right Moves*, I stayed home to run the inn. Pat traveled home off and on. He was spending less time at the inn and more time in Hollywood. He had escaped from the inn in a way that was helpful. Finally, he truthfully admitted that he didn't want to be an innkeeper any longer. It made me sad. I had asked him to be honest when we bought the inn. Perhaps in his defense, he didn't know until he tried it.

One day the phone rang. It was Laurie, "Mom I'm pregnant." I was thrilled. "Oh Laurie, I'm so happy. Who's the dad? When are you due?" I was ready for grandchildren. The sooner, the better. She explained that the father was a grip she had worked with on *Poltergeist*. Unfortunately, he wasn't ready to become a father and Laurie was heartbroken.

Laurie came home and jumped right into our life at the inn. Being a great organizer she was a welcome part of our lives. She wore brightly colored sweat outfits and she was so slim we couldn't imagine her being pregnant when we saw her from behind.

That year Max decided to sell the twelve, forested acres right across the road from us. We wanted to buy it because we didn't want anyone building there and ruining the look of our inn. It was tough on us because we were barely getting our payments made on the inn. We purchased the land, putting $10,000 down and we were short of money that spring.

Laurie had decided to have her baby at home with a midwife. In those days it was very difficult to find a doctor who would provide back up for a midwife doing a home birth. We found Dr. Hope in Sandwich, a village about an hour away. Laurie and I drove there for her exams. Dr. Hope had a beard and was nearsighted and so he took his glasses off and sometimes his beard tickled her during the exam, making her laugh.

Laurie got bigger and bigger. Her due date came and went and the midwife was worried. She told us that if one more day passed Laurie would have to go to the hospital for the birth. That day her water broke. It was exciting! We had the delivery room all ready, upstairs. After her labor began, we made some phone calls and a few hours later the midwives arrived. Strangely enough one of the midwives was a relation of a friend of Dick Hart, the gaffer who I'd met on my cruise.

Watching the birth was the most exciting experience of my life. I'd had three children, but when I was the one having the baby I'd been so involved in the pain that it was very different. Seeing the next generation of my family being born was a peak experience and I can hardly describe it. Watching a human being appear for the first time, hearing that cry of life and knowing it was a part of me, was beyond anything I had felt before. As the pains came, I held Laurie's hands willing the pain to pass to me. Finally, a tiny head appeared and soon after a little baby boy was placed on Laurie's chest. Nobody told her it was a boy, but when she felt his tiny body and realized he had a penis, her face broke into a huge smile.

The midwife cut the cord, waited a few minutes, and then drew a bath. She handed my grandson to me and told me to bathe him. "Me? Are you sure?" Gosh, was that wonderful! They cleaned up the room and, just like in the old days, all our friends were waiting downstairs. They came up to congratulate Laurie and to meet the little fellow who was to be called Patrick after his grandfather. Our friend Norman brought Dom Perignon champagne in a huge bottle and we all celebrated. I was in heaven.

That was May and by July we were again hurting for money. Bob Norin, a makeup man who had visited us at the inn, called me to go to the Pocono's to do a television show with Andy Griffith and Katherine Helmond called *For Lovers Only*. He figured I could use the extra income and he was right. I hated leaving in the summer season. In June, Laurie had flown to Los Angeles to introduce her son to his father hoping he'd have a change if heart. He didn't and so she came back home to the inn. She offered to run the inn for me so I could take the job. She always seemed to be there for me.

The Pocono's were very different from our mountains. The area was designed for honeymooners and in many ways very bizarre. We stayed at a resort. My room was all decorated in white carpet with roses on it. The carpet not only covered the floor, but also the walls. My bed was round and there were mirrors everywhere. The bathroom had a huge sunken tub surrounded by mirrors and the toilet was placed so that you could sit there and look at yourself in the mirror. How inviting!

I had the best time at night. After finishing dinner, I'd put my room service tray outside and little skunks would come looking for food. I could lie on the floor and, carefully pull the drapes aside from the floor to ceiling windows, and watch the little fellows munching their dinner just inches away.

We shot in a place called the bunker. It was a round building and each suite had its own pool for honeymooners to frolic in. Activities were happening all the time. Girls on their honeymoons were very dressed up, trying to look good while walking up the hills in their high heels.

It was wonderful working with Katherine Helmond again. She knew where I lived because she had a relative going to Waukeela, the girls' camp at the bottom of our hill. I enjoyed working with Andy Griffith, too. He was just as charming as he appears on the screen. The crew, however, was not friendly and when the show finished I was happy to return home.

Little Patrick became part of our lives. He rode on our backs as we worked around the inn. Pat would sit him in his little chair at the kitchen counter and talk to him while he cooked. I'd have him on my back when I

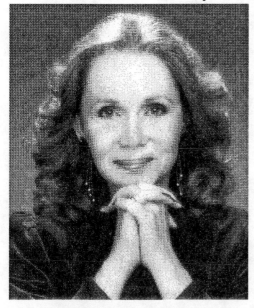

Katherine Helmond,
For Lovers Only

tended the bar in the evenings. Sometimes he would reach for the bottles and I had to be careful or they would go crashing to the floor.

In time, he no longer needed to be carried. He'd toddle into the living room in the evenings and visit with the guests, joining them while they had drinks, cheese and crackers in front of the fireplace. One evening he came crying into the kitchen because a guest scolded him for sticking his fingers into the cheese, but normally he was very happy. We found out why he was so happy one night when the waitress caught him emptying the dregs of the drinks the guests left behind when they went to dinner. A Typical Taurus, but no harm had been done so we got a great laugh out of it.

That was a good year. I had my first grandchild and we made our first profit - around $750. Xochi had started college at University of New Hampshire and was eligible for college loans and grants. Even though we brought in plenty of money, most of it was spent keeping the inn going.

Through trial and error we discovered there were seasons when tourists came and others times when they just wouldn't. For instance, I tried Memorial Day specials and early June and July specials, but nobody came. I finally realized that I would have to work in the film industry during the slow times to make ends meet.

I began to realize that many of the people, who came to the inn, really wanted to know about our experiences in the movie industry so I moved our photos to our bar cum den. They looked great and everyone enjoyed them. Once a woman reporter from Boston interviewed us for television. Her helicopter landed by the tennis court. Helen Gruzik, the hairdresser I had run into in Paris, just happened to be visiting and ended up in the segment. They photographed our pig, Gracie, and we talked about the changes in our lives. When the spot came on television, it began with a shot of Crystal Lake with "Hooray for Hollywood" playing in background.

Laurie stayed with us for the rest of the year. Pat got a call to go to Austin, Texas to work on a film called *Songwriter* starring Willie Nelson, Kris Kristofferson, and Leslie Ann Warren. Almost immediately after he left, I also got a call asking if I could do the hairdressing for the film. Once again, Laurie said she could manage. By this time I had a wonderful assistant manager, Jane Ross, who took the weight off my shoulders and gave me the organization I needed. I agreed to go.

Chapter 59

SONGWRITER
Austin, Texas

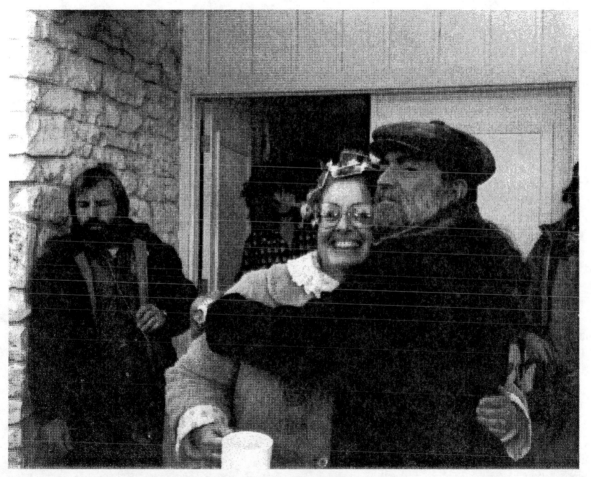

Sugar with Willie Nelson, *Songwriter*

I was back working in the movie industry. I didn't want to be there, away from the inn, but Pat was in heaven. He'd always loved Willie Nelson who was the star of *Songwriter* along with one my favorites Kris Kristofferson. It was autumn when I left for Texas, the weather crisp and clear at home. Upon my arrival in Austin, I was overwhelmed by the heat and humidity. I had left behind, the autumn weather that I loved and the heat was dreadful. My body was not pleased either. It had been getting ready for winter.

Pat and I took adjoining rooms. We could have saved money by using just one room, but getting ready in the morning, at the same time, was too difficult. We turned his room into the kitchen and everything else. We had a table built to hold all our stuff - the coffee pot, vegetable steamer, and electric frying pan. We were going to be there too long, not to be able to cook something at home, even if our home was a hotel room. We also had a little fridge. The setup worked well. My room, where we slept, was the pretty one with candles, incense, and nice decorations.

Kris had written so many wonderful songs that moved me. I was anxious to meet and work with him. Leslie Ann Warren, our female star, was quite a handful and the crew didn't care much for her. She never made an effort to be liked. She didn't need support from me and I was glad not to have to share her emotional baggage. She was close to Ed Ternes, the makeup man and more intimate with him. If she needed to communicate with me about something, she did so clearly and I felt we worked together very well. Ed Ternes had worked with her often and he gave me hints about how to get along with her which was helpful. Greg La Cava came to be the assistant makeup man.

In the beginning we had the sweetest director, Steve Rash. He was from Texas and had directed the *Buddy Holly Story*. We all loved him, but the producers weren't pleased with his work and they fired him. Alan Rudolph replaced him. Alan worked out well for a replacement. During the change over we had a few days off and I spent much of it walking in the park next to the river. I'd put Julio Iglesias tapes on my Walkman and start off. Soon I'd be singing happily along with Julio, getting strange looks from others on the trail. I lost a pound a day walking and was not really anxious to get back to work.

Willie Nelson was a far different person than I expected him to be. He had such charisma, and his hair was beautiful, so long, soft, and shining. The first time I began to work with him, my heart began to beat fast and my hands shook. I realized I was in the presence of someone very special. The more I was around him the more I grew to respect and love him. He was generous with his friends and so kind and talented. Before long, I joined Pat in his love of Willie. Kris was a different story. I had put him on a pedestal because he had written such wonderful songs and I assumed his songs were an expression of his inner person. I was wrong. My first disappointment came when I saw how slight he was. In film and photos he looked larger. His unbuttoned shirt in the photos made him look like he had a nice, broad chest. Not true. And his skin was shiny and tight, and his eyes deep set. Of course it wasn't his fault that my expectations weren't fulfilled.

My job was to stand by on the set and go in when someone's hair needed attending to. Kris didn't want that. If I went in to fix something out of place he shouted at me to leave him alone. He didn't want to be disturbed, even between shots. After that I just did the minimum for him.

Willie, on the other hand, was charming. Even though he was very capable of doing his own hair, he came to me to make me feel good.

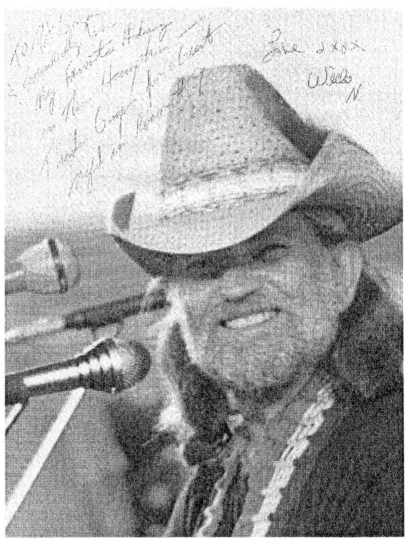

Willie Nelson

In actuality he preferred to stay in his bus with the boys. A woman entering that male domain just didn't feel comfortable. Eventually he did his own hair, coming to me before the shot, so I could make sure he had the correct rubber band on the end of his ponytail, matching it for the scene. For instance one day he'd have a band with plastic marbles, and the next a different color band without the marbles. He kept me on my toes. It was a game.

We were a real family, all of us working together. Most of the drivers were Willie's boys and really great people. They traveled with him when he toured and he always tried to keep them working. We became friends with the lighting man, Burdock who worked with Pat. Burdock also did something called "Bad TV". The guys would get together and do the raunchiest things. One day they convinced a good-looking girl to take her shirt off for them. She was willing and happy. This was typical. After all it was "Bad TV" and they gave her a free T-shirt.

We went to concerts where Willie played and other talented musicians came up on the stage and joined him. It was like a carnival at times.

Although Leslie Anne was not very well liked and difficult at times for the Production Department, she was actually quite nice with me. When the makeup man wasn't in our trailer she and I would talk about life. I liked her and her hair looked great after we figured out what she wanted. I must give the credit to Ed because he suggested how to get the look we wanted and it worked. I used the same look on other films to my advantage. I was always happy to take good advice.

One evening Willie threw us a party at his place. He had a whole studio set up, a club of sorts - almost his own little village. The party started out great, good food, great music. Patrick even ended up playing a kazoo duet with Willie - we still have pictures of it. But about two hours after we arrived there was a commotion and a man fell to the floor. It was Woody, Willie's friend and driver, one of the sweetest men ever. An ambulance was called. They tried to revive him, but it was too late. What a tragedy. We all went outside as they loaded him into the ambulance. It was foggy and I remember the bright blue lights going round and round. It was so very quiet and all those big old cowboys just stood out there with tears running down their faces. Woody had written a song for Willie to sing at his funeral. The opportunity came all too soon.

Mike Moder was our unit manager. He had been a fantastic first assistant director. Although he was making more money, and the unit manager position was a more prestigious job, he wasn't as happy as he used to be. He missed being on the set and the camaraderie that went with it. Sometimes he'd say to me, "Come talk to me," and I'd keep him company. He'd play his guitar and sometimes and we'd just talk. He was one of my favorite people. We knew his whole family. He never did go back to first assisting. Instead, he rose even higher in his career. Although he became important in the industry, he has stayed the same friendly Mike.

Kathy and Ernie, our wardrobe people, were in love and decided to get married on our set. They planned it for right after Christmas. It was great. They had food prepared and champagne. At lunch time, the whole crew stood around, upstairs and downstairs in the house where we were shooting, and joined them in their wedding and the celebration afterwards. Willie played and sang for them. It was a true first for me.

The movie business was slow and I felt lucky to be working even if I'd have preferred to be home at the inn. The money was excellent and I appreciated it. Our honey wagon driver obviously wasn't happy to be there and his attitude drove me crazy. As usual, makeup people had to be on the set early. We'd arrive at the honey wagon early in the morning to do our work and he wouldn't have the room ready. The heat wouldn't be on or he still had to sweep it or something to cause a delay every morning. It was frustrating. I'd rather have stayed in bed longer.

Finally one day I had enough of it. The weather had gotten increasingly cold, much colder than expected. By lunch it had dropped to seventeen degrees. There was no place for us to go inside for lunch so we headed for the honey wagon with our trays full of food. When we got there, he was changing the oil - something that just had to be done in that room. He'd had all morning to do it, but had decided to eat his lunch early and do it while we were eating. I blew up. I told him he should leave and send someone to take his place. He was so negative. If he didn't want the job why was he there? That afternoon, I complained to Mike Moder about him. As Mike had never heard me complain before, I guess he got after the head of Transportation who told the driver to shape up. He was distressed. Mike must have come down really hard on him. "Sugar," he begged, "will you ask Mike to let up?" I didn't want to cause trouble, but I did want a warm place when I needed it and our working area ready at the proper time. We never had to wait again.

When I took the job, I was told I'd be home by Christmas. I was getting worried. The week we had off when they changed directors was putting our schedule later and later. I needed to be home at the inn for the busy Christmas holiday season.

In the meantime we were enjoying the local restaurants. Austin was a great city, small enough to be friendly, modern enough to offer great eats. Our favorite restaurant was an unusual place called Threadgills. Originally the building had been a gas station. So when we arrived we wondered if we were at the right place. Upon entering, the first thing we saw was a huge collection of beer bottles. They were everywhere - every kind of beer one could imagine. The tables were plain and close together. My mouth still waters as I describe the food. They served fried chicken, chicken fried steak, fried oysters, fried ham steak. The vegetables were marvelous, too - lima beans, peas, corn, fried and mashed potatoes, greens, and more. It was real home cooking. My favorite was chicken fried steak. It was what I ordered every time. The dessert was a huge piece of apple pie or a delicious pudding.

One Sunday we went to San Antonio. The river walk that runs through the loveliest section of town surprised me. What a classy area. We walked along the river looking up at the hotels rising above us and watched the boats move slowly along. Later we had lunch on the terrace of one of the many restaurants.

The temperature kept dropping. One day it was only fourteen degrees - unheard of in Austin. Pipes burst in the department stores and offices. It was a disaster. We were having our own problems. Christmas was coming, a busy time at the inn and I wasn't going to be finished. I was really nervous. Now the film companies usually take two weeks off for Christmas, but they didn't on this show. I called Laurie and told her we only had two days off. She said, no problem, she could handle it.

I relaxed a little. I bought a big down comforter for our room. The heating just couldn't keep up with the weather. The swimming pool was frozen solid. Back at the inn, all was going very well until one morning. Laurie called. "The well at the barn (which had been turned into guest rooms) isn't working, Mom." Only a fire would have been worse. I knew where the well was located, but it was difficult to describe over the phone. Laurie called a well digger who actually came out on Christmas to the tune of $2,000. He dug through the frozen ground and replaced the worn out pump. By then the guests had checked out of the barn because it was impossible to be there without water. It was a real stress for everyone and I was so proud of Laurie for handling it so well.

Shortly after Christmas we finished filming and I was so happy to go home. The good part was that between the two of us Pat and I had made $65,000, which enabled us to do a lot of things that needed to be done around the inn.

Chapter 60

MOVIE BUSINESS TO THE RESCUE

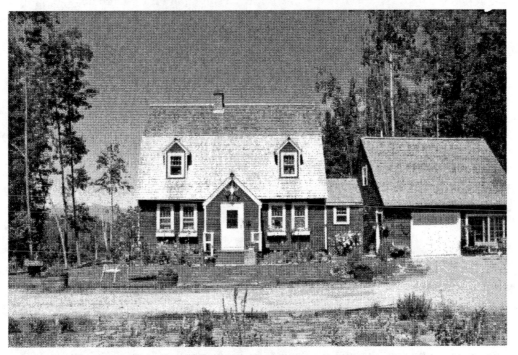

Sugar and Pat's New Hampshire Home

I stayed home at the inn for over a year after finishing *Songwriter*. Thanks to the income from the film, we were able to catch up with our bills and pay off some debts. Nevertheless, once again we put all the money we had earned back into the inn. We didn't expect it to be any different.

Having been a part of the movie industry for many years, I was capable of creating my own dramas. By now we really needed a home of our own. I'd been cutting out pictures of rooms I liked from *Country Home* and other magazines. I'd paste them on large pieces of cardboard, room by room: the bedrooms, the dining room, the kitchen, and living room. The gardens were on their own separate board. I knew that my creative powers would work, because they had before. Still, I didn't have a picture in my mind of what I wanted the exterior to look like, I just knew I wanted our home to look old. Our land across the road was available and would be a great place to build, but I just didn't know what it would look like yet.

A post and beam building with a gambrel roof was being raised in town. I stopped to watch the process. It was fascinating to watch the construction. When it was finished, it was beautiful - just what I wanted for the exterior of our home! I gave the builder Doug a call. Doug said the building was actually a copy of a 300-year-old home plan. That was it. I now had my exterior. We decided to go ahead and build. We owned the land. Now we needed a building loan that turned out to be easy enough to secure. We applied for a loan at a local bank and soon had the money for the home. We had to borrow enough to pay off the land, too.

First we hired a forester to clear the house site. After finding a site for our well, we laid out the house site tying red ribbons around tree trunks. Little Pat and I would walk across the road and make believe we were having tea in our kitchen-to-be. Patrick loved going to our imaginary home. Meanwhile, Big Pat left to work on *Weird Science*.

While the house was being built, we'd walk through it imagining what it would feel like when it was finished. A mason came and built the chimney, an electrician completed the wiring. Pat was disappointed with the plumber because he couldn't manage a swiveling toilet that would allow him to turn and look at Mount Washington while he sat there. Oh, well! We bought a wood/oil furnace so that if the wood fire went out the oil would kick in. Doug had planned for ordinary windows, but some of our guests saw the plans and insisted we install eight-over-eight pane windows instead. I bought a five and a half foot tub, painted pink with golden feet, for my bathroom and two antique sinks with brass fittings. The house, a gambrel, looked wonderful.

About the same time, I learned that I was going to be a grandmother again. I learned that Tanya was pregnant just a month before her baby was born. I couldn't imagine that I hadn't noticed the changes in her, but she had worn loose clothes. Once again I was excited to be a grandmother. Unfortunately, the father was a man who wouldn't be able to take on the role of being a father. He was a handsome fellow, a singer and if I'd been her age, I might have fallen for him, too. Rather than pressure him, she decided to take on the responsibility of her child by herself. Brittany was born on March 20, 1985. She arrived with her arm up like the statue of liberty, as though saying, "Hurrah." She was absolutely beautiful. Still is. We spent a quiet spring enjoying Brittany. It was such fun having another grandchild. She was a mellow baby and entertained herself.

While all this was going on, Patrick's drinking was catching up with him and it worried me. I knew there was nothing I could do. He had to do it himself. He was leaving for California, to do a film, and the night before his departure he asked me to walk over to the house with him. He had already had a couple of drinks and I was upset. I had begged him to stay sober this once. I cried and told him that the alcohol just put a wall between us and that he could go to the house by himself because I would not be there with him at the rate things were going. I was heartbroken, but didn't know what else to do. He left the next day to work on *Commando*.

Spring passed and the house was nearly finished. The utilities were underground, the well had been dug, and finally the carpets were installed and we were able to move. It was July and we needed to have the inn ready for the fourth of July. We moved just in time to paint our old room at the inn for the guests who were arriving the next day. We had no furniture so we slept on mattresses with our clothes piled neatly around our rooms, but it didn't matter because we were finally in our own home. Pat and I, Laurie and Patrick, and Tanya and Brittany all lived there. The house was full and it was great! My movie/life set, though, was not yet complete. The carpenters were finished. Our dream home was a reality. It was a true work of art, in spite of the fact that it stood in the middle of a barren area of the forest with nary a stalk of grass or flower in sight. As the art director, in my imagination I saw it with many varieties of trees, an English flower garden surrounding the house. At night through our bedroom window, we could look up at the stars.

I needed to cast myself a new chiropractor. The adequate, but uninspired one in town was suddenly killed in a plane crash. I wanted a spiritual friend like Dr. Hovey had been. A friend suggested Robert Johnson (everyone called him Nick) whose office was in Portland, Maine. She said he just wiggled your toe and you were better. I made an appointment.

Nick was exactly who I'd been looking for. It must have been in the stars. He had his own style of adjusting and soon I did begin to feel much better. He had shelves of spiritual books in his office and we began to have great conversations while he was adjusting me. Soon my whole family was going to him. He even adjusted Brittany. He explained how the birth ordeal often put even a soft little baby out of adjustment. He suggested I do my Transcendental Meditations to help with the stress that caused me to have a stiff neck and recommended a TM meditation course in Washington, D.C. I went to Washington D.C. for ten days. We meditated four times a day. It was a welcome rest and at the end of my retreat, I felt relaxed and restored. The next course was to take place in India. I wanted to go, but not alone, so I asked Nick if I could accompany him and he agreed.

While I was enjoying myself in Washington, D.C., Pat had a dreadful experience. The water we used for our lawn was not running. It hadn't been a dry year so Pat went to investigate. Much to his dismay he found that a baby moose had fallen into the spring during the winter and its remains were clogging up the pipe. Horrendous! It stunk and was slimy. It had to be cleaned out. Pat tried to hire someone to help to no avail. He and the handy man worked for days to clean it out. His clothes were so smelly at night he just tossed them out the back door and never put them on again.

I arrived home all happy and renewed and relieved that I had missed that dreadful experience. Still, the smell lingered and we were having a huge wedding party at the inn. We prayed that the wind would blow in the other direction the day of the wedding. Luckily it did. Eventually Pat placed the moose skull above the entrance to our house as a badge of courage. I thought he deserved that.

The house was finished and Doug presented us with the final bill. Expecting it to cost just what we had procured for our loans, we had a huge shock. It came to $30,000 more than our loan. I was shocked and frightened. How were we to pay him? We had no more money. I had not worked nor did I expect to. Pat and I were at a loss.

I don't think I've ever been so frightened. Even when we were broke in West Virginia, I always felt we could go back to work in films. When we moved to Snowville, I hoped I would never have to do that again. I kept my union dues current though, but I didn't know what to do. I took a walk in the woods by myself. Scared and in tears, I talked to God. I vowed that I would do anything to earn the $30,000. "Show me the way," I said, "and I will do it." I finished my prayer and walked back home and went on with my life. I am now aware that I totally surrendered and turned my life over to God and got out of my own way.

Amazingly, things began to change. We had tried to refinance the inn with the bank that gave us our first loan. No luck. Then I talked with a friend who worked at another inn who knew about a bank up north in Littleton. They were interested in getting business in our valley. I called and set up an appointment and we started the procedure to refinance the inn. About the same time Pat got a call to do a job in Japan - a film called *An American Geisha* starring Pam Dawber. They offered the crew an airline ticket for their wives as part of their pay. I was psyched. I was ready to go. My crew at the inn felt fine about my leaving so in early August, so off we went to Kyoto.

I felt very strange as we waited in Tokyo for the plane to Kyoto. It was the fortieth anniversary of the atomic bombing of Japan. All throughout the airport televisions ran films of that awful day and the aftermath of the bombing. There I was, an American, watching all those Japanese people looking at the horror. I wondered what they thought of me at that moment. I think I would have wanted to do away with me if I had been them, but there was no sign of anger. Perhaps they were just too polite. I was very uncomfortable.

Although at the time we were unaware of it, the Japan Airlines plane that took off right before ours crashed that afternoon killing nearly everyone. I remember watching it take off. Their insignia on the tail remained imprinted in my mind. We didn't know it had happened until the next day when we were looking at the news. It never occurred to us that perhaps our family might have thought we were on that plane. We hadn't told them which airline we were taking. We called home and Tanya broke into tears, hysterical, telling us how she had been so frightened and worried. Before we left, we had given her our power of attorney and she worried that perhaps we had a premonition of a crash. She was so relieved and happy when she knew we were safe.

We stayed at a first class hotel in Kyoto. The weather was hot and humid and I wanted to stay in my room all day long wearing only the cotton kimono that was put on the bed each day and drink the wonderful Japanese beer from my little fridge.

I did go out though and I shopped in the areas where there were huge rain covers between buildings that were opened when it was nice weather. I got frustrated in the grocery store because I knew nothing about Japanese food. It was so different and of course all in Japanese.

The people were always polite. They bowed to me and I soon learned to do the same every time I met someone. We traveled to see the huge golden Buddha at a deer park. Even the deer bowed when I gave them something to eat. The Buddha was amazing, so big and all gold.

One evening a local crewmember invited us to his home for dinner. What a meal! He must have spent a whole month's salary on it. There was shrimp, beef, chicken, wonderful liquor, and everything else one could imagine. He cooked our meal on a large hibachi in the living room. It got hotter and hotter as we sat around the fire; the only outlet for the smoke was a small hole in the floor above us. While the meat cooked, we drank and talked and all the while sweat ran down our faces. Our host told us the Japanese couldn't own a car unless it could be parked off the street at night. So people often used their living room as a garage. I began to realize just why the people were so polite - living so close together, one had to be polite or it would be impossible to live. It was quite an evening. The food was wonderful even if I did wonder if I was going to faint from the heat.

Eventually Japan started to wear on me. I was sick of the hot weather and I'd seen enough of the sights. Me, who loved to talk and communicate, was unable to speak Japanese and most people didn't speak English. They didn't need to. The food had worn out its newness and I realized I preferred Chinese food anyway. I didn't want to be ungrateful for my trip, but I was ready to escape.

And escape I did. Lee Harmon called to ask if I wanted to work on a film called *Running Scared*. It was starting in two weeks. "Of course," I said, "I'll be there." And do you know how much I made working on that film? $30,000! And to boot, by the time I got home the inn had been refinanced so we had some extra money and I was able to pay off the $30,000 debt on our house.

Chapter 61

RUNNING SCARED

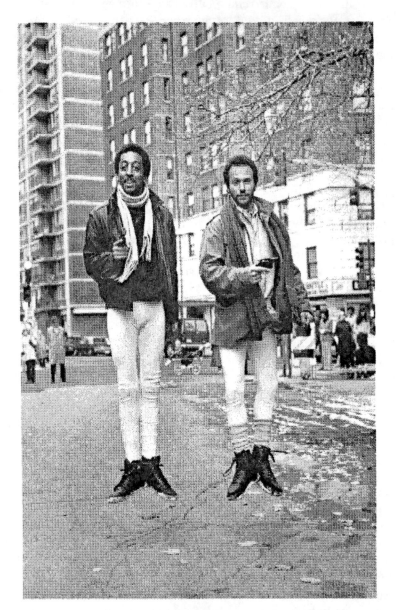

Billy Crystal and Gregory Hines, *Running Scared*

The trip home was a marvel, sort of like traveling through space. I had wanted to experience the Bullet Train that ran from Kyoto to Tokyo - it's supposed to be quite an adventure, but there were no reservations available and I was in a hurry. Instead, I flew from Kyoto to Tokyo and then to Los Angeles. My plane from Tokyo was so late that I had to run through customs and I barely made my connection to Philadelphia. Once there, I had to run to catch the last plane to

Boston. I needed to call Xochi, who was in Boston. She was going to pick me up at the airport, but there was no time. I asked the attendant at the desk to call her so I wouldn't miss my flight.

In Boston, Xochi picked me up and took me to her apartment that she shared with an artist. I slept on a bed in the artist's studio and the next day I drove three hours north to New Hampshire.

At home, in another whirlwind, I threw all my work things together, did some work at the inn, and two days later I was back in Boston to catching a plane to Los Angeles. Fortunately I had made arrangements to rent a room in a condo in Marina Del Rey for my stay in Los Angeles. I rented a car at the airport.

From the moment I left Kyoto I hadn't had a second to relax. The following morning I reported to work in MGM's production office. I was waiting for Peter Hyams, the director I'd worked with on *Peeper,* when my exhaustion finally hit. I began to wonder if I'd be coherent enough to deal. Peter greeted me with a huge hug. I felt much better immediately and I knew I was going to make it. After all I'd prayed for it, right?

Lee Harmon, the makeup man who'd called me for the job, had always been one of my favorite people. We had worked together on *The Other Side of Midnight,* but I hadn't heard from him in years.

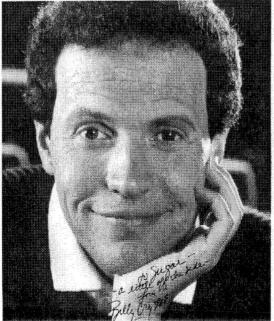

Billy Crystal

Usually he worked with another hairdresser and I was very happy he had called me this time. In the years since I'd seen him, he'd divorced his actress wife and was now married to a nice woman he had met while on location in Arizona. She had a daughter whom he was fond of. His new wife wasn't the fantastic beauty-type he usually was attracted to, but a real person with normal needs. It seemed Lee had finally found someone to have a normal relationship with, rather than being in the caretakers' role that he usually chose.

Billy Crystal and Gregory Hines - what a duo! It was entertainment from the moment they walked through the makeup trailer door. Billy is always so bright, and Gregory not far behind. I had to order a wig for Joe Pantoliano who played the weirdo. His part was that of a creep. I designed a wig with a red flat top and brown sides. It looked great on him. Jimmy Smitts played a bad guy. He was very attractive and I loved talking with him.

Joanie, the script supervisor, was a piece of work. She loved sports and always came into our trailer while we were doing the makeup. She loved to talk sports with the guys. Mornings were filled with conversation about whatever game had been played and games in the past, too. The sports talk didn't interest me. What did fascinate me was the way Joanie just pushed right in. Usually the makeup man prefers to have a quiet

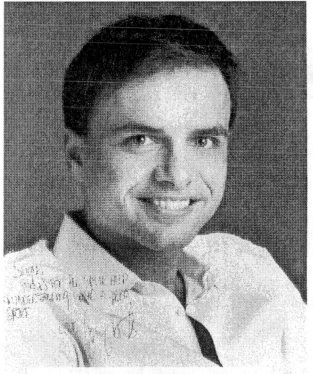

Joe Pantoliano

time with the actors, but Lee didn't seem to mind, at least not until he realized she had a huge crush on him. Then he had a hard time getting her out of there.

Gregory is such a wonderful dancer. One day he came in and took his shoes off for some reason and I just had to ask, "Are those the wonderful feet, I see, that do that fantastic dancing?" He laughed, "Sugar, it's all in the hips."

At the time Billy was doing lots of bodybuilding, lifting weights. He got Gregory started and as the film progressed their bodies became quite attractive with muscles beginning to develop. It was a major change for both of them. Later I saw Gregory in *Tap* and was amazed how muscular he had become.

The condo was comfortable and I didn't have to do anything, but keep my room clean. For dinner I'd bake a potato in the microwave or heat up something simple. I didn't have time for much else because we worked long hours.

Peter Hyams not only directed, he now also did the photography. He loved making films. He had endless energy and seemed to go for weeks without sleep. Sometimes it was difficult to keep up with him. Being close to where we worked and having little other responsibilities was perfect for me.

Steven Bauer and Jonathon Gries played a couple of sidekicks in the film. Jonathon was the son of Tom Gries who had directed *Helter Skelter*. A few years earlier Tom had dropped dead of a heart attack. It was a real surprise because he seemed to be so healthy. At the time, Steven was married to Melanie Griffith. I think their marriage was just about to end. Steven was very handsome, tall and dark and sporting a full beard. Since the beard covered most of his face doing, his makeup was fairly easy for Lee.

Easy, until one Friday night while we were working on *The Queen Mary* in Long Beach. Lee's wife was still living in Arizona and he had planned to sneak out early to get a flight home to be with her. We came into work, got the trailer set up, and then in came Steven - bare faced, no beard at all, not even a mustache. "What on earth happened?" shrieked Lee. I think Lee could have happily killed the guy at that moment. We didn't even have a double beard for him. How could Steven have done that, especially right in the middle of the scene we were shooting?

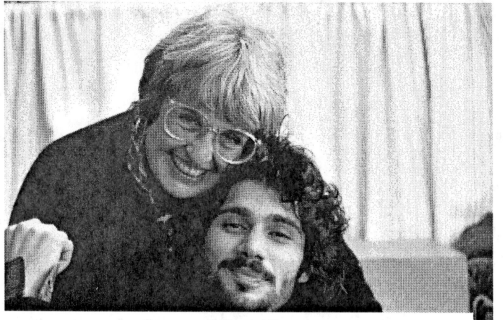

Sugar and Steven Bauer

Steven explained that he had been a little high (on goodness knows what) when he decided to shave. He made a mistake, tried to correct it. He had made such a mess that he decided to take the whole thing off. It seemed logical to him at the time. I'm sure he wished he hadn't done it though because Lee never let up on him during the rest of the film. Lee liked to belittle people and when he found a soft spot he dug right in and never let up.

Lee couldn't leave for home that night which made it even worse. Here he was just married and wanting to be with his bride and as far as he could see this jerk had made that impossible. In a way it was funny, but I didn't laugh because I wasn't the one who had to recreate the beard. Lee got out his beard hair and did a great job. Nobody ever noticed it on the screen.

A strange thing happened to me that evening. I had often worked at the *Queen Mary* with Natalie, but never in the bowels of the ship. This night we went under the decks where there was a huge swimming pool and even farther where all the pipes and machinery for the ship was located. It was dark and sort of scary. As I sat there, it began to feel familiar. It reminded me of a dream I had when I was a little girl where a man was taking me away, down to a place that looked just like the bowels of the ship. I'd wake up and my father would come in and comfort me until I went back to sleep. I wondered if I'd been down here in another life. It was eerie.

We finished up on the set and took off for Key West, Florida. I'd never been there, but I'd heard a lot about it. We were booked into an awful motel that was damp, smelly, and musty. I was glad our stay would be short.

The town of Key West, where we worked, was very commercial just like any tourist town. I'd pictured Hemingway-type houses with writers drinking mint juleps on their verandahs. Maybe that was somewhere else. One of the great places was the Half Moon Pier where people came to watch the sun set over an island. There were many characters selling souvenirs and food. One lady who rode a bike and sold brownies stood out. She looked as if she needed a bath and her curly hair looked as if it hadn't been combed for months. The crewmembers warned me, "Don't buy a brownie." I wasn't tempted. I did buy some conch salad from a reputable stand and it brought back nice memories of the Bahamas.

We did car run-bys near the ocean where a couple weeks earlier a hurricane had come in. There was a still lot of debris lying around. The warm breeze caressed me and I longed for another stay in the islands of the Caribbean. Our last location was going to be in Chicago, in November and December. I wanted to keep the warmth in a little pocket, just in case I needed it later.

We finished up in Key West and went to the little airport

Peter Hyams, Director of *Running Scared*

for our flight to Chicago. Our gaffer, Johnny Baron, was a drinker and a terrible person when he was drinking. I didn't trust him; he'd already once turned on me and he could be vicious. As we were leaving the airport Johnny, drunk as usual, started walking through the clearance place where the metal detector buzzes if you have metal on your person. Every time Johnny tried to go through, the buzzer went off. It happened over and over again. All he had on were shorts, a T-shirt, and sandals. He emptied his pockets and took off everything he could. Still, the buzzer kept going off. We laughed and laughed. It wasn't the metal detector at all. One of the guys could imitate the sound and kept doing it each time Johnny tried to go through. It couldn't happen to a better person, I thought to myself. I am sure I wasn't the only one. When we reached Chicago, it was cold and rainy. There was good old Johnny, still tipsy, but now freezing, walking around in his shorts, T-shirt and sandals, looking for his baggage.

We stayed in a huge Holiday Inn. My room was large, warm, and cozy. I had been planning my trip to India so while I'd been in Los Angeles I had paid a visit to the Indian consulate and had found loads of fabulous posters. They were of the Taj, the countryside and various market places I had also bought saris and incense. I hung my posters all over the walls, put the sari's around, and burned incense. It was so nice to come home from a cold day's work and open the door to my warm room, full of great smells and bright colors. When I ordered room service the waiters, who were often from the East, loved the incense and often it inspired them to tell me about their homeland.

We made snow the first day, but it was cold enough to really snow. My boots from home were not adequate. My feet were cold and hurt by the end of the day. After work I, along with about half the crew, hit the Eddie Bauer shop in the Water Tower Shopping Center. We spent hundreds of dollars on boots, long underwear, jackets, snow pants, hats, and mittens. It was a necessary investment if we were going to make it through two months of shooting in Chicago in the winter.

In the morning I had a routine for dressing. First I took a shower. Next I put on silk underwear, then regular long underwear, then a turtle neck, a woolen sweater, sweat pants and over pants, and finally two pairs of socks, one for wicking the moisture away, the other for warmth. All this was topped by boots, my big coat, and a beaver hat with flaps that covered my ears. I was comfortable, but looked like the Fridge, the football player so popular at the time. If I had fallen down, someone would have had to pick me up. I was so bulky, but I wasn't cold. I felt sorry for the guys who had to be out on the camera, or camera crane, or moving lights because they couldn't dress so warm. They had to be able to move about quickly. I didn't.

Sometimes the wind blew so hard that the waves on the lake froze in the air. It was a beautiful sight, but one day the weather caused a real dilemma for me. Two of my actresses were supposed to walk into a bar from outside. We had already shot the interior of the bar scene in Los Angeles; this was the exterior of that scene. In the film we shot in Los Angeles, they had walked into the bar looking quite lovely, their hair in perfect shape. But as they walked down that Chicago street the wind blew so hard there was no way for their hair to be neat as they entered the bar. I got pretty tense while trying to think of how to make it match. Finally I asked the actresses to act like they were smoothing their hair as they went through the door to the bar. Of course, it was impossible for it to look as good as it had in Los Angeles, but no one seemed to notice the discrepancy.

One night the crew decided to meet at a jazz club and stay up late so we would be able to sleep in and change our schedules around. We were changing to night shooting in the middle of that week. Someone had told us about a great Blues club so we all decided to meet there. When I entered, I was asked for my ID. "You gotta be kidding." I had no ID with me, but the guy let me in anyway. It was obvious I was more than twenty-one, but he explained that if the cops came they would check everyone to make sure he had checked all IDs.

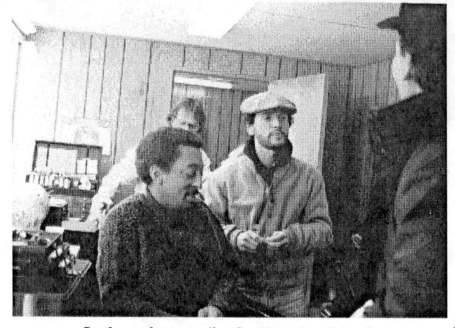

In the makeup trailer for *Running Scared*

We stayed at that club for a while and then went across the street to another bar. It felt wonderful, so dark with the music playing and everyone sitting or standing close to one another. Gregory Hines asked me to dance. I was entranced as he held me in his arms and we hardly moved, the floor was so crowded. The way he moved his body was something like I'd never experienced. Wow! Later I told Pat I had danced with Gregory and he asked, "Is he a better dancer than I am?" I carefully replied, "He dances differently than you do," so as not to hurt his feelings. Thanks for the dance, Gregory.

I began having a real problem with Billy's hair. It was getting thin. To camouflage it I painted his scalp dark brown. It was a great way to make hair look thicker, but it was a slow, tedious process. I had to part the hair a little at a time and paint the scalp and then part it again. Because you couldn't see the scalp, it looked fuller. One morning Billy remarked, "Sugar, do you realize that each day it takes you a little longer to do this?" It hadn't occurred to me, but it was true. I laughed it off and then, moments later, I began to wonder what if he was losing his hair that quickly. I hoped it wasn't possible. I also wondered how I could ever get him a hairpiece to match what he had naturally in the middle of the film. Fortunately I didn't need to.

Xochi came to visit for Thanksgiving. While she was there, I went to Northwestern Medical Center for my shots for India. As a result of the shots, I felt awful and so she spent the day watching me sleep, recovering from the shots. Great vacation for her. Actually she did get to know Steven Bauer and Jonathon Gries. They all went out one night, so she did have some fun.

One day we shot in the huge glass government building. The floors were reached by a glass elevator and it was all open - quite impressive. We had guys dropping from the ceilings and chases all over the building. It felt great to be in out of the cold for a while.

I was walking down Michigan Avenue when a tall, black man dressed in a long overcoat and hat jumped out in front of me. I stopped and he began to sing to me, "I love you, I truly love you." I laughed and continued on my way. He followed, jumping in front of me and singing all the way. I kept laughing until after I crossed the street and he began to walk closer. I wondered if he was okay or if he was going to grab my purse. Fortunately I saw the Benetton Store in front of me and dashed through the door. I told the clerks what happened and later the police took him away. I guess he was a fixture around there, harmless, but still scary. Later at work I told everyone how I'd been sort of mugged by a man who said he loved me.

By now Lee was unhappy. He wished he hadn't committed to this film. He wanted to be home with his new wife. He was sleeping a lot, eating lots of desserts and was totally depressed. He was also mean at times, taking out his frustrations on me. Because he worked in the trailer with me, he heard everything I said. He began holding up a finger for each time he heard me tell a story. I probably told my mugging story five times or more. He held up five fingers. Then he got the whole crew to begin holding up fingers and soon I was afraid to say anything. After a while I didn't think it was funny and felt like crying.

Pat came to Chicago to visit me and drank the whole time, embarrassing me on the set. After he left, I wrote him a letter telling him I loved him very much, but I could no longer sit by and watch him kill himself with booze. I was planning to live a long life and didn't want to spend it with a pickle. I didn't even want to go home when the film finished. It was sad, but I just couldn't stand it anymore.

We worked all night underneath a building in a parking lot. It was a long night, but we had entertainment. Since leaving Los Angeles, the script supervisor had to share the room at the other end of our trailer with Production. She wanted it to herself. That night there was a war. After Production put their papers and things in the office and had gone to work on the set, she came in and heaved everything out into the parking lot. Later Production returned and put it all back. Lee and I stood by watching. We laughed and laughed at the drama. It helped keep us awake that night. I don't remember who won the war.

After work that night, I called home to tell my family not to call me the next day at the usual time because I'd be asleep. Pat answered. I was in a hurry, but he said, "Please take a moment and listen to me." He told me that after visiting me he had gone home and seen just what a mess he was. He read my letter plus all the staff let him know, too, so he had to admit it wasn't just me. Barbara, our assistant innkeeper, had found him a rehab and he was going there on Jan 2. He promised he'd stop drinking by December 21, before I was supposed to get home. I was so happy I cried and cried.

We filmed a car chase on the elevated railway tracks of the EL. There were two cars going down the tracks chasing each other in and out of tunnels all over the place. We could only film the scene on Sundays. It seemed that every Sunday the weather was freezing. The days were long and things didn't always work out like they were supposed to because special effect's crew didn't get their act together. The stunt men were going crazy trying to make up for their failures. It was tense and dangerous. One day we had a train working with us. It had to come off the track and turn on its side after hitting a car. It was quite an undertaking, but it turned out great despite the problems.

The filming was taking so long we thought we might not make it home for Christmas. Yet we did. The last day I was up on the EL looking down at all the trucks and the equipment and the crew and began to imagine, once again, how Peter was feeling. I never felt that way about other directors, just Peter. He'd been the master of us all. Now the film was finished and soon all of this would no longer exist. The circus folds up the tent so to speak and the director is left to work with the editors. Walter Hill once remarked that he liked postproduction best. I am not sure Peter did. I had the feeling he loved the filming part best of all. His wife and I had a good laugh once picturing him as a very old man, in a home being pushed around in his wheel chair, still crouched over the camera, with some old grip pushing the chair as he filmed the home.

We did leave for home on Christmas Eve and Pat picked me up at the airport, sober as could be.

Chapter 62

MY OWN PASSAGE TO INDIA

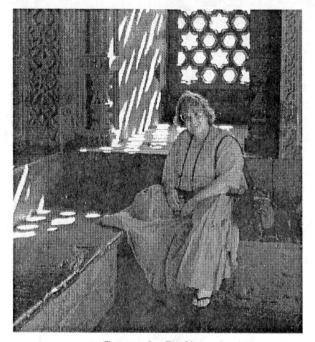

Sugar in India

It made all the difference in the world to me to know that on my return home Pat had decided to make the changes in his life that I longed for. He quit drinking on December 21, 1985 and actually bartended at the inn during the holiday season. I admired Pat's ability to stick with something once he set his mind on it. I was the sort of person who starts out with great enthusiasm and determination and then I lose interest and don't always follow through.

Christmas that year was perfect. Our finances were in good shape with the inn refinanced and some money in the bank. The $30,000 we owed on our house was paid off and, best of all, Pat was sober. What more could I ask?

Nick and I had bought our tickets for India and planned to leave for our meditation trip on January 3. On January 2 Pat was set to check into the rehab. That morning, I drove Pat down to Seabourne in Durham, New Hampshire. He would be there during a four-week stay. All the way down to Durham that morning, Pat was angry with me. Angry, because he felt I was forcing him to quit drinking although he fully understood that he had to. The power of denial still had a strong hold on him. He accused me of driving him down to Seabourne because I thought he might not go otherwise. In reality I took him because I loved him and wanted to say good-by.

Despite his anger, Pat's humor was still intact. As we walked up to the door of the rehab Pat looked at me asking, "Shall I stagger in so I don't disappoint them?" After he checked in I went with him to his room and met his roommate. I'm sure Pat was scared, but assured myself that this was the only way for him to get well. Tearfully I kissed him good-by and left, relieved knowing that he was going to get the help he needed. I made it home in a snowstorm safely, but I was totally exhausted from the stress.

The next morning the blizzard had passed and it was the kind of bright, sunny day that only happens after a snowstorm. After what seemed like forever, Nick was finally ready to leave. He had a flat tire, but we figured we could make it to a gas station for air. We kissed everyone good-by and off we went.

We barely made it to Boston on time. After we boarded the plane to New York, buckled our seat belts, and the plane took off I began to relax.

In New York we boarded the plane to Bombay. It was a twenty-four-hour flight, but luckily it wasn't crowded so we had plenty of room to stretch out. Settling back in my seat, on my way to India, I began to think about what I was doing. I hadn't had time to think about it before leaving. Everything had been so hectic. The whole year had been hectic, actually. What was I doing? I realized I hardly knew Nick. Yes, I was a patient of his and he had been to our house. We had great conversations, but now I was going to be alone with him for six weeks. What kind of a wife was I? I had just dropped my husband off at rehab and here I was taking off with another man on what felt like a spiritual adventure. I knew Nick and I were just good friends, but still I began to wonder if it was too weird. I knew Pat wasn't sure about what was going on either. He had to be a little nervous, too. It was probably the first time I'd ever done anything that I really wanted to do without considering everyone else.

Well, I knew worrying wasn't going to do any good and I believed this trip was meant to be. So I decided to relax and enjoy myself, taking things as they came. It was going to be wonderful to be able to spend hours talking about some of my favorite subjects - Nick's too; I knew he and I were very different, but very compatible. He was thirty-eight and had never lived with a woman although he had many girlfriends. I was fifty-one and had my family. I loved people and enjoyed sharing my home with others. I trusted everyone. He trusted very few. He was a Scorpio and I was a Gemini. He was very careful with his money. I was extravagant. It was going to be interesting.

We were supposed to land in Cairo, but it was fogged in so we landed in Athens then flew back to Cairo when the fog lifted. They opened the plane and I could feel the warm air. A couple of flies flew in and buzzed around. It felt good after the cold and snow at home. From Cairo we went on to Kuwait and then Dubai. We arrived in Bombay at three in the morning. It was a long trek through the airport to customs and immigration and it took forever to get through. Everything was written by hand, no computers there. Finally two hours later we came to the head of the line at immigration. We couldn't find our luggage and were told it would be three days before the next plane with luggage arrived. The airline officer told us to stay in Bombay. They would notify us when the luggage got there.

Great. Here we were dressed in heavy clothes suitable for a New England winter and Bombay was warm even in the middle of the night. Luckily I had packed some extra underwear and cosmetics in my carry-on.

We walked outside where we were besieged by what seemed like hundreds of taxi drivers yelling, trying to get our business. I was ready to hire one when Nick, upset, pulled me back. He'd been warned about the taxi drivers who took advantage of tourists. Eventually he made a deal with one of the drivers and we set off for the Taj Mahal Hotel. It was one of the best hotels in Bombay and we had been told we might get sick eating in less reputable places.

Day was just beginning to break as we drove along and everywhere we saw little hovels and other signs of poverty. I had read *City of Joy*, which described India, plus I had talked to a friend who warned me about the poverty - and the heat. She told me a story of how she had seen what looked like piles of rags get up off the sidewalk and walk away. It wasn't rags, but homeless people who had spent the night on the sidewalk.

Nick hadn't done any research and he had no idea how it would be. He was getting worried. He began to picture us living right next to these poor people. There was no plumbing in the neighborhood and we could see people squatting over ditches relieving themselves. It wasn't like anything we had ever experienced.

At last we came into Bombay proper and Nick breathed a little easier as the driver let us off at the Taj Mahal. It was quite lovely and a real contrast to the poverty we'd seen earlier. We walked in and headed for the restaurant. The menu was in both English and Indian, the food very traditional, and I loved it. After ordering breakfast, I walked down the hall to the bathroom. Looking out the window I saw Queen Victoria's Gate looking as I had seen it in *Passage to India*. The image had stuck in my mind. Above it raised the orange sun, diffused by dust, bright and dense. I took a deep breath. I knew I was going to have the time of my life.

Years before, when I decided I was going to be a writer, I found it was helpful to look at my life from the perspective of a writer. That way, no matter how difficult, or easy, happy, or sad things were, I could look at it as gathering information for my future career. Seeing my life that way often made a difficult situation more bearable. Now here I was in India on the other side of the world and this trip was to be my own "Passage to India".

During my life, the movie business had more influence on me than I had realized. I knew anything could be produced in the studio and I began to imagine that the same thing happened for me in real life. I know every film began as a thought in someone's mind, eventually coming to fruition, just as my ideas culminated in my adventures.

In truth, I never expected to find myself in India. I didn't think I'd be able to handle the poverty and the everyday difficulties of life in that country. But since I had come to believe in reincarnation, I could accept that these people had chosen this life for whatever reason. So acceptance became my way in India. Reading books about India, before hand, helped, too. So did a conversation I had with a man I met in Ojai before I left. He was married to an Indian woman and after moving to India he had wanted to do something to make things better. Finally he realized it was impossible. "Just remember you cannot help, or change things," he told me. "It's just too big. Don't feel guilty." I took his advice and observed without judgment. I did give some money to the beggar children, though, and while I often felt for the plight of people, I looked at them with love and allowed them their own lives. Perhaps mine was no better than theirs, just easier.

That first morning after Nick and I finished our tasty breakfast, we walked down the street looking for a place to stay because the Taj Hotel was far too expensive. Thank heavens there were no beggars on that street or Nick might have caught the next plane home. We found a small hotel that was quite nice on the same street. For thirty-five dollars a day we found a room with two beds that faced the ocean. We took it.

We hadn't discussed whether we would share a room or not, but now it seemed silly to pay for two rooms. We carried what little luggage we had upstairs. From the window in our room I could see Queen Victoria's Arch. I was very happy.

By this time I was ready to sleep for a while, but Nick wanted to be on the go and acclimate to the new time zone right away. It was obvious I needed some cool clothes, so after a shower and underwear change we left the hotel to find a marketplace that sold saris and other warm weather clothes. Marketplaces were everywhere and many stores sold saris. Nick changed some money with the illegal moneychanger in the street. He had been told that was a good idea. I bought two saris, but wasn't able to find one of those little blouses that show the midriff. Anyway, I wasn't ready to show my round, white belly. Finally I found a place that sold T-shirts and bought a couple of white ones to wear with my saris. I bought a pair of sandals that kept falling apart so eventually I just went barefoot. Nick thought that was not a good idea and was sure I would get some sort of worms by going barefoot. I was too tired to care.

Back at the hotel I changed into my sari. I wasn't quite sure how to wrap it, but I felt far more comfortable than I'd been in my winter clothes. We decided to go see the caves on Elephanta Island that was right off the coast. The boat to the island departed from the end of our street. As I sat in the boat, the motion of the sea was so soothing and I nearly fell asleep. I watched tiny women carrying loads of various kinds of goods on their heads down to the boats. They seemed so strong for their size.

When we docked, I bought some bananas and before I knew it a monkey came up and snatched them out of my hand. What a surprise! I wasn't about to fight with a monkey over a banana.

The caves were incredible. There were ancient carvings everywhere on the chalky walls and there were figures of people and columns carved right into the rock. Nick had brought a very large video camera and taped the caves. I acted as his assistant carrying his gear, but at times I wished he had forgotten to bring the camera, it was so heavy.

On our way back, I did fall asleep in the boat. After landing we went directly to the Taj Mahal for dinner. It was delicious and very spicy. I ordered a beer and relaxed even more. Finally as it grew dark we went home to sleep. At last.

Bombay was beautiful and the weather was perfect as it always is in January. We took in museums and gardens and saw a cobra, a dancing monkey, and a Jain Temple. We watched vultures flying above the houses where the dead of the Zoroastrian faith stayed for four days before their remains were kept out on top of tall towers to be picked clean. We ventured deep into the city to Mutton Street where antiques were a real buy. I wondered how we would ever find our way out of there.

Getting around Bombay was a real adventure. The traffic was thick and the noise volume was always high. Everyone was honking, screaming and in a hurry. Cows wandered about in the streets as cars dodged around them and men pulled flat wagons piled high with goods. It was an amazing sight. Sometimes I just closed my eyes and prayed.

After three days, we were notified that our luggage was there. We went back to the international airport and had to go through customs again to pick it up. Finally, we were able to report to the domestic airport for our flight to Delhi. After retrieving our luggage, we spent twelve hours waiting for the fog to clear in Delhi so we could take off. By the end of the day we arrived in the capital of India.

New Delhi was very different from Bombay. While Bombay was full of brightness, thanks to the brilliantly colored clothes people wore and the beautiful weather, Delhi was colder and the colors of clothing muted. I was sorry we hadn't spent more time in Bombay. We decided to take a taxi to a government hotel that our guidebook had suggested was reasonable and comfortable.

The hotel was huge, dark and noisy and everyone seemed impatient. Our room was dreadful. It appeared to be made of disintegrating cement and there were huge blots on the wall. The beds were thin mattresses on a platform. The shower had two faucets, one at shoulder height and one at knee height. There was no pressure in the higher faucet so I found myself on my knees under the lower faucet taking a shower. The towels were about the size of a large washcloth and thin. Oh well, it was cheap. We didn't plan to spend much time in our room anyway. I tried to call home from the phone in the lobby, but the connections were almost non-existent so I gave up. A postcard had to suffice.

We settled in and got on a schedule of sorts. Meditation first thing in the morning, then breakfast, then touring around the town. We found a driver named Bakshi who came for us each day. Sometimes we walked to Connaught Circle where there were hundreds of restaurants and shops.

Nancy, who was a friend of Nick's from Portland, was staying in Delhi for a few days. She was on her way up north to study with a guru in Kulu. She and I had fun together while Nick did his long meditations. (I only meditated for twenty minutes at a time.)

One morning we came upon a temple where girls were painting designs on people's hands and feet with henna. I sat right down and four different girls began to work on me, each taking a different limb. They squeezed henna from a baggie (just like decorating a cake!) and applied it in designs. Such artists. When they were finished, I had to sit in the sun for a half hour for it to dry then the henna was brushed off and I was left with beautiful designs on my palms and feet.

A real highlight of our trip was the Taj Mahal, which was about four hours from Delhi. We took a wild cab ride to get there. The driver passed everyone, narrowly missing oncoming traffic, honking every few seconds. It was truly worth the trip. The Taj Mahal has to be experienced. Words and pictures don't do it justice. As we walked through the entrance, I couldn't speak, I just breathed in the grandeur. Nick felt the same way. He put his arm around me and we walked toward it. The building was truly a work of art, but the feeling it invoked broke my heart right open.

Across the way from the Taj Mahal was the Red Palace where Shah Jahan, the emperor who built it lived. He could gaze out at the Taj where his beloved wife was buried. Now the Red Palace is empty. As our guide described the past, I could imagine what it must have been like when people lived there. There had been piles of jewels in the basement, the Persian carpets covering the marble floors, filmy curtains blowing in the wind, dancing girls and spicy food piled high on huge trays. This was my movie set and I was the decorator, even though it was all in my mind.

Old Delhi is aptly named. The streets are narrow and dark. We walked along smelling the huge baskets of herbs and spices, peeking in windows displaying silver jewelry. We followed a man up a back alley where we were shown into a silk showroom and offered tea. Everyone in India was a salesman.

We decided to go to a famous Ayurvedic healer, Dr. Triguna. His clinic was way out of town. Bakshi took us. We drove past fields, crossed over railroad tracks and finally came to a muddy road at the end of which was a small building. We entered the building, taking Bakshi with us. Once inside we were instructed to sit on a bench. After waiting a short time we were shown into the doctor's office. He took my pulse and dictated his conclusions to a secretary. Then he explained to us what he told her - that my weight was no problem and Nick needed to laugh more. He then sent us to the pharmacy across the way where we bought what he prescribed. The examination was free. We were sure the pills were some form of goat turd. At least that's what they looked like. We bought them anyway and convinced ourselves they would make us healthier.

Each morning when Bakshi, a Sikh, arrived to pick us up in his little three wheel vehicle he had a flower stuck in his turban. One morning his flower was missing. When we asked him why, he explained that he was late and hadn't taken the time to go to the temple. We told him to go and he took us with him. At the entrance we took off our shoes and followed him inside. The temple was beautiful and very peaceful. There were numerous statues and fragrant incense was burning. We knelt in front of a priest who placed a chrysanthemum Mala around our necks and a spot of red on our foreheads. I was taken with the ritual. Outside many devotees were meditating by a large pool with a fountain. It was very appealing to me.

We saw lots of temples on our trip, but many were empty except for a statue or two. I began to wish I'd read more about religion before I came.

One afternoon we went to the library to check something out and were shocked to see the headlines. The Challenger had exploded a few days before. It was strange. Although we were sad, it didn't have the same impact as it would have if we'd been home watching as it happened.

We planned to go up north to Rishikesh where the Maharishi had lived, when the Beatles had gone to see him. Before we left, we found the Blue Triangle YWCA where we were able to store our luggage. We planned to stay there on our return to Delhi.

We bid Bakshi good-by after deciding to take a bus. It was a long trip and we arrived in Rishikesh after dark. Nick hadn't been to the bathroom for the whole trip. He wasn't comfortable going by the side of the road with all the other men. When the bus stopped, he rushed out to take a pee. In the meantime I found a taxi. Nick didn't trust the driver, but he took us to a decent hotel with no problem. We checked in and were served dinner in our room because a big party was taking place downstairs and the place was full. That night we made a new friend of our waiter, Khemlal, whom I still write to these many years later.

The first morning in Rishikesh I woke up and looked out the window to see a sawmill and there were a dozen monkeys roaming around on the roof. In the street below was a water pump where people patiently waited for a cow to finish drinking before getting their own water. Pigs rooted in the ditches along the road.

The first thing Nick wanted to do was go to Maharishi's ashram across the Ganges. He took off on his own. Nick was always restless and kept me moving. I was grateful for the time alone to rest. He found only two caretakers at the ashram. Maharishi was living outside of Delhi working on world peace. Later that day Nick took me there. As we passed by the beach, I saw a leper with no fingers and many beggars. They were the only people I noticed who had any body odor. They didn't have a place to bathe. We gave them money because that is the way it is done.

We climbed up to a cave that had been the home of a saint called Tatwallababa who had been killed outside the cave a few years before. We met his devotee who still watched over the cave and served the sacred space. He told us how he had left home at the age of seven in search of his master. After wandering all through India he had found him here. Now that the master was gone, he watched over the cave. Now that's real devotion. His story brought tears to my eyes. I'd never felt passion like that. I wondered if I ever would.

After we crossed the Ganges again, on our way back to the hotel, we went into a small bookshop and met a man named Kant who offered to take us up a mountain the next day. We met him at six in the morning. I had a cup of chai (tea, sugar, spices, and milk all boiled together) for breakfast. A bus dropped us off at the foot of a four thousand-foot mountain. I barely made it just trudging up the road, lagging behind the two men. It was worth the effort. At the top we could see the Himalayas in the distance. There was a small temple and a woman with silver jewelry all over her body. I learned that some Indian women carry all their wealth on their bodies.

That night Kant invited us to hike to an ashram. I, who seldom exercised, walked seven more miles that evening to the confluence of the Ganges and another river. It was difficult, but I pushed and made it. After a dinner of bread and cheese and talk I found myself trying to sleep on a plywood platform, thankful for my beloved sleeping bag. Sleep did not come easily and I began wondering about myself. What was I doing here with two men? I hardly knew one. Yet the confluence of the two rivers was a powerful place and I felt wonderful and free. I never expected to be doing anything like this at the age of fifty-one. I could hardly walk the next day.

We spent three weeks in Rishikesh with a side trip to Jotermath further north and then returned to Delhi. The Blue Triangle was nice and clean and our room was pretty and finally I was able to call home. The ladies helped me pin my sari so I would look nice when I went out. We found Bakshi again and did some more touring. When we checked on our tickets to Nepal we found they were not good and we couldn't use them. There was a problem with the travel agent who sold them to us. We hurried to American Express to cancel payment then bought new tickets home with a stopover in London.

I was enthralled by my experience in India and imagined spending more time there some day, perhaps in my own little place. But by the time we left I was ready. I longed for peace and quiet, fresh water and toilet paper. I had been warned about the lack of toilet paper so I brought small packs of Kleenex with me, but I'd be glad for the real thing.

The day before we left India, I wanted to have the henna designs put on my hands as it faded after about a week. Bakshi took me to a friend who ran a beauty school. I had a ball. The girls gave me every treatment possible. A facial, hair treatment and shampoo, massage, makeup, manicure, pedicure, and, of course, henna designs on my hands and feet.

That evening, back at the hotel, Nick took one look at me and remarked, "You look like a whore. Let me take a picture." I guess I did. The girls had piled on the makeup. They were having such a great time and I'd given them a free hand. My face was very white and I had a red part in the middle of my hair. But Nick was used to me without makeup and was utterly shocked.

We left for London and once there stayed in a cozy little hotel, all chintz and flowers. Nick had a tiny room next to mine, happy to finally have some privacy. He finally confessed that all during the trip he had been observing me to see if a woman could actually be happy. His mother was always unhappy; perhaps that was why he never married. He had seen me crying or upset once in a while, but underneath it all he realized that I was truly happy. It relieved him to know happy women existed.

We walked around London looking for antiques. Each time we passed an Indian restaurant my stomach turned. I'd had enough Indian food to last a lifetime. I soaked in the wonderful bathtub, drank water from the faucet, and most of all loved having toilet paper right at hand when I needed it.

We returned to Boston in the middle of February. It was snowing. My movie was finished and now it was time to make more changes in my life.

Upon my return, people would ask me if I had any spiritual experiences. What came to mind was my fear of falling off a cliff, hating to look down from high places. I realized I had finally turned that over and let it go during the frightening bus rides in the mountains. If I hadn't, I might have died of a heart attack. I had often thought that nobody in the world knew where we were and if anything had happened to us, I wondered, would anyone ever know about it?

A few years later I discovered that on January 10, 1986, while we were there, some very potent things were happening on an island in Fiji, which were to influence my future. But at the time I had no idea. I began to realize that everything is planted within us and our experiences enable us to bring out what we need in life. India had more influence on me than I realized and as time went by the gifts began to reveal themselves in my life.

Chapter 63
END OF MY DREAM

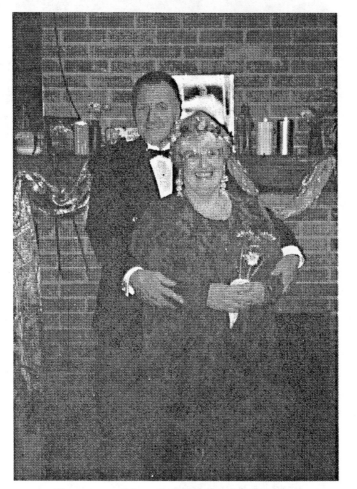

Sugar and her husband, Pat Blymyer

Pat was now sober and loving it. He was on the perennial pink cloud, where people who quit drinking find themselves. They are warned to be careful that it won't last, but for Pat it has lasted for over fifteen years. It was a wonderful home coming for me.

While we had been in India, Nick once asked me how I would feel if when Pat sobered up, he no longer wanted to be in our relationship. Just the thought, the possibility, had brought tears to my eyes and a pain to my heart. Still I realized that whatever made Pat well was the most important thing. I needn't have worried; Pat was overjoyed to see me.

Pat was in such great shape. I was amazed. Everyone was enjoying his recovery. We went to AA meetings at Seabourne where I learned that only a small percentage of people actually stay sober. I believed Pat would be in that small group. He had made some good friends while there and had even done a couple of oil paintings. He was ready and willing to let go of anything in his life that interfered with his recovery and sobriety.

Nick came to live in our unfinished basement. I had decorated the bare cement walls for him with my saris and did my best to make it livable. Nick had been seeing Sheila O'Connell, a psychologist in Maine. He told me that he wanted to learn to understand women. I thought he was a very unusual man to want to do that and I decided that I'd go to see her, too. I realized that it was time to clean up my act, now that Pat was sober. For many years I had distracted myself with work and other things knowing I couldn't stop his drinking. Now that he had, I wanted to be able to be more available for him.

Right after I met Sheila she announced, "This is going to be fun." And it was. She helped me learn to be kinder to myself. When I said I hoped Pat would become more spiritual she said, "Don't ask Pat for anything, just make space in your life for what you want." So I proceeded to do just that. And wouldn't you know it, a couple of weeks later Pat and I had a very spiritual conversation! It worked.

Pat left for location in El Paso to do *Extreme Prejudice* with Nick Nolte. It was the first real test of his sobriety. Nick had drinking problems himself and between Nick and the makeup man they got into a great deal of trouble, thanks to booze. It was instructive for Pat to observe how he'd once been. Pat had been a hero to many men in the business. When he drank, they drank, following his example. Now Pat was sober and things were changing. Many of his friends decided it was time to quit too - or maybe die. One by one they became sober. Unfortunately, some of the men who didn't quit are either no longer able to work, or dead.

Laurie and little Patrick left for California. Nick headed to Fairfield, Iowa to join the Transcendental Meditation settlement out there. They had a university and Nick had decided to open his practice there.

I decided it was time to hire assistant innkeepers so I could be with Pat more often. I put an ad in the paper and two people, recovering alcoholics, who went to AA, applied. I hired them assuming they were wonderful like Pat. What a mistake!

Pam and John arrived and proceeded to drive me - and everyone else - crazy. John was so lazy. He'd see me carry things never offering to help. Pam was a snob, talking to our guests behind our backs about how badly the place was run. Jane, my assistant, had problems with them, the cook hated them. Jane and I went to see Sheila and we talked the whole hour about our awful innkeepers. Finally, Sheila said she was going to come to the inn and fire them herself if I didn't. In fact, she eventually found me a woman who ended up taking their place.

I found the courage to fire them after July 4. Every year on the Fourth, we had a traditional Lobster Bake, served outside, if it was a nice day. I had made a list detailing everything that had to be done and ordered, including the seaweed, the lobsters, clams, corn, and potatoes. The morning of the big day, I came over to the inn to find the cook chopping wood. I was stunned. Cutting the wood was John's job, but he didn't see it that way. I had asked John to get the big metal barrel with legs in which we cooked the lobsters. He couldn't find the legs so I used some from a metal table. While setting the barrel up over the logs I noticed there were holes in it so I lined it with foil. I layered in the food. Seaweed on the bottom followed by the potatoes, then the lobsters and corn. Finally, clams were piled on top. In no time, the fire was nice and hot - but quickly the table legs melted and collapsed spilling food everywhere. The poor lobsters were still alive and they started crawling all over the lawn. The only thing I could say was, "Shit". One of the guests heard me and laughed, then he came to help gather up the lobsters. I gave up on legs and just set the barrel right on the rocks that surrounded the fire. It almost worked, but because of the holes, juice kept leaking out, threatening to douse the fire. I sat there most of the day with a hair dryer acting as a bellows to keep the fire going.

Finally, the food was done. By this time, I was exhausted and wreaked of fish and smoke. John and Pam appeared, looking very fresh and clean. I didn't dare react, I was so very angry and I said, "You handle this, I'm going home." I walked across the road to my house and took a shower. Then I sat down with a pint of Ben and Jerry's Toffee ice cream to comfort myself. I didn't go back to the inn that night. John and Pam were fired soon after. The rest of the help was overjoyed.

Shortly after this incident, my cook fell ill so I had to become the cook, which didn't thrill me. Cooking didn't leave me enough time to be a good innkeeper, but I had no choice. It was the middle of summer and all the cooks in the valley were working. It was hard to get other reliable help, too. The outlet stores had come to town and hired the women who previously would have been working at the inns. It was a difficult time. When Pat would call, I'd cry to him about all the troubles I was having and he'd ask, "Are you ready to sell? It doesn't sound like much fun to me."

That spring I had attended a seminar for innkeepers. Bill, the facilitator, said that anyone who had intentions of selling their inn should call him and he'd come and talk to them. So I did. He came and stayed for a couple of days to see what could be done. His take was that I was great as an innkeeper, but he could tell I wasn't interested in making the kind of cost-cutting changes that would make our business profitable. He also felt my clientele was too mixed. He thought innkeepers needed to specialize in a certain kind of client in order to make it. It was definitely time to sell.

I didn't like what he had to say, but I knew he was right. We'd been struggling for eight and a half years to make it work. The kids were on their own now, Pat didn't want to be an innkeeper and I couldn't get help. I told Bill to find us a buyer. By the end of the year, new owners took over.

While they were moving in, Trudy, the new innkeeper asked me if leaving the inn upset me. I honestly told her "No, not at all." I had let it go and had no regrets. She invited me over for New Year's Eve, but I thanked her saying I had waited all these years to go to sleep early on New Year's Eve.

The next spring when I saw the food trucks pull up, I was so relieved to know that I didn't have to unload them or worry about how to pay for all the food. We were great innkeepers and had made many people happy. Now, as Max told us when we were looking to buy an inn, it was time to close the Chapter and tie it up with little silk ribbons.

1987 arrived and I felt freer than I had ever been in my life. My kids were grown and living their own lives. We had some money from the sale of our inn and our finances were in good shape. I decided it was time to launch my writing career. I was ready to be serious about it. The first thing I did was order a Macintosh computer. Next, I signed up for a Proprioceptive Writing Weekend in Portland, Maine. I reserved a room at the Marriott Hotel a couple of blocks from where the class was held. As I checked into my room, I began experiencing my freedom for the first time. I unpacked, called room service and ordered my favorites, a glass of white wine and a dozen raw oysters. I indulged myself all weekend - a gift I deserved.

Proprioceptive Writing Classes taught by Toby Simon and Linda Trichter-Metcalf were unlike any writing class I'd ever taken. We lit a candle and listened to Baroque music and wrote whatever came to mind. I was utterly surprised at what came up as I wrote. The last instruction we received before heading home on Sunday was to light a candle, listen to classical music, and write each day.

Winter weather was pleasant and I enjoyed my freedom, but I found it hard to relax. I'd start to take it easy, then I'd lapse into "martyr mode" because I was so used to doing something every minute. I stacked wood when my body told me to relax. I was burned out, but didn't want to give in to it. At one point I fell on the ice and hurt my knee. That made me sit still for a while anyway.

Pat was getting itchy. He could only take winter for so long. Matt Leonetti, his cameraman, called and offered him a job on *No Secrets*, a movie of the week. It was to be filmed on Catalina Island and they offered me the job of hairdresser. I was still weary, but it sounded like fun. Besides I'd get to see Laurie and Little Pat. Tanya and Brittany decided to come, too. Xochi quit her job in Boston and came too. The family was going to be united again.

Xochi had finished college and had been working at the Better Business Bureau in Boston running their computer room. She was bored. She realized that she wanted to be in the movie business. Her father Bill still owed back child support and I had put a lean on the house he owned

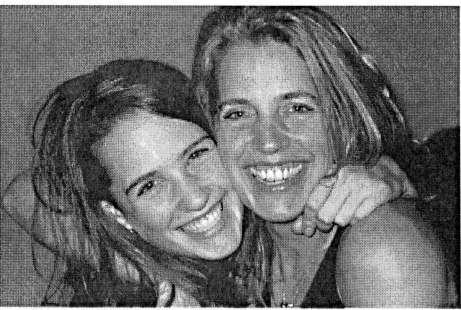

Sugar's daughter Tanya (right) and granddaughter Brittany

in Palm Springs. He decided to sell it and called asking what I wanted to remove the lean. I suggested he pay off Xochi's college loan and he agreed. With her bills paid, Xochi was free to try something new. She gave her notice and Pat hired her as a stand-in for the movie.

We all arrived in California and piled into Laurie's apartment in Huntington Beach. It felt so good to be together again. I wasn't very peppy, but that was okay. Off we sailed to Catalina. Catalina in March was perfect. The weather was lovely, there were virtually no tourists, and it was so pretty with the springtime flowers in bloom.

We had two rooms in a lovely pink hotel. There was a Jacuzzi bath in our room. Pat and I stayed in one room, the kids stayed in the other. Looking back, I realize I shouldn't have tried to work. I was still suffering from burnout and my leg hurt so badly I limped. To top it off, the first day I got sunburned and suffered with sun poisoning for the next three weeks. I wondered if I'd ever get through it.

I met River Phoenix's family because his brother, Joaquin (Leaf at the time) Phoenix, was working with us. Kellie Martin was our female star. She was a great little actress and her career went up from there. She continues to work in television and has grown into a lovely person.

I adored the Phoenix family. River's mother told me how she had grown up in a family where everything seemed to go drastically wrong and so had her husband. They finally decided to disown their lives, walk to a different tune and build a new life apart from their families. They took new names and lived like vegan gypsies. They had several children and River's success meant a lot to them. They loved their children so much, trying to give them the best life tools they could. I followed River's career from then on.

Sadly, River died so young and under circumstances that didn't have to be. I couldn't understand why and I am still sad. I wrote a poem to his family, which I never did send. All I could think about was how his parents had done everything within their power to keep their children from the family history, but it seemed there was no way River could escape it. It's hard to understand.

FOR RIVER PHOENIX

It's all bullshit.
You can't run away from karma.
Your parents tried so hard,
changing names,
changing places
instilling decent values,
respect for life,
love,
Family together.
You had talent, beauty,
fame, something to do.
But karma got you anyway,
and who knows why.
Your family, who loved you
tried to keep it away
But it caught up with you anyway
so soon at twenty-three.
I cried when I heard the news.
Although I'd never met you
I felt as if I had through your family.
What was it you had to learn?
What was it you needed to know?
What was it God took you from
before it became too much?
The universe unfolds as it should,
everything is absolutely correct in
the big picture.
Yet for us, still left here in the middle
it seems like such a waste.
Damn it.

After finishing the film, we traveled to Guaymas, Mexico where my 78-year-old half brother, John Zuckerman, spent his vacations in a fabulous home. I hadn't seen him in almost thirty-five years. He surprised me, greeting us at the airport accompanied by Cecilia, his seventh wife. We stayed at his place that was situated on the highest hill in the area, in our own guesthouse. We sailed across the bay in his beautiful boat and ate the delicious food he cooked in the evenings. Listening to him was a wonderful experience. He talked about life with my father. I could see so much of Daddy in him.

Chapter 64

THE PRESIDIO
Fall, 1988

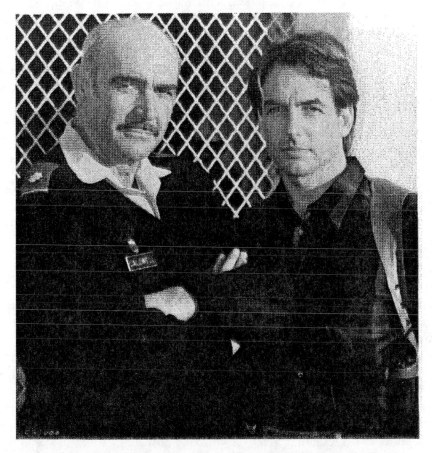

Sean Connery and Mark Harmon, *The Presidio*

In the fall of 1988, I got a call from Peter Hyams's office to do a film called *The Presidio*. It starred my all time favorite, Sean Connery along with Meg Ryan, Mark Harmon, and Jack Warden. What a great cast! I could hardly wait.

The Presidio was a story of an army officer (Sean), his daughter (Meg), and a policeman (Mark) and the many problems between them. Much of the shoot was going to take place on *The Presidio*, the army base in San Francisco, one of the loveliest places in the area.

Pat was now working often in Los Angeles and he had found his "dream" cottage, a little place to stay when he was there. It was really tiny - fine for one, crowded for two - but it didn't cost much and he could afford to keep it year round so now there was always a place for us to go.

At first I was told to fly into Los Angeles and then we'd fly to San Francisco a couple of days later. Next I received a call telling me to report straight to San Francisco, which was fine with me. At that time Pat was in Chicago working on *Red Heat* with Xochi, who was now a production assistant. There was really no need for me to go to Los

Angeles and upon my arrival in San Francisco I found out that a good-sized earthquake had occurred in Los Angeles that very day. Oh my God! The angels must have been watching out for me.

I was picked up at the airport by a driver with a sign that said "Sugar" and taken to the Holiday Inn at Fisherman's Wharf. I checked in and then reported to the Production office. Peter Hyams - my friend the director - was sitting on the floor sorting papers. He got up and gave me a big hug. I have a great fondness for Peter. I always felt rewarded when I worked with him on a film. He infuses me with enthusiasm by appreciating all I do for him.

Next, I was introduced to our producer, Dino Conte, an Italian guy and a real character. Alan, the first assistant, shook my hand and another assistant handed me a script. Peter described how he pictured Meg Ryan and a few minutes later Dino put forth his ideas. They were not in accord and I was confused. The director wanted a sweet Goldie Hawn-look while the producer wanted Kim Basinger. I wondered how I was going to please them both. Personally I leaned in Peter's direction.

It turned out not to be a problem, mainly thanks to Meg Ryan, the goddess herself. What a great lady. How cute she was, a tiny woman with thick, shoulder-length, blonde hair, bright blue eyes and a darling little face. She was dressed in the baggy clothes that became her trademark, a style that would later land her awards for the worst dressed.

She stepped into our trailer and announced, "I'm ready for the Goddess to appear." It was very funny. She knew that out of this little character she presented to us we could create something wonderful for the screen. I told her what Peter and Dino had said and asked if I could just work with her hair a little bit. Ideas never come clearly to me right off, but once I put my fingers in a person's hair my creativity comes to life. Sometimes I've had an idea of what I wanted to do, especially if I was working on a period picture and I'd done research, but I still had to have my hands in the hair before I'd know for sure.

Thinking of what Peter and Dino wanted, I closed my eyes and said a prayer to myself, "Please, dear God, work through me." Then I relaxed and began to work. I remembered the technique I used for the hairstyle on *Songwriter*. I took a small iron, heated it up, and began to crimp Meg's hair, back and forth, strand by strand, in small sections. It took a lot of time, but in the end it was perfect. It looked permed, but more attractive. After Steve Abrums did her makeup, we presented her to Peter. Success! He loved her look and so did Dino. To brag a bit about myself, I think that was the best her hair ever looked for years.

My next job was to meet with Sean Connery about his hair. As the production manager drove me downtown to Sean's hotel, I sensed his nervousness. I wasn't worried because I had known Sean from *Meteor*. We knocked on his door and he opened it. A few people were just leaving. I shook Sean's hand saying, "We worked together on *Meteor*. He seemed to remember. We talked and I saw that Sean needed a haircut because he was playing a military man and needed to look very neat. He wasn't wearing his hairpiece in the film. He didn't need it anyway; he was beautiful as he was.

The production manager, relieved to see I was at ease and capable of handling the situation, left. I was alone in the hotel room with Sean - a place that probably millions of women dream to be. We went into the bedroom where Sean had set up a place for me to cut his hair. Then he excused himself to change his clothes so as not to get hair all over himself. He came out of the bathroom wearing nothing, but a towel.

As I began to cut his hair, he said "Not too short, especially in the back." As always, I was a little nervous at first. I wanted everything to be perfect. I kept trying to get it a little shorter and cleaner in the back, but he insisted it wasn't necessary. He said I could keep after it on the set. So that's the way it was. I wasn't about to argue. He asked me to trim his mustache a little while I was at it. Of course I didn't say no. I loved listening to Sean's Scottish brogue and enjoyed the afternoon with him. I was laughing to myself thinking how lucky I was to spend time with him wrapped only in a towel. I don't think he thought anything about it. He is not a modest man and it was natural to him. I like that in a man.

Next was Mark Harmon. Now how could one improve on that perfect face? I gave him a trim and found him to be polite and considerate. I felt this film was going to be very enjoyable.

Brad Wilder was our other makeup artist. It was interesting to see the contrast between him and Steve Abrums's. Brad was a very attractive, sensitive man. I've always been sure he had been a prince in a former life. Steve on the other hand was a strong, muscular man who wore starched white shirts and stood ramrod straight. He was quiet and liked doing his makeup by the numbers. He enjoyed my conversations with Sean (unlike most makeup people who don't appreciate someone chatting with the actor they're working on) because then he didn't need to make conversation and could concentrate on doing the makeup. He did an excellent job, turning Meg into the

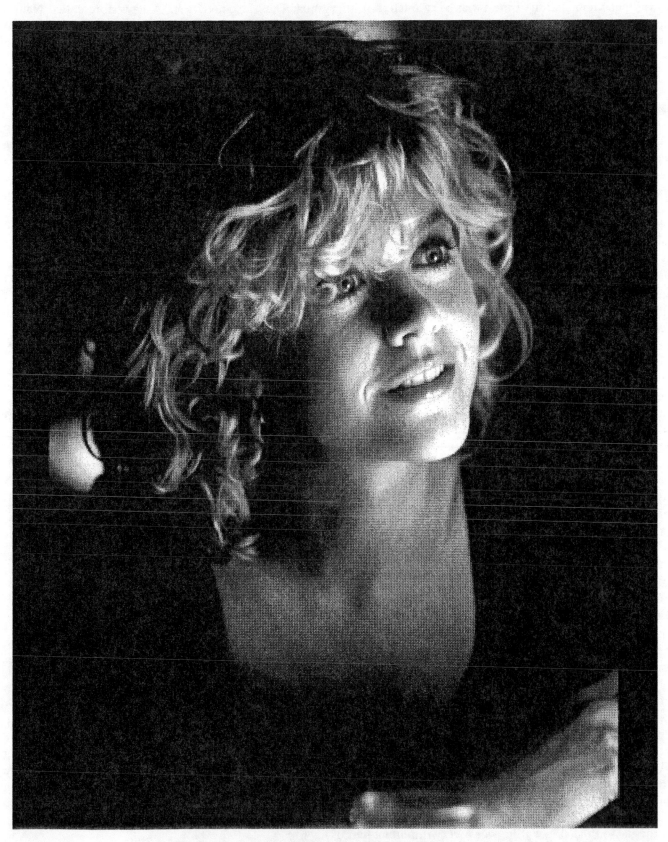

Meg Ryan, *The Presidio*

Goddess and shadowing Sean's face so it was even more attractive.

Fisherman's Wharf was a perfect location for our hotel. There were so many places within walking distance to spend my per diem. At this time I was very interested in crystals. They fascinated me. A new store called Nature Company had opened in Ghiradelli Square and I'd walk over there and buy beautiful crystals, some of which I gave to the crew. I also bought books to read about their powers. Peter was trying to quit smoking and I gave him an amethyst and a rose quartz. He laughed at that. He didn't really believe in that stuff, but took it anyway. He later said, "Stay away from my family Sugar, they could go your way and I wouldn't like that."

The Presidio was a fabulous place to work, so beautiful and elegant. Being in the army must have been okay if you were an officer stationed there.

One afternoon we were shooting a scene where Meg walked out of an office building. The crew had been told to stay inside. It was crowded in the hallway. I leaned back against the wall to get out of someone's way and all of a sudden the fire alarm went off. I had goofed! Big! All the bells were going off and the whole building began to empty I was so embarrassed. I wanted to disappear. It took over an hour for the firemen to make sure there really wasn't a fire and for everyone to get settled. I confessed to my sin to Peter even though I wanted to forget about it. He laughed, not mad at all. Now whenever I lean against a wall, I always look carefully for an alarm.

On Veterans Day, the Navy came to town. It happened every year, but I had never seen anything like it before. From where we were shooting we could see huge ships and aircraft carriers sailing into the harbor. We even staged some shots with them in the background.

Most impressive were the Blue Angels in their planes. Being the Navy, they wanted to show up the Army. I have always loved those daredevils in their fast, little jets. They buzzed us time and time again with their crazy antics. I was thrilled right down to the pit of my stomach. Later the pilots came to visit the set and I was surprised to see that they looked like ordinary guys. Not a Tom Cruise in the bunch.

In the movie Jack Warden died. His funeral was filmed in the graveyard where soldiers had been buried for more than two hundred years. While they were setting up the funeral scene, I wandered around. Many of the graves were for men, boys really, only sixteen-years-old - so very young.

The funeral scene was heart wrenching. Each time Taps played I cried. It was only a movie, I knew that, but I couldn't help it, the scene was so moving.

We flew back to Los Angeles to begin the stage work at Paramount. It was fun to be back at my favorite studio, the one where I had grown up. It had changed and I hardly knew anyone.

Sean hadn't let me cut his hair short enough in the back, so before each shot I had to comb it carefully so it wouldn't hit his collar and look too long. He was very patient. I think he enjoyed the attention. He was a real pro - more so than any other actor

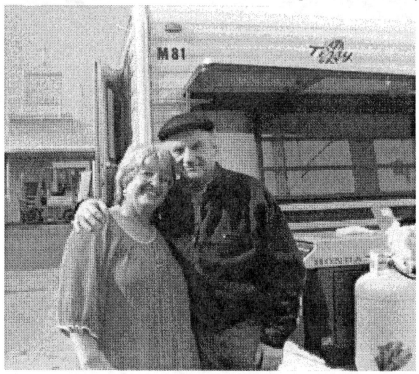

Sugar with Jack Warden, *The Presidio*

I've worked with. He allowed people to do their job even if that meant disturbing his concentration at times.

Sean loved to talk about nearly anything and I loved to listen to him. He told us about his adventures being Bond and described how he decided to quit when someone in Japan crawled under a toilet stall door to get a look at him. He confessed he wasn't nearly as brave as Bond. His wife, Michelene, was far braver. She was just a little bit of a thing, but powerful. One time in the Bahamas, he was doing a diving scene and wasn't enjoying it at all. Suddenly, his wife appeared in the water, not a bit fearful. He told us how he loved to sit in the ski lodge enjoying the warm fire while she spent the day on the slopes. She was a very important part of his life.

He described his childhood days in Scotland telling us about how his family had been poor and how he felt when his siblings arrived. We asked him questions about everything, but he said he didn't like to remember the past. However, Michelene was putting together a scrapbook about him. She actually knew more about his life than he did. I felt privileged to have this time with him.

In one conversation, Sean said he didn't like playing golf with women. I figured that was okay. He should be able to play with whomever he wanted. This was around the time of the interview with Barbara Walters in which he expressed his opinion about playing golf with women. During the interview, he had made a remark about hitting a woman that was taken the wrong way. The next day, everyone who knew him was appalled about the interview. We knew his remark had been misinterpreted. He would never hit a woman. That afternoon, I was walking to the commissary for lunch and he caught up with me. He had gone to the golf club that morning wondering how the women would receive him. He found that they seemed to actually respect him more. In reality, Sean wasn't concerned about anyone's opinion. He is a very secure person.

One day, Mark Harmon asked me to shave his back because it was too hairy. He was going to do a bedroom scene with Meg and was concerned about how he would look. At the appointed time, he came into the trailer and took off his shirt. I got my clippers and began to clean the hair off his back. We took it off up to his shoulders and he did look more attractive.

Sean was in the trailer getting his makeup done at the same time. A few days later he asked, "Sugar, do you think you could thin out the hair on my chest? I get so hot." "Sure," I replied, "I'll be glad to try. I've never done anything quite like it before; except for the time I shaved my father's chest so he wouldn't see his gray hairs." We set a time for the next day.

He walked in wearing the Snowvillage Inn kimono I had given him after he mentioned that he loved light cotton robes. He took off the kimono and sat there in his jade-green silk shorts. Once again, I had to laugh at the funny situations I found myself in. I began to clip the hair on his glorious chest, being very careful not to take too much off. We worked together. I'd clip and then comb his chest. He'd look in the mirror and then "Take a little more off." Finally, he was quite satisfied. That was a once in a lifetime experience. That and dyeing Redford's eyelashes were the two extraordinary experiences in my movie career.

At the time, Meg was going with Dennis Quaid. She was concerned about his drinking and we discussed it often. I shared my experiences with Pat, how I had felt about his drinking and my joy when he quit. Dennis, as she described him, was a lovely, wild character, but she had reservations about spending a lifetime with him because of his drinking.

At Christmas, Meg's mother came to visit her. Meg was shocked. Her mother had had all sorts of plastic surgery done since the last time Meg had seen her and no longer looked like the mother she knew. Meg was appalled. It seemed to me that Meg was taking care of her inner life and working toward wholeness while her mother was dedicated to her outer life and staying young. It was hard to believe they belonged to the same family. I felt for Meg and told her if she ever needed a mother figure, she should give me a call and I'd come and give her a big hug.

Much of the same crew that worked on *Running Scared* was working on this film, too. Even though they had heard that I had gone to India, not one of them ever asked me about my trip. Once in a while someone would say, "Oh Sugar, tell so and so about your trip to India," but not one of them showed any interest. One day we were standing around, waiting for a shot when it dawned on me that they had done this on purpose. I decided to let them know I had caught on and was not amused. "I get it now, you rotten people." I raised my voice. "You made a pact didn't you, to not ask me about India?" They all stared at me with a blank look on their faces then they slyly smiled. I figured it was their loss.

Christmas arrived and I decorated our trailer. Peter Hyams came in and said he felt most at home in my trailer. We had an espresso machine and other home comforts. But whenever Sean wanted an espresso, I had a difficult time making the milk foam. He once told me that only men could do that well.

For Christmas I gave Sean a card that said, "Few things are better than Christmas," and then added "But you are." He was touched.

The last scene took place in a factory where they bottled water. The set was about a foot deep with water and we all wore high rubber boots. That day I wore a skirt that was above the waterline and panty hose. Unbeknownst to me, Sean sneaked up behind me and began running his hand up my leg. I couldn't feel his hand at first because of the panty hose. When I finally felt his hand, I jumped. He laughed and remarked, "She didn't even tell me to stop." I didn't want him to know I hadn't felt his hand, so I retorted, "I didn't want you to." He got a kick out of it.

That last day I was in tears knowing he was leaving and I might never see him again. He was and is my favorite. He gave me his address in Spain and told me to visit if I was ever there. I think he really meant it.

We returned to San Francisco in January at the end of the first unit shooting to do a second unit, which consisted of lots of car chases and wrecks. It was like a gift to the crew. We worked nights and the weather was mild. I got all dressed up in my warm clothes and walked the streets, imagining myself to be a well-dressed bag lady. I scouted out likely places to sleep knowing in reality I had a warm hotel room to return to. Yet it was instructive to imagine how it might be.

The last two weeks passed quickly. Brad and I had a delicious French dinner on the last night to celebrate the wrap. The last day was my anniversary and to my surprise when I returned to the hotel, a huge, elegant flower arrangement in a lovely vase awaited me. It was a real surprise because Pat was in Budapest working on *Red Heat*. He had arranged with Laurie to send them before he left. I carried the flowers home with me on the plane the next day.

Chapter 65

TURNER & HOOCH
Spring, 1989

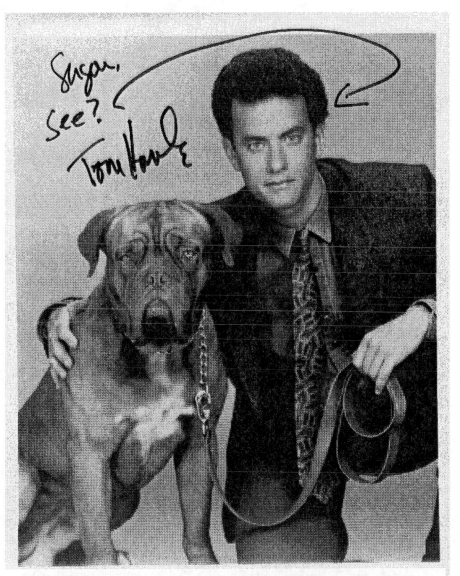

Sugar,
See?

Tom Hanks

Tom Hanks (with a comment on his hairstyle) and Hooch,
Turner & Hooch

The Presidio finished in the spring of 1989 and I decided to stay on in Los Angeles to be with Pat who was there working on *Johnny Handsome,* a film about a deformed petty criminal being transformed by surgery. It starred Mickey Rourke, Ellen Barkin, Elizabeth McGovern, Morgan Freeman, and Forrest Whitaker. Walter Hill was directing and working on his films was always fun. Xochi was a production assistant on it.

I thought working with Ellen Barkin and Mickey Rourke would be really difficult for makeup and hair. They were something else, quite a pair. Nevertheless when I got a call to be Mickey's hairstylist on one of the makeup tests, I went. Mickey's makeup was difficult. His hair was not the important thing in this test. I was sort of nervous. I didn't fit in with his crew and it was very apparent. Mickey was patient and kind, and although he had another hairdresser from "the outside", I was not asked to leave. Still, I did very little. I didn't get the job, which I later discovered was a good thing. A friend, Donna Turner, ended up working with Mickey and he drove her crazy. He was impossible, lying on the counter at times, while she tried to do his hair. She was often near to tears.

Ellen Barkin was a real piece of work, too. Peter Tothpal, who usually did Arnold Schwarzenegger, did her hair. Suddenly Peter's mother fell ill and he was called to go home to Europe. He asked if I could cover him for a week. I was available and therefore happy to do it. Xochi was working on the film and Ellen liked her. Xochi told Ellen to be good to me and not make me cry. Ellen turned out to be great.

I loved working on Elizabeth McGovern. She was so lovely, sweet, and genuine. One day she was playing in a difficult scene. She had psyched herself up for it, getting emotional and was ready to shoot. All of a sudden the cameraman and his crew stopped and began talking about technical stuff breaking Elizabeth's concentration completely. That lovely woman got very angry and upset. The crew was dumbfounded. They couldn't understand where she was coming from. I wondered how the crew could be so insensitive. I think they sometimes forgot about the actors.

Years ago someone told me, "Actors are different from us. Their emotions are right at the top of their heads,

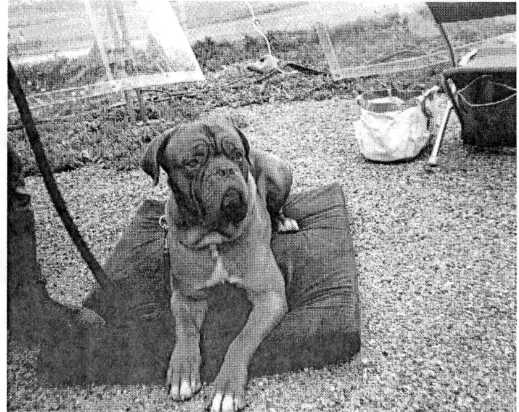

Hooch at rest

so they are capable of pulling them out at will. Ours are buried much deeper. We cannot act."

Personally, I've noticed that actors can be like children in many ways and sometimes need to be treated as such. Of course, it has to be done in a subtle way. I felt I had a talent for it. Being able to act is a gift, but it doesn't make it easy to get on in the real world. Sure, I'd get fed up at times when an actor became ridiculous in their demands, but people who did not understand where actors were coming from caused the most problems.

I was still working on *Johnny Handsome* when I got a call from Disney. Danny Streipecke was about to start filming *Turner & Hooch* and they needed a hair-stylist immediately. Something had happened with Danny's usual hairstylist and all of a sudden they were in a bind. Another hairstylist recommended me. I was uncomfortable about replacing a friend (as always) so I went and talked with Danny about it. I'd known him for years although we had never worked together. He convinced me that he was fine with it, so I took the job. The film starred Tom Hanks, Mare Winningham, Reggie VelJohnson, Craig T. Nelson, and Hooch, otherwise known as Beasley. Mare played a veterinarian with whom Tom Hanks, a cop, meets and falls in love while she cares for Hooch.

The producers had already decided the look they wanted for Mare - actually the producers' wives had decided - and Mare wasn't too pleased with their choices. At the time she had five children and was nursing the youngest while we were shooting. She reminded me of hippies I'd known and I liked that. Mare is an amazing, independent woman. She didn't like any artificiality and was not pleased with the changes they wanted her to make. I was told to take her to the hairstylist that the wives had picked to have her hair streaked. Her hair was so heavy and lank. It did need livening up, but they put a hair product called "mud" on it that it took all the life out of it. It looked dull and dead.

I had never met Tom Hanks before, but he and Danny had worked together for many years. I observed as Danny showed me how Tom liked his hair. Tom had a quick, funny sense of humor. When he first met me, he kept to himself, but as soon he realized he could trust me he opened up. When he left our trailer for the set he tended to put on a different face and used his humor to keep people at a distance. I valued the time in the makeup room with him.

Last, but not least was Hooch, a French Briard with short, beige fur who reminded me of a boxer, but different. His trainer was Clint Rowe, Disney's pet. Clint did most of their animal films. The first time I saw him I had this vision of a clean cut, lovely man who had just come strolling out of the hills of Scotland. Boy was I wrong. Clint was a complicated human being. He cared so much for his dogs that he took it personally when they were treated like animals. He considered them just as important as the other actors, and he was right.

I loved animals so Clint and I became immediate friends. He had two assistants, Madeline and his brother Scott. Actually there were three Hooches, each with a different talent, but Beasley was the main star. I loved watching Clint train Beasley to drag himself across the lawn, rehearsing for the scene where he gets shot. His acting was so convincing that it brought me to tears.

Henry Winkler was our director, a charming person. He brought in delicious pastries for everyone and smelled so good when he gave me a hug each morning. The trouble was that he didn't seem to be able to direct. In his defense, he never had a chance. It was direction by committee. A group of producers, from Disney, were always looking over his shoulder. It was an impossible situation, yet comical too. I remember the first shots at an old, white farmhouse in Pasadena, the vet's office. There was a monitor so we could watch a scene when there was no room for us on the set, or in case the director wanted to see the scene played back. The monitor was set up out in the orange grove. Four producers sat there in directors' chairs watching the scene being filmed. There was no way we could see anything. After each scene they drew Henry aside and discussed everything with him. The script had been rewritten numerous times and the latest writer was on the set in case they wanted to make changes. It was very strange.

Later, I found out that Mare's wardrobe had even been picked by committee - one that included the wives. Their choices weren't appropriate for Mare at all. I wondered about working at Disney. It wasn't like the old days.

We put our heart and soul into the first two weeks, work. The days were grueling with long hours plus the drive out to Pasadena every day. Things were not going well. Tom was distraught. He'd come into the trailer and described Henry's direction. For instance, as Tom walked into a scene where Hooch is dying. "Crisp as an apple," was Henry's direction. Frustrated, Tom moaned, "Now what in the hell does that mean?" He had just gotten great reviews for *Punchline*, now he was picturing his career going right down the tubes.

Mare felt the same way, uneasy in her part by now. She had gotten the part because Tom admired her acting and insisted on her being in the film. Disney agreed to Tom's demand, but Mare wasn't the usual run of the mill bimbo actress Disney execs were used to dealing with. They didn't know how to treat her so they avoided her.

Even Clint was at his wit's end. One time he came to me nearly in tears, upset at the way things were going. All the actors were depressed and nobody knew what was going to happen except that it couldn't continue. I'd never seen this happen on a film. The actors, whose faces were seen on the screen, felt totally helpless.

Finally, the executives got the message. They gave us a week off while they regrouped. The first thing they did was replace Henry. I was sorry because I liked him. Rodger Spottiswoode was hired to take his place and suddenly the film took on a new life. We resumed filming at an entirely different point in the film - the beginning, and Mare was put on hold.

We shot in San Pedro at a grungy area with a pier and some moorings. The drive home was so long and the San Diego freeway so hectic at all hours, that I decided to stay down there. We had to work six days a week to make up for the delay. The film was already booked into the movie houses by a certain date. I found a small, cheap motel to stay at. I bought a pretty quilt for the bed, and decorated my room so it looked attractive. I hung some black cloth I'd gotten from the grips on the windows so I could sleep during the day when we worked nights. Once Pat came to visit, but he finally decided that it wasn't worth the long drive down there, just to watch me sleep.

In our first scene, Hooch needed to look dirty and scraggly, a real junk yard dog. He lived with an old man on the pier played by John McIntyre. We all knew John because he'd been in films for years. His wife, Jeanette Nolan, was a wonderful actress, too. She was on the set all the time to make sure he was okay. John was very fragile and she took good care of him.

Making Hooch look dirty was no easy job. Clint brought him in so we could experiment. Hooch seemed to have self-cleaning fur; it was so difficult to get anything to stick to it. Eventually we found a non-toxic solution and he began to look somewhat filthy. Hooch was patient with us all through our experiments.

One afternoon, while we were shooting, a boat pulled up at our pier and a familiar face appeared. It was Paul Lohman, the cameraman from *Meteor*. He lived on the boat docked out in the harbor beyond the set. It was just like him to be so unconventional. He invited us to visit. Next door to us they were shooting *The Abyss* in a huge hanger with a gigantic tank built inside. Never had I imagined San Pedro would be such a busy place.

Rodger Spottiswoode brought new life and creativity to the film. For example, he had the cameraman use the steady cam (the camera they use to follow people so they can film from the person's point of view) down low so they could film from a dog's point of view. That way people could see what the dog saw. When I saw the movie, I realized what a good idea it was.

Clint had the dogs doing remarkable things. The greatest trick was drooling. In reality, the dogs didn't drool as much as it appeared in the film. Clint gave them meat to increase their drooling. When his dogs did well and it was time to stop he would gently tell them, "That'll do," and they stopped. He never shouted.

Tom Hanks was having a wonderful time. I had brought in Angel Cards that have sayings like Love, Think, Meditate, etc. on each card. We picked one for the day to give us a theme. Tom loved it. While Danny applied his makeup Tom told us how his career got started, about his first marriage, and how much he loved and missed his kids. They had moved north and he saw them as often as he could.

Tom was so happy in his marriage to actress Rita Wilson. Her energy, liveliness, and outgoing personality attracted him. At heart Tom is a simple and quiet soul, although intelligent and clever. Rita balanced him. He hoped to have children with her and was waiting for her to take time off from her career, which she eventually did.

Mare and her way of life fascinated Tom. He liked how she handled her family, which included five children, with such ease. She also had a band. Tom didn't like the way Disney's executives treated her. They had put her on hold until the end of the film and, in fact, had someone else waiting in the wings. Still, Tom insisted Mare be his co-star.

Reggie, now of *Family Matters* fame, played Tom's sidekick. What a lovable, good-humored man. One morning Reggie arrived all flustered and upset. He had made a stupid mistake and almost gotten in trouble with the law. He was so upset, but most of all he was worried his mother would find out, which I thought was remarkable. The problem was resolved and I felt he learned a lesson for his future. He had just been signed to do a pilot for *Family Matters* that turned out to be a great success.

During the filming, Tom gave the crew a remarkable gift. He hired a masseuse, Diane, to come to the set three days a week to massage the crew. We could sit in her special chair to get our shoulders rubbed. Sometimes she would give a whole body massage in our trailer. We all appreciated his gift.

Danny Streipecke and I often talked together. Once he had produced a film called *SST*, about a snake. He told me about his efforts to make a living in other ways, too, but he always came back to being a makeup artist. He advised me not to write until I was more than sixty because the money we made in films far surpassed what I could earn as a writer. It worked out that way for me in the end.

Danny wasn't used to anyone so spiritually inclined and I'm sure he often thought I was a flake. Tom, on the other hand, became interested. He asked me to bring him reading material to acquaint him with my beliefs. I chose *Science of Mind*. I don't know if he ever read it, but one day while we were working in Monterey, he came in with the front page of the paper that had a photo of a rainbow. Pointing to the end of the rainbow he said, "That must be where you live."

A couple of months later when we came back for retakes, he told me a funny story. He and Rita were vacationing in the Caribbean. A sudden storm came up while they were sitting on the beach. When the storm was over, they saw a rainbow on the island across the way. He told Rita, "I know Sugar is over there watching us."

Working on this film was fun and I loved going to work each day. There were fights with doubles falling off the pier into the water and lots of action. The dogs performed wonderfully, but Clint would often get upset because production insisted on treating them like dogs instead of actors. In reality, Clint was the actor, but people generally didn't see it that way. Clint didn't appreciate the second-class treatment and often threatened to quit the business.

Hooch was supposed to fall in love. They had originally chosen a dog Rodger didn't approve of. Clint brought in the most wonderful dog of all - his favorite - Mike of *Down and Out in Beverly Hills* fame. What a perfect dog/person. He was wonderful. I had to spray him black for a test and he stood there so calm and patient for me. I fell in love. Mike didn't work out, though, and Hooch eventually fell in love with a dainty collie.

Finally, Mare came back for the last ten days of the film. She was angry because Disney had denied her the opportunity to do a prime part in the television film *Roe vs. Wade* even though there had been plenty of time for it while she waited to finish our film.

I notified Production that I wanted time to work with Mare's hair. I wanted it to look right this time. The costumer also insisted on time to dress her properly. When we finished with our work, everyone was delighted. We all agreed that production hadn't been fair to her earlier. In my opinion, the biggest disgrace was that the executives had never taken the time to meet Mare face to face. In fact, when she expressed her dissatisfaction at how she had been treated their response was basically, "Don't be a hard nose about it. It isn't important." It underscored the fact that actors have to look out for themselves because nobody else will. Both Tom and Mare learned a lot on this film.

The best part was saved for last. We went on location to Monterey and Carmel where I'd worked years before on *Soldier in the Rain*. We stayed in a lovely motel. Most of our locations were on the beach, but we also filmed a dog show, and had a day at the aquarium.

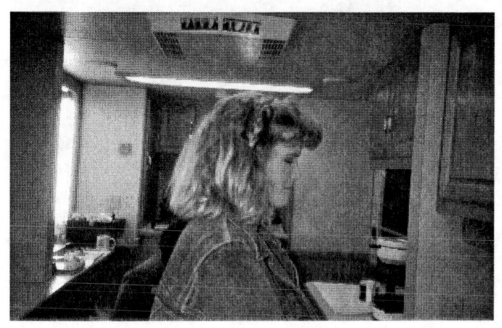

Mare Winningham, *Turner & Hooch*

Diane, our masseuse, went with us and, since we all had our per diem, we booked her for whole body massages in the evenings. She had lovely music playing in her room, which smelled awesome. After my massage, she rubbed me with salt. When she was through my skin was soft as silk. Back in my room, she rolled me in a sheet and sprayed lavender all over it. I was in heaven. I called Pat and told him I was sorry he wasn't there to enjoy my silky body.

We had a great time together those last days of filming. Tom had enjoyed the Angel Cards so much that on the last day he decided to sacrifice them in a little fire to celebrate our finish. I was touched by his gesture, but then he never ceased to surprise me.

The last night Production booked a party at Clint Eastwood's hotel. Mare's band played and she sang. Beasley came with Clint and for the first time we were allowed to pet him, but he only had eyes for Clint.

It was May, a perfect time to return home to New Hampshire. Tanya was getting married at our house and she had done all the work, arranging for the tent rental, the caterer, the church, and the music. She was the most un-nervous bride I'd ever seen.

It was good she had everything under control because I got a call to go back to California to do a few days of retakes on *Hooch* right before the wedding. It was fun to be together again. Clint, who trusted nobody human, finally admitted he had begun to trust me. I was a mother figure to him. In fact he told me he would have been a much happier person if I'd been his mother.

It was a fun if rushed trip and I hurried home for the wonderful wedding on my fifty-fifth birthday, June 17. I never forget their anniversary.

Chapter 66

HAVANA

We called it The Perfect Summer. From the day of Tanya and Tom's wedding on June 17, 1989, the weather was gentle, beautiful, and sometimes misty. It continued like that all summer long.

I wanted to stay home. I began thinking about what I could do when I really retired. I'd always loved books, especially metaphysical subjects. I began to think. There was no bookstore of that the sort in our area. I figured it would be wonderful to have my own store, just like The Bodhi Tree in Los Angeles. Maybe a little smaller.

Ever ready to support me, Pat went with me as I began looking for a likely location for a bookstore. We had a great time looking here and there, wearing out our kind realtor. We considered putting the store in our garage in Snowville, but we lived too far out of town and the road to our place was steep and mountainous. No one would venture up that hill, especially in the winter. Finally it dawned on us that we could use the little store that was attached to the house we had bought in Conway. We had thought that the girls were going to open a Mexican restaurant. It hadn't happened and so an air-conditioning business was renting the little store attached to the house. They had outgrown the building and were ready to move to a larger space. They were happy to get out of their lease early.

Now that the store was available, I became serious about creating a bookstore. In my ignorance, I figured it would cost less than $10,000 to set up a nice little bookshop. What an optimist. Bette Snow, a good friend, was also very interested in having a bookshop. She didn't have the cash, but she had what I needed - balance. Bette was orderly, bright, and cautious with money. We decided to work together. To learn the ropes, she took a job at a local bookshop and I decided to return to the movies to make the money to fund the shop. Meanwhile, we sent away for catalogues for all the things a bookseller might need.

In September, I got a call from a hairdresser named, Susan Schwary, who was preparing to do *Havana*. Obviously, it couldn't be shot in Cuba, so it was being filmed in the Dominican Republic. The film starred Robert Redford and Lena Olin and was going to be directed by Sydney Pollack - my old buddies from *This Property is Condemned*.

Susan's husband, Ron Schwary, was the producer. He had hired her as head hairstylist and she wanted to do her best. Susan and I talked for quite a while. She told me stories of many hairdressers who she felt had done her wrong in the past. She mentioned some of my favorite people. I should have listened closer, but I was so excited about the opportunity to work on the film and earn the money for my book shop that I only heard what I wanted to hear. I wanted the job. The day after I talked with Susan, her husband, Ron called. We had worked together years before and he knew I was good at what I did. He was aware that Susan would need some high powered help to make the film work, it was going to be a huge undertaking and he didn't want anything to go wrong. Ron basically hired me. I suggested that he also hire my friend Barbara Lampson, who did wonderful period hair work. He took my suggestion and we were both hired. We were happy to be the workhorses Susan needed. She was lucky to have us.

My job didn't begin until the end of October and neither did Pat's. It was a rare opportunity for us to enjoy the gorgeous fall together. Our schedules didn't often coincide. I felt secure knowing I had a great job waiting for me. When the time to leave for Santa Domingo rolled around, Pat saw me off at the airport in Portland, Maine. A couple of days later he headed out west to do *Another 48 Hours*. We were going to be apart for a long time, but we had plans to come home for Christmas.

First of all, I boarded a tiny commuter plane in Portland, Maine and flew to Boston. There I transferred to another tiny plane for New York. From New York to Santa Domingo, I flew on Dominican Airlines. Normally we are supposed to fly first class when we leave the country, but there was no first class on Dominican Airlines. It was full of happy Dominican families on their way home. I didn't mind. I'd made that trip once before.

Although October, it was sweltering upon my arrival in Santa Domingo. I was met by Sergeant Pete from the army, who still ran the country just as it had years before when we were there during the filming of *Sorcerer*. Sergeant Pete was very helpful. He loaded my luggage into a car and took me straight to the Jaragua Hotel. What a surprise. It was one of the most magnificent hotels I'd ever seen. It had certainly changed since I had been there before. Completely rebuilt, it was a city unto itself with its own power system, a casino and several incredible restaurants. There were the most lovely, feminine women walking around in gorgeous outfits. I was impressed.

My room was large and lovely, all done in soft turquoise with touches of coral and furnished with white wicker furniture. It had everything I needed including a refrigerator, a desk, and a sitting area. The windows looked out to the ocean so I could see the sun set in the evening. Seeing as this would be my home for the next five months, I had brought my typewriter with me so I could write home. It cost over a dollar a minute to call home.

After unpacking, I walked to the production office where I was delighted to find Nanette, my favorite production secretary from the *Sorcerer* and other films I'd worked on. We had originally met on *Day of the Dolphin* in the Bahamas. She knew the ropes better than anyone. Nanette introduced me to the people working in the office.

I looked up as a woman came around the corner. She stopped, smiled, and said questioningly, "Sugar?" I hesitated for a moment. Something about her appearance made me think to myself, "Beware." I was surprised. I hadn't pictured her looking like this. "Yes?" I replied. "I'm Susan." my new boss announced. We hugged, and then she explained that our hair supplies things had just come out of customs and soon we'd be able to put everything in the makeup trailers. There would be one star trailer for Susan and Gary Liddiard, who did Redford, and another for us because we would be doing the extras.

Gary wasn't coming down for another week. Barbara was also coming the next week along with Kathy from Chicago. Susan and I began getting the trailers ready. I was so excited about being there that I never paid attention to the subtle warning bell in my brain telling me Susan might be impossible for me to work with - something about the way she took control. Had I been aware, I would have given my notice and gotten on the next plane home, but I didn't.

Susan's husband was busy most evenings with Sydney Pollack so she and I began eating dinner together. It wasn't really what I wanted to do. I like having my evenings to myself. I'd lost some weight that summer and I would have preferred to skip dinner. But Susan was lonely so I kept her company. I did enjoy having a couple of my favorite El Presidente beers along with my meal. It was just as good as I remembered.

Finally, we were able to stock the makeup trailer and I learned the true meaning of "honey dos" as Pat calls them. By now I realized Susan demanded total control, so I did as she asked. I lined all the boxes up according to numbers she had written on them. I was allowed to clean the drawers and counters while she unpacked everything she had brought, putting supplies here and there. She unpacked Gary's supplies and when he arrived he was not pleased. I'm sure she thought she was doing him a favor, but he was also a person who demanded control. I laughed to myself thinking each had met their match. Two bosses in one trailer - what fun.

Finally, Barbara and Kathy arrived. I was relieved. Kathy, who would do anything to be liked, took over my dinners with Susan and I hung out with Barbara. We were both low-key and didn't care much about the nightlife. We'd had enough of that already in our lifetimes.

Now that we were all there, we began cutting the extras' hair, fitting wigs, getting the extras ready. We had a couple of weeks to prepare before shooting started. We worked in a huge warehouse where the wardrobe was being fitted. The extras came to us, dressed in their costumes and then we'd figure out the appropriate hairstyles. Seeing as it was the Sixties some of them needed wigs. The styles had to be appropriate for the period. The men's hair had to be short and greasy. Susan wanted all the women to be wigged. She thought it would make things easier. I thought it was a crazy idea.

Two fellows from the army helped us cut the men's hair. They were fast and did great work. I appreciated their help. I wasn't great with the clippers, just adequate. At the end of the week, I gave the soldiers an extra ten dollars for helping us. I had made a mistake. Susan reported me to Ron, the producer and he called me into the office explaining that, if I gave them money, they'd brag to their buddies about how much more they were making and it would start trouble. I hadn't considered that aspect and apologized. He said I could give them a bonus at the end of the film if I wanted to do it.

Lunches were wonderful. Our assistant directors lived locally and knew all the best restaurants. One of them had grown up in Argentina and had a diplomat for a father. Another had attended film school in Chicago. They were bright young men and we had incredible, worldly conversations over our meals.

Robert Redford arrived, but I didn't see him right away. One afternoon, I ran into him in the hall as he was on his way back from a tennis game. "Sugar," he called, "how are you? It's been so long." He gave me a big hug, apologizing for being sweaty from his game. He looked terrific. It had been such a long time since we'd last worked together on *Barefoot in the Park* and many things had changed. Natalie was gone now. Robert had made his first important film with Natalie, *"Inside Daisy Clover*, and Sydney Pollack had, too - *This Property is Condemned*. We shared a lot of memories.

We talked about my life in New Hampshire and he was delighted for me. He had moved to Connecticut. He said that Sundance had grown too large and busy for him to continue living there. I felt a kinship with this fellow Californian having moved to the East Coast. In parting I said, "I think we're gonna have a good time." A bit more cautious, he replied, "We'll see."

A couple of days later, Kathy was in the main trailer dyeing the hair of Redford's double. Bob walked by and I asked him if he would mind stepping into the trailer so Kathy could see his hair color that she was matching. He happily complied and I introduced him to Kathy. Later, when I told Susan about it, thinking she'd be pleased, she snapped, "I had pictures. She didn't need to see him." Oh my!

At a production meeting for all the department heads (which included my friends Sydney, Bernie Pollack, Sydney's brother, now a costume designer, and Redford, conversation got around to our experiences on *This Property is Condemned*. It was the film where Bernie got his start in the Wardrobe Department. Since I had also worked on that film, my name came up. They talked about how I'd surprised them by being so wild, leaving my husband for an electrician or something. That didn't sit well with Susan. Even though I wasn't at the meeting, she felt I was somehow stealing her glory.

My next mistake - and I was beginning to think that everything I did would be a mistake - was trying to help Susan engineer some unusually complicated hairstyles. I talked with the special effects fellow who was happy to see what he could do to help. He figured out a simple way to engineer the hair dos with some base that he created out of thick wire. Because consulting him hadn't been Susan's idea, she resented it. All I did was to try and get the job done in the simplest way that would make Susan look good in the long run. Oh well.

One hairstylist who worked with us was Dominican and Susan treated her as though she was beneath her. I spoke Spanish, so we had many conversations. Unfortunately, Susan was not making any friends and goodness knew she was going to need them once production got underway.

By this time, it occurred to me that perhaps I should quit, but I didn't. After all, they had flown me all the way down there, and although Susan was difficult, I loved getting to know the Dominicans. They were such fun-loving people.

On my days off, I took walks by the ocean. Next door to our hotel was a place that sold exotic, colorful Haitian paintings. I wondered how people, who were so mistreated in their own country, were still able to produce such wonderful art. I bought many paintings to take home.

The beginning of the end for me came with the start of production. In the first scene, a group of people were dancing on a boat. Susan wanted every person's hair to look alike. Some of the extras had been fitted with wigs so she told us to set them all exactly the same way. I knew it wouldn't look right. I pointed it out to her and said, "The reason for hiring many hairdressers instead of just one is so the hair doesn't look as if it came right out of the factory. We have different talents and you need to use our artistry." Wrong thing to say. I also had learned how to bring some of the person's own hair out at the hairline of a cheap wig, so it didn't look so wiggy. She didn't like that idea, either. Even though I had been nominated for an Emmy for my wig work, I couldn't please her.

Production began in a hot, stuffy building with a tin roof. Redford looked just as appealing as ever, although there were more lines in his tanned face than when I'd first met him. There seemed to be a little tension between him and Sydney, the director, at times. Gary assured me that was the way things usually were whenever they worked together.

One day, Redford was sitting behind the set and expecting him to be as friendly as he had when I talked with him before, I began to engage him in conversation, but he was different and sort of shut me out. It was strange.

To add insult to injury, when I was working on the stage Sydney sometimes called for me when he wanted a hairdresser, instead of Susan. The final blow came when Gary was having trouble with Redford's hair and asked me for advice. I told him what I thought would work and then gathered up some supplies. I put them in his makeup chair. Susan was incensed. "I had all those supplies. Why didn't he ask me?" They didn't get along very well either.

Next, Susan banned me from the set. She had me make up hairdressing kits for all the hairstylists for the big scenes. I made bundles of pins, combs, and other necessary things - seventy of them in all, even though I knew we'd never use them all. I gave up when I realized that it was just an exercise to keep me off the stage. I couldn't help being me and that wasn't good enough for Susan.

One day when Barbara and I were putting up Christmas bells up around the walls of the trailer, Susan called me into her trailer. As I walked through the door, she announced, "I'm letting you go." I wasn't really surprised and yet, I was. After all, I had considered quitting. I'd even talked to Pat about it. At that moment, I realized I should have heeded my first reaction to Susan and beaten it right out of there.

Still, I thought I deserved an explanation. "Why are you firing me?" She wouldn't answer stating simply, "I have my reasons." That wasn't enough. Later, she admitted my resume intimidated her. How strange. She should have used my talent to make herself look better instead of fearing it.

Even though I was relieved, I walked back to my trailer in tears. I'd never been fired before. Barbara was great. Immediately she began taking down the Christmas ornaments, packing them back into the box. At that moment, she decided to quit, too. She could see the writing on the wall. She didn't want to wait to be fired, too. Susan lost her two best workers. When I talked with Ron, he was surprised at Susan's actions. I told him I felt his wife was an arrogant bitch and he was going to have trouble all through the film. He did, too.

Two days later, Barbara and I packed up and went to the airport. I kissed everyone goodbye including the maids, bellboys, and the doorman; they were all so sweet.

After we checked in at the airport, I gave all my Dominican money to Sergeant Pete. We were scheduled to take off in an hour and I didn't think I'd need it. Wrong. Barbara and I waited all day for our plane to board. They told us there was a problem and we wouldn't be leaving that day. We had to re-book for the next day. Luckily, I spoke Spanish, so I made the new arrangements after spending hours in line. Through it all, the Dominicans remained good-humored and so did we. They put us up at a hotel for the night and paid for our meals and room, which was fortunate because I didn't have any cash left. The next day, I flew out with only ten American dollars to tide me over until I reached home. I arrived to a snowy winter. I was disappointed that I hadn't been able to save all the money for the store, but relieved not to have to endure the stress.

Years later, in the fall of 1996, I was in Wales with Pat who was working on *Mortal Combat Annihilation*. I sat down at the breakfast table with him and Lee, the first assistant on the film, asked, "Is your name Sugar? Did you work on *Havana?* "Yes," I replied, "and I got fired." Laughing, Lee said, "I remember you now. I was just a second assistant then. I start all my stories about *Havana* with you. "It all started when Susan fired this very nice hairdresser named Sugar." Lee told me Susan fired thirty-five people after I left. He said it was the kiss of death if anyone of importance paid more attention to any of the hairdressers other than Susan. I laughed because it was funny, but at the same time I felt sad at the way things had turned out.

Chapter 67

REVELATIONS

I'd been trying to quit the movie business ever since we moved to the farm in Appalachia in 1969. I never seemed to be able to; it always lured me back. This latest experience on *Havana* was one more push in the direction I'd been trying to go for almost twenty years. The business was no longer kind and friendly. Now it seemed to be a "gotcha" business, with people trying to catch people doing something wrong and blaming, instead of supporting, one another. I'd seen others get fired and I always felt bad for anyone who was fired. Sometimes a lot of people got fired on a film. Other times it never happened. But the fact was, increasingly, more people were sacrificed instead of the person who was really at fault. Now that I had experienced it first hand, it didn't feel good. I'd been replaced before starting a film because somebody asked for someone special. That was disappointing, but not like this. Now I'd been fired for the first time in thirty years. I knew it was because my resume intimidated Susan. I knew I did good work, but I was devastated anyway. I began to doubt myself. Was she right? Was I really incapable? I went back and forth in my mind trying to make myself feel better, but no matter how I looked at it, the event had affected me deeply.

A woman at our union was sympathetic. She confided that she wished it had been possible to warn me about Susan, but it wouldn't have been legal. She had a feeling there might be trouble, but she couldn't do anything. My friends were in shock over what had happened and shared their Susan horror stories with me.

In the following months, I was called many times by hairstylists who were considering working with Susan to find out what happened. I told them exactly what happened to me thinking that if they were forewarned, they might work out. Some tried and got fired anyway. Even the spiritualist I saw before I left for location told me there would be many different people in Santa Domingo who would seem as though they were from outer space. That sounded quite strange. When I returned home, I saw her again and she confirmed she had seen trouble, but because I had been so excited, she hadn't wanted to discourage me.

Before I left for *Havana*, I took a course called YES. One week I was given a wooden coin that said, "This is the greatest thing that ever happened to me" on one side, and on the side it said, this is the worst thing that ever happened to me. I didn't think I would be able to finish the class because of the film. I was back in time for the last two classes. The group was surprised to see me. I told them my story and then quoted my coin - losing the job was the greatest thing that ever happened. And it was when I looked at it from a larger perspective. The pain I felt at being fired caused me to seek a deeper meaning.

Upon my return home, I learned that my friend Barbara Leonetti, the wife of Matt Leonetti, was dying of cancer. I'd planned to send her a book I'd found called *Deathing, A Conscious Approach to Dying*, but I wanted to read it first to be sure it would be okay to send. I called her and asked how she was. "I'm still here," she said. I decided to quickly read the book, but sadly, Barbara died before I could send it to her.

After reading the book, I began to understand that most regrets at death come from a life that is unlived. Personally I knew I didn't want to die curious.

I began to sense a change in me. I wanted to know more. A recommended reading list at the end of the book, suggested reading *No Boundaries* by Ken Wilber. I ordered it immediately. I gobbled that up and then looked at the recommended list at the end of his book. He suggested a book called *Enlightenment of the Whole Body*, by Bubba Free John. That very book had been sitting above my bed for more than two years, just waiting for me.

The prayer I had said that summer was being answered. I'd always studied spiritual teachings and each time I'd finish I would be disappointed. All the teachers were dead. I had said a prayer, asking for someone who knew more about God than I did to come into my life. I asked that this teacher be alive. I wanted a living God Man.

Now He is called Adi Da Samraj, but He had many names in the past. The moment I began to read Adi Da Samraj's writings, I knew in my heart it was the Truth I'd been searching for. The uneasiness and the longing I'd felt within all during my life had finally come to the fore and I understood that my search was over. It was as though He had been waiting for me to "remember". From then on, I knew that I no longer needed to look anywhere else.

I had many things to learn about a spiritual relationship. It wouldn't be an easy thing to do. Adi Da Samraj wasn't going to be like a parent telling me what to do. I was going to have to take responsibility for myself. I read His Teachings and learned how he guided his devotees and showed us that we are not separate from one another. He showed me how we were pinching ourselves and complaining about the pain, when all we had to do was stop pinching. He explained that we couldn't become happy. We are already happy and all we need to do is to remove the barriers to feeling that. We are not separate from one another. One of my favorite revelations was "Dead Guru's can't kick ass." I knew that and it was why I fully understood that it was so important for me to find Him to be alive. I truly needed a teacher. My ego could justify anything the way I wanted it at the time. It was no friend of mine if I wanted to evolve.

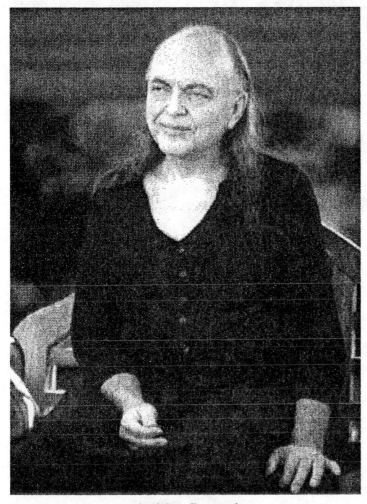

Adi Da Samraj

His writing, His wisdom, His truth poured into my brain like liquid gold. My whole world became bright. Somewhere, inherently, I had always known He existed. When doors had closed in the past, I'd wondered why. Now I understood where I'd been heading all my life. Getting fired had been a wonderful door to close while opening an extraordinary new one.

A couple of years later, I ended up working with Susan on *Death Becomes Her* as an extra hairdresser. I ran into Susan and at first, I was polite, but uneasy. Later, she came over to me and asked, "Are you still angry with me?" I could truthfully tell her "No." I explained that when I was fired, I had stayed home feeling vulnerable. In my reading, I had found the teacher I'd prayed for. Between Susan and Barbara, I'd been led to my future and a Living God Man. This was the most important thing that had ever happened in my life. I tried to explain that to her. I'm not sure she understood, so I gave her a hug. I also wished that good things would come into her life. I don't think they did.

I'd taken to Transcendental Meditation in 1974, but that had only been a technique. Adi Da Samraj offered a relationship to me, a communication from the heart, and that was what I'd longed for. Relating to the nebulous God of my imagination just hadn't cut it for me.

My friends were concerned. They asked if this might be a cult. Of course it wasn't. In a way, I sort of resented their questions. I wasn't mindless. Adi Da Samraj was my teacher. He put no unreasonable demands upon me. It was my responsibility. To put it simply, I began to see how I needed to peel off all the layers that prevented me from feeling my inherent happiness, just like the skin of an onion.

I finally began to understand how I was contracted, as we all are. I had cut myself off from the God I longed to know. Although my life had been so full of wonderful adventures and I had so much love from people, somehow I'd never really had a true spiritual foundation. When the high times were happening, I didn't have to think about that, but when things were quiet, I'd had no place to turn until now. I no longer felt alone in the many ways I had during my life. The loneliness, which I'd never really admitted to myself, was gone.

Chapter 68
ROCKY V

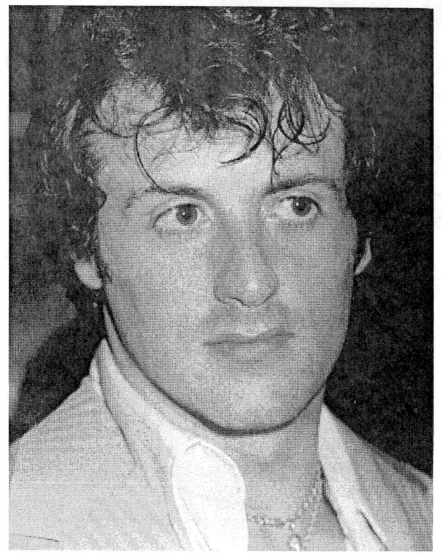

Sylvester Stallone, *Rocky V*

Although my spiritual life was looking up, as far as work went, doubt assailed me, I wondered if I'd ever work again. I had just about given into my fears, when I got a call from Shirley Dolle, my hairdresser friend. She was on location in Philadelphia. "Would you be available to work with me, on *Rocky V?*" she asked. We began to talk about my being fired and she bolstered me right up, reminding me how much she had looked up to me and admired my work when she was just starting out at Paramount. There was nothing wrong with me as far as she was concerned. I really needed that.

She told me she'd call as soon as they returned to Los Angeles. I was very happy to be wanted again. You know, like getting up on the horse after you fall off. I headed off to Los Angeles a few days later. The day before Shirley returned, I got a confusing call from Production saying that I might need to come in and do Sylvester Stallone - Shirley might be quitting. I was quivering in my boots. I knew Sly, as he was called, wasn't easy to deal with. Luckily, Shirley worked everything out by the time she came back. I remained her assistant, which was just where I wanted to be.

What a great crew we had. There were two hairdressers: Shirley and I, three makeup people, two women and one man complimented us. Frank Perez who did Stallone - one makeup man had already quit that job and Frank had taken over. Plus two makeup ladies - Carol Schwartz, a gentle English woman, and Katalin Elek. We became good friends.

We were like a family in our trailer. Each of us came in with our problems and among all of us, we got them solved. We kept after Frank relentlessly. His soon to be ex-wife was driving him crazy, running up credit card bills. He never knew what the total at the end of the month would be. He drove an old car and hardly had anything for himself. Our advice was simple, "Dump her."

Shirley had done Sly's hair on other films. It was a prestige job. I did Talia Shire, Sage Stallone (Sly's son), and Delia Shep. Her part was of a beautiful woman who courts Tommy Morrison, the fighter who Rocky encourages and trains.

Talia actually had a hairstylist from New York, but he couldn't work on the stage because he wasn't in our union. He'd do her hair in the dressing room and then I'd stand by with her on the stage while he watched to see that the hair stayed as it should. It wasn't as easy as it sounds. Talia would arrive on the set all coifed and then moments later, Sly would walk over and begin to play around with her, messing up her hair. Her hairstylist stood in the background, so nervous, always hoping I could get it back into the shape. I usually succeeded.

I'd never worked with Sly before. His reputation preceded him. I didn't think I'd care for him, but I was wrong. I grew to like him a lot. I found him quite beautiful in many ways, so healthy, shiny, and clean looking. He wasn't really tall, but had worked on his body so he appeared bigger than he actually was. He was a cocky man, and seemed to love all women in some way. Yet he appeared to be unable to trust them. The exception was his partner at the time. Jennifer was a sweet woman and is now the mother of his children. I guess he finally realized he had a treasure. He created her look, sort of like Rex Harrison in *My Fair Lady*. They must have had some sort of an agreement because sometimes he showed up on the set with a woman who looked like a barmaid. He seemed more at ease with this kind of woman. Who was I to judge? It often occurred to me that although he was very bright and successful, he might still have felt that he had a lot to prove to himself. I could understand that, knowing how far he'd come and how hard he had to fight to get the first *Rocky* produced with him in the lead role. When he played the part of Rocky, he really touched my heart. I believed in his character and wanted Rocky to succeed.

Our schedule was erratic. The director, John Avildsen of *Karate Kid* fame, often seemed unprepared. Most mornings, upon his arrival, he'd come in and change the set-up he had given the night before. Then he would go to his trailer to figure out what to do in the scene. We seldom got our first shot before lunchtime, but nobody seemed to care.

Nobody, that is, except Mike Glick, our production manager. Mike was tight with the pennies and was having a difficult time. He was under a lot of pressure, caught in the middle between the producers and Production and who could talk back to Sly? Once I asked for an extra hairstylist for a large scene and he blew up at me. After I explained the reason behind the request, it was fine with him and we ended up good friends. I would never want to be in his shoes.

Besides Talia, I had to do Delia Shep, the glamorous actress who courts Tommy, the new fighter. She was a tall, fabulous-looking, Norwegian woman with a voluptuous figure. Shirley and the New York hairstylist had designed her hairstyles when they were on location. I had to have Shirley's help on one hairstyle that was particularly intricate. It took hours to do.

In one scene, Delia was supposed to be wearing the difficult hairstyle. We hadn't been informed about that particular scene being shot that day. Shirley had the day off. I tracked her down and she agreed to come in. All of a sudden they needed Delia right away. "Sugar, you do it yourself," Production demanded. I realized they didn't understand why I needed Shirley and I resisted. Eventually, I agreed, as long as the script supervisor recorded that we weren't given enough time to do the hair properly. I wanted it noted in case there was trouble for Shirley when they edited the film.

I knew my hairdo wasn't as good as Shirley would have done, but when I saw the film I couldn't tell the difference. It was a bit disappointing when I realized how much work we could put into something and that it would never be photographed closely enough to be appreciated.

We had plenty of time to sit around and talk about life in general in our trailer because we seldom got a shot before noon. Kathy complained that at home she had to do all the work - cooking, washing, cleaning, etc. on top of her makeup job. We all agreed it wasn't fair, her husband, also a makeup man, should have helped. Then she confessed that although he wasn't willing to do the housework, he had always asked to her to hire someone. Then she finally confessed that she was never satisfied with anyone and therefore chose to do it herself. We began working on her to delegate more.

Everyone except Frank and I had elegant cars. Shirley drove a Mercedes and was thinking of upgrading to an $85,000 one which she did. Stallone had just bought a Mercedes just like it for Jennifer as a birthday present. When he found out Shirley had the same model, he was surprised. On the other hand, I drove an '85 Honda Civic that I loved, dents and all. I was saving my money for a bookstore, not a car. We talked about how, because we worked such long hours in the business, we bought things to make up for it. Trouble was, sometimes the things cost a lot and eventually paying for them often kept people from taking off much needed time for themselves. It was very common in the movie business to live beyond our means. I had done it myself.

One day while we were working at the airport, the radio show guys, Mark and Brian, of Southern California fame, came in to get their hair done. They were funny and obnoxious and really panned me on the radio. They said what a terrible job I'd done on their hair, but what they said wasn't really true and I just laughed. Thank you guys - or should I say jerks?

During a bedroom scene with Talia and Sly, they exchanged words. I don't know what she said, but it seemed that somehow she had severely wounded his manhood. They had worked together in so many films (this being *Rocky V*) that she knew how to push his buttons. He was very angry with her and from then on, he treated her terribly. She didn't know when to quit. She should have known better, but perhaps she wanted to be finished with him.

Stallone had bodyguards. The nicest one was Gary, a big handsome man. They weren't there to protect him from harm rather to protect him from himself. He tended to blow pretty easily if someone offended him. The bodyguards would put an end to a fight before it began.

Sage Stallone, at fourteen, was already a handsome boy and so bright. He was curious, always asking questions. "What's this for?" or "Why do they do that?" He was affectionate and liked a hug. One day I asked him what he liked to do in his spare time. "Oh, go to the mall and hang out." I was appalled. Here was this kid who could afford anything and he still did what ordinary bored kids do. I told him he should spend a summer with me in the mountains and see what that was like.

One day he was playing on the prop truck, looking around, asking questions, and he fell off the lift. After that, he was banned from the truck. The prop men didn't want to get into trouble with Sly. Sometimes it was hard to get Sage to let me brush his hair, which was very curly. One morning, he appeared on the set a bit disheveled. Sly took one look at him, grabbed my brush, and proceeded to brush Sage's hair into shape. Sly had been a hairstylist before he began to act. He was quite good, too. He had a mean brushing style.

Tommy Morrison played the man Rocky trains. He was young and very tough. We were working downtown in the Olympic Auditorium filming try-outs with different boxers. Tommy was supposed to be climbing up the ladder of success. One fighter whom nobody liked much began to fight in the scene and Tommy actually hit him so hard he broke his jaw. Later I questioned him asking if he liked hitting people and he replied, "Yes." I guess a boxer has to feel that way. Years later I read in the paper that he had killed someone. Too bad he didn't learn to control that power. Burgess Meredith came in for a cameo appearance. What a dear man. I remembered him from my first location in Pasa Robles on *Rawhide*. He had aged quite a bit, but then, I had too.

Paul Monte was Sly's stand-in. He was a relative who looked remarkably like Sly - perhaps a little handsomer. Paul took a liking to me. We talked a lot and he wanted me to meet his mother. He was comfortable with me. Sometimes he sat with his head in my lap. Ah yes, another son.

After wrapping in Los Angeles, the plan was to go back to Philadelphia for two weeks of location work. Shirley didn't want to go because she had been newly married just before the film began and had made plans for a honeymoon cruise at that very time. She asked if I would do Sly. I said I would as long as it was okay with him. He agreed. In the middle of May we left for Philadelphia. I had never been there. We were scheduled to work many nights and one day recreating the scene where Rocky runs back up those famous steps again.

I was astounded at the first location site. It was underneath the tracks of the train in a rough area where every last inch of the buildings was covered in graffiti. Shirley told me she hated it when they filmed there last winter. There had been needles lying in the snow. Every time she saw kids wearing expensive dark glasses like hers she was bummed thinking they probably got the money in drug deals.

The spring was more pleasant and warmer, too. Industrious neighbors set up card tables near the sets and sold gum, candy, and soft drinks. Most of these folks were just poor, not druggies, and I had fun getting to know them.

We stayed in a comfortable hotel and my room was very quiet. I had to sleep all day because we worked at night. Around 4:00 p.m., I'd wake up, order breakfast and a cappuccino and then head into work around 5:00 p.m. Stallone treated me well. Actually, he liked to do his own hair. I usually just made sure it matched on the set. The first time I did his hair, I was nervous. He was impatient when he wanted something. He'd ask me for the brush and always wanted to look in the mirror. At first, I had a hard time finding the brush instantly, so after the first night I went to Banana Republic and bought a vest with lots of pockets. From then on, he could reach into my pockets for whatever he wanted. He thought that was great.

One day standing on the set, Sly and I began talking about Sanpaku - a weird thing where you can see white on three sides of a person's eye. Sal Mineo, James Dean, and Natalie Wood all had it and they all died in tragedies. Sly said, "I have that, too." "No," I said hopefully, but then I looked into his eyes and he was right. It made me feel sad.

Every morning, around 5:00 a.m., someone sent out for pretzels and mustard. I loved eating mine because it meant it was nearly wrap time and very soon I'd be crawling into bed.

Delia, our glamorous actress, was in only one scene those last two weeks - dressed in a low-cut dress and furs. We had a new cameraman for this part of the filming - Victor Hammer. He was so short that he could lean on her and happily nestle his head right between her breasts. He was always in seventh heaven when he leaned on her. Fortunately, she thought it was amusing.

We worked on top of the famous steps Rocky had run up in the first *Rocky*. The view from there was spectacular looking down the long avenue below us. They brought the Rocky statue all the way from Stallone's office and put it there for the last time. Shucks, I though it was a permanent fixture there.

The last night we shot, I saw Sly sitting alone on a pile of wood. I went over and told him I appreciated working with him on the film and thanked him. I told him that the work had made it possible to get my bookstore started. He was pleased and seemed surprised by my thanking him. I guess no one had ever done that before.

I flew home to New Hampshire, all excited about getting the bookshop ready to open by the middle of July.

That September I got a call to do two days of retakes at Goldwyn Studios with Delia. I was heading west anyway, so I agreed. Delia hadn't kept her hair color up because the film was finished. When she arrived, her hair needed to be tinted. Trying to save the company money, I did one of the dumbest things I'd ever done in my career. I had the formula for her color, so I went to the supply house to get the tint. They were out of one of the colors, but the sales person gave me something else, assuring me it would do just fine. Wrong! Wrong! How could I have been so stupid?

The tint turned her hair more brown than red. I hoped it would look better after it was washed, but the next day when she reported to work it was even browner. I panicked. Luckily, the other hairstylist had the presence of mind to remind me of Laurie Davis, our famous Hollywood hairstylist who tinted like a magician. She could do anything and had been called all over the world to fix color mistakes. I called and fortunately she was at her shop. Delia and I drove to Brentwood and an hour later, the color was perfect. I was so relieved. God was watching over me

That afternoon, Stallone walked by me and strangely enough he held out his hand and caught mine. It was very sweet.

Chapter 69

THE JUMPING OFF PLACE

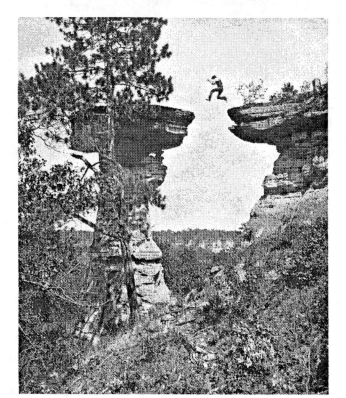

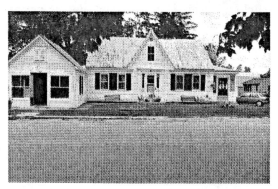
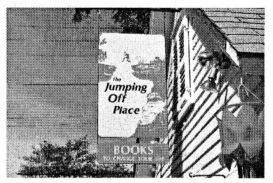

Photos of Sugar's Book Store in New Hampshire

After *Rocky V* wrapped, I rushed home from Philadelphia. I wanted to begin to create the bookstore. We had decided on a name. My Guru Adi Da Samraj had written a book called the *Holy Jumping Off Place*. On the cover of the book was a photo of a man leaping from one cliff to another. In the photo, he was suspended in mid air. It was a fantastic, provocative photo. Taking a spiritual leap was what our bookshop was about so we decided to call it The

Jumping Off Place.

It was convenient having the store in the house where Tanya and her family lived. We were able to use the bathroom and we could make coffee in the kitchen. We had so much to do to get ready. The building was only a shell. First the builders put in new walls. Next they built bookcases on all the walls. We painted the shelves. It was a big job. Bette wanted to paint the shelves a very light blue, which was lovely, but then she suggested we paint the front of the shelves white. Pat, who up to this time had been very patient with us, put his foot down. "We're selling books, not shelves." I had to agree. We had enough to do as it was.

The space was divided into two rooms with a little office in the back. Shelves were everywhere. We carpeted the floors and I brought in curtains from home for the front windows. We had a sign designed and painted and hung it over our front door. We designed a counter and had it built. We bought a cash register, fax, extra phone, and file cabinets. I brought the copier from the inn and I already had a Mac Computer.

Bette had put together a business plan before we started. We would have to gross at least $96,000 to cover our estimated expenses for a year. Bette would draw $2000 a month to run the store. My job was to earn the money for the books and improvements.

Looking back, I have to take the blame for not being realistic. Our New England town was very small and not ready for this kind of a bookstore. I always tended to be about five years ahead of the times. One time my accountant told me I should have gone into business in the west, but I had no desire to live out west. So we looked at the plan, ignored it and went ahead anyway. I was in creative mode and wanted a place to work when I retired. I was afraid of being bored; I had plans live to be very old, at least a hundred and five. I didn't want to ever completely retire.

It was a real laugh, but not funny, when we added up the expenses for our store. Pat and I took a mortgage on the twenty acres across from our house to carry us through that year. We took a lot of time off to build our store. Even if wasn't turning out exactly like I imagined, I was optimistic.

Bette went through all the book catalogues and marked what she thought we needed. We agreed almost one hundred per cent of the time. We decided to use New Leaf Distributors out of Atlanta because they supplied the kind of book we wanted to sell. Bette had planned a fantastic inventory. Pat loved the Twelve Step books with affirmations that had been so helpful to him in his recovery. They were hard to find around our area. We ordered those, along with self-help books, books of all different religions, health items, herbs, crystals, oils, and candles.

The books began to arrive, carton after carton. It was a fantastic experience watching my dream becoming a reality. We had ads in the paper and magazines for our grand opening on July 15, 1990. We made it and everything looked fabulous.

Our store was beautiful and we offered many items that nobody could find around our town. We burned incense and played new age music. When you walked in through the door, it smelled great and had a different atmosphere from any place in the area. A woman from Los Angeles visited the area and told me the shop reminded her of The Bhodi Tree in Los Angeles. What a compliment! It was exactly what I was aiming for.

Amidst all this success and happiness, I suddenly began having a problem with my right eye. I began to see bright shooting lights in front of my eye. I figured I was having a high spiritual experience as a result of what we were doing. Next, a darkness appeared at the top of my eye. I thought it was because my bangs were too long, but it wasn't that at all. I had a detached retina. Pat drove me to the eye doctor up north in Berlin and the doctor had Pat rush me to a doctor in Lewiston, Maine. I was admitted to the hospital that afternoon and was operated on by dinnertime.

It took six weeks for me to return to normal. At first, I was a dreadful mess and my sight did improve in that eye, but I couldn't read for a long time. Fine thing, here I owned a bookshop and I couldn't even read.

Chapter 70
THE DOCTOR

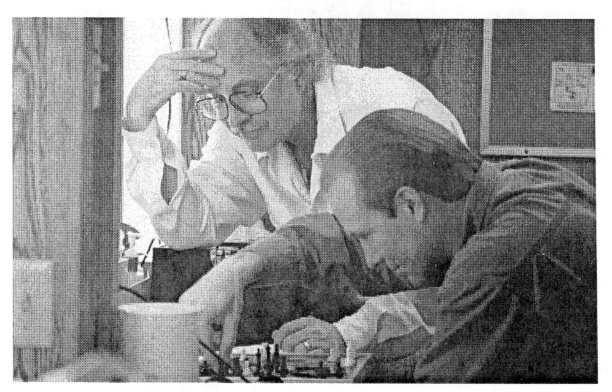

William Hurt playing chess with Leonard Engleman

Shirley Dolle had another film in the works, *The Doctor*, a Disney film starring William Hurt, Elizabeth Perkins, Christine Lahti, Mandy Patinkin, and Adam Arkin. We'd had such a wonderful time working together on *Rocky V* that Shirley wanted to work with me again. We were scheduled to go on location for a few days in San Francisco in the beginning and at the end of the film to Reno to shoot at Pyramid Lake. The script, about a repressed surgeon with no regard or compassion for his patients until he has to go through surgery himself, was actually a fabulous true story.

Our stage was way out in the valley near Magic Mountain, in a new area full of stage cum warehouses. *Terminator 2* was also shooting out there. Working at that location meant that I would always be driving the opposite of all the traffic. Perfect for me.

Pat, in his no friction paranoia, threw me for a loop. When he learned that his old friend Bill Hurt was on the film, he reminded me of a letter I'd written Bill, years before, after Bill had come out of a rehab in Minneapolis. At that time, Bill had sent Pat a letter telling him about his recovery. The letter sat on the desk for the longest time. Finally, knowing Pat never wrote letters, I wrote a long letter to Bill, and we hadn't heard from him since.

"Remember when you sent Bill that letter and we never heard back from him again?" Pat questioned. I did. The letter had been very long, but my intentions were honorable. I'd told him how happy I was when Pat had quit and now I was happy for him, too. I invited him to visit whenever he had time. I even suggested he change his name because names can affect our lives and Hurt isn't a kind name. I went on and on. Sometimes I didn't know when to stop.

Now, Pat was reminding me of this. "He might not have liked you writing to him. After all, AA is supposed to be anonymous." I began to get concerned, too. Maybe I had interfered when I shouldn't have. I hadn't seen it like that. I just figured I was a friend writing to a friend. I began to get paranoid myself. When I told Shirley about it she said "Forget it." Still, I was worried.

I was at work in the trailer when Bill first came in to do some tests. Elizabeth Perkins was in the chair by the door. She was having her wig cut and fitted and the makeup person was trying to see how she would look in a bald cap. I was sitting behind Elizabeth and my heart started to beat fast when I first heard Bill's voice. The night before I had a dream where Bill came on the set and he wouldn't even look at me. He just motioned to his assistant to get me off the set. When Bill glanced over and saw that I was there, he was so happy that he came over and gave me a big kiss and a hug. Then right off he said, "Thanks for your letter Ginger. Sorry I never answered you, but I saved it. Please don't ever send me such a long letter again." I giggled and began to get annoyed with Pat for putting me through all the needless worry.

We did the makeup and hair tests and when they were completed and approved, we took off for a short location in San Francisco. We stayed at the same Fisherman's Wharf Holiday Inn, the same one I had stayed at on *The Presidio*. We shot many exterior scenes and later used Malibu locations to tie in with San Francisco.

We had another great crew. Leonard Engleman and Mathew Mungle were our makeup men. I met John Seale, the Australian cameraman, for the first time. He became one of my favorites and I made a friend of his grip, Robin Knight. What a crazy fellow. He lived in Sedona and discussed metaphysical things with me at times, but he made me promise not to tell his grip crew that he ever talked about such things. His wife, Margaret was interested in all that stuff, so he had been exposed to that sort of thinking. His grip crew was a riot. They all wore shorts and had shapely calves. They would stand in line and flex their calves for us if we asked.

Bill Hurt was in nearly every scene, every day. He had rented an apartment nearby and only visited with his family on the weekends. Each morning he got up early to run, hoping to stay fit, but it was a strain. As the hours got longer and longer it began to take a toll on him. He was very intense and was never easy to work around. Randa Haines, our director, had directed him in *Children of a Lesser God* and was well aware of the difficulties. She knew it was worth it. Bill was a wonderful actor who never failed to give a great performance, but he sometimes was hard on the crew. The actors, on the other hand, loved working with him because he gave them one hundred percent.

Our producer, Ed Feldman from Disney, was an old timer. He was always around the set making sure everything went as well as possible. Our unit manager from *Rocky V*, Mike Glick, was on the film too and he was happy to see me. He reminisced about the past. He remembered Pat when they both were starting in the business. By this time we had become good friends.

We finished location, returned to Los Angeles, and began shooting in the hospital set which had been built on a huge stage, originally a warehouse. The hospital set was very unusual. The production designer had planned it very cleverly. To the eye it made the actor doctors look huge and the patients smaller. There were all sorts of psychological things going on inside the set and they were very subtle, but the camera picked them up. The crew had problems because it was terribly stuffy in the set. There wasn't any ventilation and it often made us so sleepy that it was hard to stay focused. There were lots of lights and sometimes the heat was unbearable. They'd fan cool air in when a scene wasn't being shot, then turn it off during the shooting. Another ventilation problem was caused because the sets were built and painted at night so the fumes hung around the rest of the day making the air quality even worse. Sometimes I wondered how much the movie business has shortened our lives with all the guck we breathed in during our careers.

The opening scene of the film took place in an operating room just as the doctors were finishing an operation. Bill Hurt, playing the surgeon, tells his assistant to take over. Next he makes a rude remark to the patient lying unconscious on the table, and walks over to turn on the stereo. Jimmy Buffet's "Let's Get Drunk and Screw" began to blare. I could hardly believe it. I asked Donna Cline, our head technical advisor about it and she told me that it was an accurate portrayal - surgeons all have their favorite music ranging from rock to classical.

Years before I had learned that although a person may be unconscious, he still hears and understands what is being said around him. You should never say, "He looks like he's gonna die," or anything like that. That was one of the points of the story. In the script, another surgeon, Adam Arkin, whispers encouragement to his patients under anesthesia and they recover in a better frame of mind than Bill Hurt's patients. Bill Hurt's character thinks that is downright stupid.

Elizabeth Perkins played a woman dying of brain cancer. Bill treats her and she softens him up a bit. Bill's wife, played by the excellent actress Christine Lahti, cannot get through to him. He shuts her out until he contracts throat cancer and has to go through the ordeal of being a patient of himself.

During the hospital scenes, there were lots of extras on the set playing nurses, doctors, and patients. Once in a while, an extra would speak to Bill saying, "Good morning," or something mundane and he'd get very upset. He was quite unreasonable at times.

Seeing as our hours were outrageous, Production suggested it might be best if we worked French Hours. I remembered working like that in Paris and it wasn't great. It meant that the crew would work from eight to five without a lunch break. Food would always be available on the set and we could eat during our breaks. It sounded great in theory, but in Paris I had seen that it didn't always work for everyone. Hair and Makeup and the actors came in earlier than the crew. It made for a long day for them. I didn't trust that it would necessarily work to our advantage this time. Some of the crew was concerned that they would miss the overtime they depended upon.

Bill was all for it and I couldn't blame him. Ten hours of shooting sounded great to him because he was really worn out. Each day he'd get on a rampage and fuss and fume, on and on. He was driving everyone crazy. He didn't stop to think his pay was in the millions. None of ours compared to his. One day Shirley made the mistake of having an *Inquirer* paper on her dressing table when Bill arrived. When he saw it, he jumped up, and rushed out of the door. Poor Shirley, she had meant no harm. He had become impossible.

I found myself more and more upset about his behavior. I think I felt responsible because he was a friend. Finally, one night during my meditation I asked Adi Da Samraj to help me with Bill. I didn't want my mind to be filled with him at work or at home either. I let go and let God, so to speak.

The next morning once again there was Bill, sitting in Shirley's chair, griping about this and that. She finished with him and he got up. He had to pass by me to get to Leonard's makeup chair. We were face to face when he made some remark, I don't even remember what it was, but I began to yell, "Bill, you are driving us all crazy. I happen to like working on this film. I'm enjoying myself. All you think about is yourself. Why don't you quit blaming everyone and handle your own stuff?" Finished with my outburst, I rushed out the door not wanting him see me break into tears as I was prone to do when I got so angry. I didn't know if I would get fired or what. I just couldn't stand it anymore.

What happened right after that was amazing. Production heard about my outburst right away and they were thrilled. Every one of them, right up to Ed the producer and Randa the director had longed to do what I had done. Mike Glick, the unit manager, even said I should get a bonus though that never materialized.

What happened later that day was even stranger. I was back in the trailer with Bill and Leonard and I began looking at some beautiful post cards of paintings by Nicholas Roherich, an artist I admire. I walked over and showed them to Bill and asked if he'd like one. "Pick one out for me," he said. He wasn't angry at all. In fact, I think he appreciated me blowing up. Perhaps it was proof that I cared about him. Afterwards, he invited me to his trailer to talk. We discussed my teacher Adi Da Samraj and I gave him some of His books. A few days later Pat came to visit. Bill and he had a wonderful time reminiscing. Pat had the ability to perk Bill up. They could laugh at themselves, which was something Bill seldom did.

One day when Bill was very tired, I asked why he didn't have his agent put in a ten-hour maximum of daily work in his contact. He said he didn't want to make waves. I was definite, "But if you don't protect yourself in the beginning, see what happens? It's stupid not to ask for what you need." I think he fired his agent after that film.

One beautiful morning on the drive to Malibu, I was listening to Al Green sing Gospels. I arrived at work high with my joy. The producer made the mistake of asking how I was. I assumed that he wanted to hear the truth. I told him just how happy I was since I found my teacher, Adi Da Samraj. After he had listened for a few moments, he remarked. "Don't ever tell me about your teacher again." I was stunned. I wanted to share my spiritual happiness. I later realized he just wanted to be the center of attention. He wasn't interested in what I had to say. I never volunteered information like that again. At the end of the show he apologized in his own way, "You're in the right frame of mind," he said, "I am such a doubter." A few years later while working on *Honey I Blew Up the Kids* I saw him again and remembered to let him do the talking.

Adam Arkin was wonderful. I'd always admired his father, Alan Arkin. He told me how his father had been so miserable on the Disney film *Rockateer*. I had worked as an extra hairstylist on that show and found it very strange. Adam said his father would have enjoyed talking with me.

A year later I met Alan Arkin's agent in Montana. She told me he was planning to do a film on a psychic surgeon in Brazil and was looking for people who might be interested in working on that sort of film. I gave her my number and told her to keep me in mind. I never did hear from her. I wonder if they ever made the picture.

I'd seen Mandy Patinkin on stage in *Evita* in New York. He had such a wonderful voice, but we never heard him sing on this film. He and Bill were great friends though and clowned around together.

I was weary most nights. The days were so long and hot and Pat's Dream Cottage didn't have a bathtub to soak in at night, only a little shower. One night Pat was sitting in the living room and asked, "Are you ever going to talk to me in the evenings?" I replied from the bedroom, "Only if you come in here and lie down beside me, I'm too tired to sit up." I did buy "him" a hot tub for Christmas. Of course, I was the one who got the most pleasure out of it. I like giving gifts like that. I enjoyed it more than he did. It made such a big difference in how I felt.

It was getting very crowded at the Dream Cottage. It was a fine place for one and Pat was really happy there, but I was getting claustrophobic. Pat's clothes were on shelves built high above the bed, and he had nails everywhere to hang things on. Our king-size bed filled the whole bedroom, leaving only a foot on each side. I couldn't even get my dresser drawers completely open.

On the next street behind us was a sweet-looking, empty, little house. I began to envision us living there. I was "back" in the movie business and would be for a while, so I needed more of a home. Each day I drove by the little house and pictured us living there. Finally, I found out who owned it and asked to see it. It was perfect. I begged Pat to rent it and of course how could he not?

We didn't go home that Christmas. We had time off, but stayed in California getting ready to move. By January, we had moved in and I gave a housewarming party and invited all our crew. We bought Australian beer and even John, the cameraman came. It was fun having everyone to our new home. I was still an innkeeper at heart.

We went on location to Reno and filmed scenes with Elizabeth and Bill at the mysterious Pyramid Lake. It was the sweetest and most romantic I'd ever seen Bill act. He became so vulnerable and tender. Was that the real Bill? I wondered.

Randa, our director, was a Salsa fiend and loved to dance. For the wrap party, she hired a Salsa band to play. I was ready to party and excited, so I went shopping and bought a wild dress of orange, black, red, and yellow meant for Salsa dancing. I even bought a black hat to wear with it. Pat was on location, so I went to the party by myself. The hospital set had been turned into a nightclub. I didn't have any idea how to do the Salsa, but they demonstrated for us and so the boom man and I were dancing forehead to forehead, laughing all the time. We'd order another Corona with lime and then we'd dance some more. He left early and someone else asked me to dance. After a couple of turns, something drastic happened to my right hip. I could almost hear it tear and creak. Panicked, I found my way to a chair, wondering if I would be able to walk again. What a relief when I realized, I could, if only slowly. When it felt a little better, I hobbled to my car and drove home.

Pat called the next day and Laurie, who was now living with us, answered the phone and told him I had hurt myself. "Serves you right, going out when I'm gone," he joked. Then Laurie told him I was really hurt and he felt terrible. It took me three days to recover. No more Salsa dancing for me. Now I only wear that dress for Halloween.

Chapter 71
FAR AND AWAY

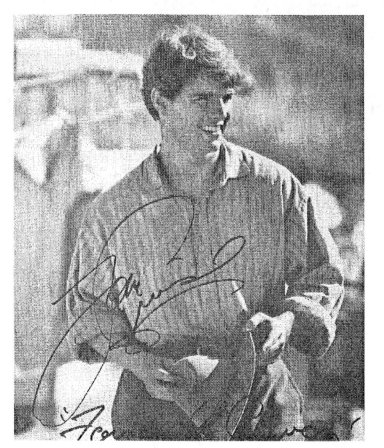

Tom Cruise, *Far and Away*

After I finished filming *The Doctor*, I hurried home to New Hampshire. I had missed my family and my home on the east coast. I was anxious to see my new book-store. I didn't mind going off to work to get the money to make it a go, but I wanted to be a part of it too.

I parked in front of the store that first morning. When I opened the door, I was delighted. It was just perfect. Bette had done a great job and customers were actually coming. Some were old friends, but there were many others also, including a few who reacted negatively. Yankees are very cautious about anything new or different. Some very religious folks assumed that our store was full of wicked things like black magic, devil worship and all. I invited people like that to come in and see for themselves. Some believed me and others didn't. Mostly they preferred to be close-minded and didn't come to investigate. But the positive comments far outnumbered the negative.

That next spring I attended a mastermind class with a small group of women meeting once a week. We would write down what we wanted to happen in our lives and work on manifesting it by releasing our wishes and picturing them coming true. Pat hadn't been working for a while. His cameraman was having a dry spell. I knew I'd better get back to work if I wanted to keep the bookshop. It didn't pay its way yet. I asked for a great job, in a great place, great people to work with, and great pay all by June 1, 1991.

The very next day I got a phone call from the production secretary on *Far and Away* which was going to be filmed in Billings, Montana and Ireland. It was starring Tom Cruise and Nicole Kidman and was directed by Ron Howard. They needed a hairstylist to oversee the extras. It would be a big job and they wanted someone who could handle that. Barbara Lampson, who had been with me in the Dominican Republic, was assisting on it. She had given them my name.

So there it was, another miracle, my wish granted immediately. I was on my way to Montana on May 20. My accountant said she wasn't surprised at all. She knew I could manifest anything I wanted. I was hired to work on the Montana segment. When the crew went to Ireland, they planned to hire Irish hairstylists. I never entertained the thought of going to Ireland. I was happy to have a job.

My equipment was in Los Angeles, so Laurie packed it up, took it to Production and they sent it up to location. One of my recurring anxiety dreams nearly came true. I used to dream that I had come to work without my case. But fortunately, my supplies arrived just about the time I did.

When I walked off the plane in Billings, the air was warm. Men were wearing cowboy boots and big cowboy hats. It was very different from New England. The crew was staying at the Sheraton, in downtown Billings. It was comfortable and my room was large.

Barbara greeted me happily and introduced Lyn Quiyou, the hairstylist in charge. Lynn was doing the stars - Tom Cruise and Nicole Kidman. She said that she wanted me to take complete charge of the extras. Recalling my experience on *Havana*, a red light went on in my brain. "What exactly do you mean, by taking charge?" I asked. "I don't want to have to think about the extras at all," she replied. I prayed that she meant that and that she'd be able to use my talent and not resent my help. I had two local hairstylists, Robin and Cindy who became my assistants. I had to teach them a lot about film hairdressing, but they were bright and capable.

The local ice-skating rink had been set up as Wardrobe and Makeup departments. There was lots of room. There were seamstresses and tailors to make alterations of the costumes. I had shelves built for our supplies, bought plants and a few other things to decorate our Hair Department. My makeup partner was Rod Wilson, a friend for forty years.

What an absolutely delicious job. I couldn't think of another way to describe it. I could really sink my teeth into it. The extras had all been cast months before giving the men time to grow long beards and hair and the women let their hair grow too. Lynn had ordered some beautiful hair lace wigs, just in case our bit

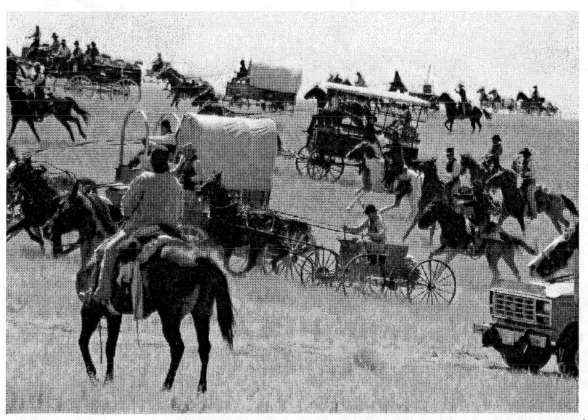

On the set of *Far & Away*

players needed extra hair.

Our schedule went as follows. Every morning our extras came in a few at a time to get their wardrobe fitted. Next they came to us fully dressed with their hats so we could decide how to dress their hair. Then we took a photo, so we could remember in our busy mornings of production what we planned to do. It was fantastic to have that time, because in our last scenes we would be dressing the hair of more than a thousand people.

Far and Away was the story of two young people who come to America, from Ireland, in 1889. Nicole is rich and Tom is poor. Under normal circumstances they would never have met, let alone have had a relationship. As it turns out, they have great difficulties and become separated, but meet again at the Oklahoma Land Race of 1890. It was a fairy tale.

Right before we began shooting, the production company threw a huge kick-off party and invited the crew from *A River Runs Through, which* was shooting in Livingston. Robert Redford never showed up, but I did see a couple of familiar crewmembers. Our set was decorated as a real western ho-down for the occasion.

Working with Ron Howard was super. There was no shouting, no tension and much of that was due to Aldric Porter, our first assistant. I had met Aldric in Chicago on *Running Scared* years before. It tickled me when he reminded how grateful he'd been for the warm jacket I'd given him when he was just starting out. I'd totally forgotten that.

Our first scene took place in a replica of a large saloon in Boston. It was actually shot in the Billings Railway Station. The set looked just perfect. Nobody would ever believe it had been shot in Montana. This was the first place Tom and Nicole come when they arrive in Boston. Tom asks the Irish boss for a job and ends up fighting with a man. He wins and becomes a boxer to earn his living.

The first day on the set, Aldric called, "Sugar, Tom needs something to be done to his hair." Lynne was nowhere around so I walked up to Tom and introduced myself. I did what needed to be done. I was gun shy, not wanting Lynn to think I was after her job, but there was no problem. Lynn was often distant, but could be utterly charming when she wanted to be. I quickly discovered that although she had said for me to take over, she always wanted to change something. That was just her way.

The weather was hot and the saloon was nearly unbearable when the lights were on. Especially uncomfortable were the men dressed in warm woolen suits. As the day went on, the set got hotter and I could smell the damp wool of the costumes along with all of our sweat. I made sure water was available at every break for the extras, for which they were grateful. Nobody else seemed to be concerned. They were all so busy.

Frank and Michelle of For Stars Catering catered for us. Their food was rich, but there were always fresh things available. Unfortunately, I chose to ignore the healthy food, so wonderful were the dishes they prepared. One day I did myself in when I ate fish with a cream sauce and later strawberry shortcake with whipped cream. Soon after lunch I began to feel strange. First my back began to ache, and then a pain came around my right side. I tried lying down in a van, but it still hurt terribly and finally I went to the makeup trailer to tell Lynn I was sick. She took one look at me and said, "Your face is almost green. Please go home." I was able to walk to the hotel a couple of blocks away, so relieved to reach my cool room. A few moments later, there was a knock at my door and a driver had come to take me to the

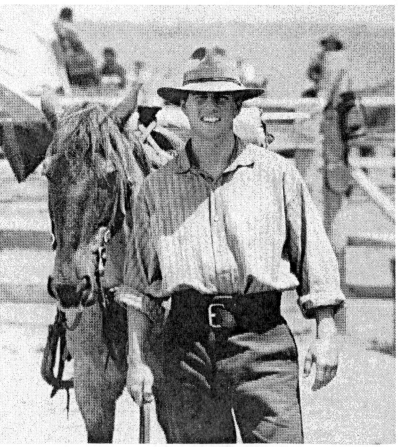

Tom Cruise, Far and Away

hospital. The first aid man had sent him and insisted that I go.

I checked into the emergency room. They gave me a gown and put me into a little cubicle. I lay there in a lot of pain, but at least I was cool and didn't have to go back to the stifling set. The doctor first checked me for ulcers and finally found gallstones. He put me in the hospital for the night. I called Barbara and asked her to bring my things and asked her to call Pat so he wouldn't worry when I didn't answer my phone. The doctor was sure I would need to have my gall bladder removed, which worried me. I needed that job and if I had the operation, I'd be off for six weeks. Besides I didn't want to be cut open. Fortunately the gallstones passed and I told the doctor I didn't want an operation, but I assured him if it returned that I'd be back. I'd never felt pain like that.

As soon as Pat found out what had happened, he called Capitol Drug Store in Van Nuys and asked for a homeopathic cure for gall bladders. A man named Sean, suggested a Chinese herbal remedy called Lia Dan, which dissolved gall stones. I took the remedy and it worked.

Since discovering Beloved Adi Da Samraj, my life had changed. Each morning, I got up early to meditate and study. I learned that I didn't need to try to control everything. No matter what problem came up, I now realized, I could turn it over to my Teacher and let it go. For the first time in my life, I never felt alone and my life felt fuller than ever before. Up until that time, I'd never had a place to turn when I was confused; I never had a real foundation. Although I'd had many exciting, high times especially at work, but when they finished, I'd feel adrift. I'd be waiting for the next excitement to come along. Now I no longer had those ups and downs. I had a direction and a foundation.

It wasn't so easy for Pat. He was worried about the expense of the bookstore. We were paying out far more than we were bringing in. Although he often joked about me supporting him for a change, he didn't feel good about not being the breadwinner. I loved being able to bring in a paycheck because for so many years he had supported my projects. I was happy to do it. Still, despite my assurances, it was hard on him. Meanwhile, he had found a set of tapes of the twelve steps of AA and he began to listen to them on his drive to Montana with my herbs. He began to realize he hadn't gone beyond the fourth step and it was time to move on through all twelve. Later I listened to them along with him and he remarked. "You were born knowing the twelve steps Ginger."

Pat arrived the day before my fifty-seventh birthday. He gave me the herbs and I started taking them immediately. We set up a little kitchen in the room, so I could toast pita bread and make tea or coffee. I had a little fridge for veggies. By then I knew that the fat in my diet was causing the gall bladder problems. Now that I was not supposed to use butter or oil, I began to long for it. But I refrained, because I never wanted to feel that pain again.

My mother who was to be eighty in August sent me a birthday card. My sister had helped her express her feelings toward me when she asked "Why do you love Sugar?" My mother had answered, "I love her, because she's always happy." This was written on the card. It brought tears to my eyes. My mother's life had not been very happy.

Montana was truly "big sky country", it stretched out forever. From my hotel room window I could watch incredible storms, with thunder and lightening shooting across the sky. It was nature at it's wildest. Sometimes there would be huge hailstones falling while we were at the rink. The noise was so loud that we couldn't hear each other speak. The hail damaged many cars, giving the car repair business a real boost.

Pat became the location housewife. He'd see me

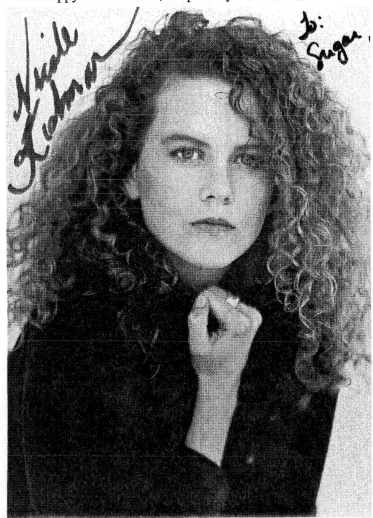

Nicole Kidman

off to work and then take a long walk. After his walk, he'd sit on the key bench, downtown, under a big tree, drinking gourmet coffee and eating delicious, fresh muffins from the bakery. He went to the library and began to study the waterways which were amazing engineering feats located all-around Billings. In the evenings he was back at the hotel with something ready for me to eat, ready to give me a back rub or whatever was necessary to make me feel good. I appreciated his care yet I understood that he would have rather been at work on his own project.

As usual, I had done lots of research for this film. I'd found photos of my father, as a young man, taken in 1890. He'd actually been a sheriff in Oklahoma during the time period we were shooting on the film. In his photos he had short hair so when the extras fussed at the short haircuts, I whipped out my father's picture to let them see how "real" men wore their hair in those days. I once again began to regret that I hadn't asked more questions about Daddy's life while he was still alive.

Nicole Kidman was a Gemini. Her June birthday came along and Tom Cruise threw a huge surprise party for her. He invited the whole crew. It was held in the saloon set. We were finished with it. We all came early and hid so Nicole wouldn't see us when she entered. In walked Nicole and Tom. The music began to play and we all shouted "Surprise!" Next Tom gave her his present. He'd brought her whole family up from Australia - her parents, brothers and sisters and their children. Nicole was so happy and surprised and Tom was absolutely thrilled at her pleasure.

What a great party. There was fabulous food, free drinks, and music. We all had fun, but Tom and Nicole had the best time of all, dancing in circles with the children. I played with Ron Howard's little son Reid, who reminded everyone of what Ron looked like as a child. Everyone had their children there. It was a huge family party.

Keeping the atmosphere on the crew enjoyable was important to Ron. Every Friday there was a special theme at lunch. Frank, our caterer, would produce something unusual. One day there were magicians, another day they parachuted from a plane. One day they had a Mexican theme, but I worked my way through lunch on a second unit. I was so thirsty when I got back and so dry, that all I could do was gulp down the non-alcoholic Margueritas, one after another, forget the tacos.

The finale of the film, the big race, was rapidly approaching. Each day we dressed the extras' hair for the scene they were shooting that day. I'd send Robin and Cindy to standby on the set, while I stayed behind to give haircuts to the rest of the extras that arrived hourly.

Lynne was difficult at times. She couldn't explain what she wanted in clear terms. Maybe she only knew what it was when she saw it, but it was frustrating for me and sometimes hard not to take it personally. Many days I did what I thought she wanted, only to have her change her mind after I was finished. For example, one morning she told me how she wanted me to cut the hair of some well-dressed male extras. Thinking I was doing what she wanted, I cleaned off

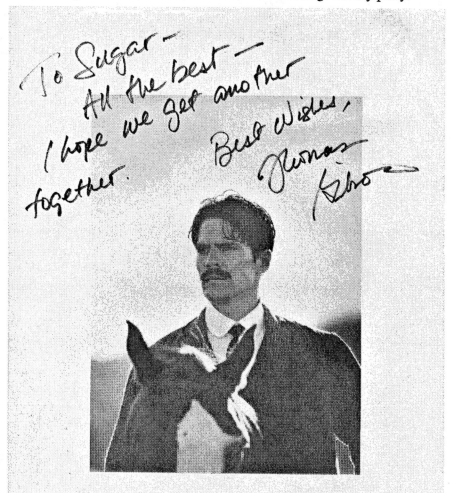

Signed photo of Thomas Gibson

the

hair on their necks and sent them to the set. Lynn called me and bawled me out for not leaving enough hair on the necks. Fortunately while she was yelling at me over the phone, a hailstorm blew in and the sound on the roof was so loud that I could hardly hear her. Later on the set, she acted like nothing had happened. One other time I had kept a hairdresser with me at the rink to help me because I had too much work to do alone. Lynn called again to yell, but this time the phone fizzled out. I was blessed somehow. I decided to just get on with it and run my department as best as I could.

There were going to be nearly a thousand extras for the race and I needed to hire more hairdressers. I called and got the list of available hairdressers from the union and began calling them. When a hairdresser said yes, I gave their name to the production secretary who called them back with the dates they would be needed. Our production manager, Larry DeWaay, was a person Pat and I had known since working on *Gaily, Gaily*. He was tough with the money and kept cutting down on my help. I tried to make him understand how having a couple of extra hairdressers would actually save time and money, but it never changed his mind. He even balked at Lynn buying extra bobby pins.

Our second assistant, Cheryl Ann, just didn't cut it as far as I was concerned. She never communicated with us and as we were always miles from the set, it caused many problems for me. Often I had to take responsibility for decisions that shouldn't have been mine to make. I had found during my many years in the industry that I was willing to take responsibility, if nobody else was willing, when perhaps I should have stepped back. But, in my mind, production came first and I didn't want to sit around and watch problems develop just so the person who should have taken care of things would get into trouble. I think Cheryl Ann just never considered us important. She seemed to forget all the work we did behind the scenes.

Oh, it was hot out on the prairie and we stood in the broiling sun for hours. Trying to keep cool, I'd put a wet cotton scarf beneath my hat. I constantly dipped in water both hat and scarf, but it dried so fast that, I had to do it often. At the end of the day I could hardly wait to get into my air-conditioned room and shower off the accumulated dust.

More stunt men arrived for the big race. I saw a familiar name on the call sheet; Jerry Gatlin. He had been the young stuntman who had fed me the jalapenos along with his friend Chuck Hayward so many years before in Tucson on *McLintock!*. When I saw him, I was amazed. He appeared to have lost all his energy. The sparkle he'd had in his eyes when he was young had disappeared. He looked worn out and it made me sad. I thought about so many of my favorite stunt men that had lived and played hard. Now they were dealing with their aches and pains and limped a lot.

After finally identifying Jerry, I walked over to talk with him. That day the horses were running wild and so I asked him a stupid question. "Where do you go, when a horse runs toward you?" For the first time, I saw the old sparkle come back into his eyes as he answered. "Out of the way." His humor still surfaced. He told me that now he preferred the simple life. He was happiest when he took off with his two mules into the mountains of Wyoming where he lived all alone.

We were filming a scene where Tom Cruise stopped in a bar and has a few too many. I was standing by on the set, behind the tent when Tom walked back toward me. He stood beside me. I figured it would be okay to talk with him. I asked if he was having a good time. He smiled, "I'm having the best time I ever had on a movie." He was so happy working with Nicole and Ron and it showed. Tom had so much enthusiasm. He had learned to ride a horse like a real trooper. With it all he was just as nice as he had been when I met him on *All the Right Moves* in Pennsylvania, years before. Now he did keep more to himself than he had at that time, but I understood it was for his own self-preservation.

The Reinactors arrived. They are folks who do everything they can to simulate a certain period in history. They dressed completely in styles of the period they preferred. They had the correct weapons and transportation. Reilly Flynn was the man who arranged for hundreds of people to take part in the race. They were a great boon to the film.

A village had been set up where they would live, including a huge meal tent and an amazing truck that held toilets, showers and sinks. It was very clever. The truck was filled and emptied daily. Our hair and makeup tent was set up right next to the village so we were able to watch as they began to trickle in. First a couple of trucks arrived, pulling horse trailers. They began to set up house. Soon more and more people began to arrive from all over the country. There were covered wagons, other wagons, oxen, horses and many means of transportation used in the 1890's. They were unloaded and it was an incredible sight. Within a week the whole campground was filled with people who came to work in the race scene.

The Reinactors came to us and we fitted some for hair, but mostly they were used to dressing in the proper time period. In reality the men would not have had time for haircuts so we didn't have to be too picky ourselves. Many of the women were used to doing their own hair and some had their own costumes. It was amazing.

I had a great hairdressing crew. My friend's Shirley Dolle, Vivian Macateer and Cheryl Ross all came to help. My local girls, Robin and Cindy, had become very capable, but were not used to this kind of huge set up. I was happy to be working with friends, professionals who knew how to deal with such a big crowd. Hiring more local hairdressers, just wouldn't have worked. I needed experienced people.

The big day arrived and with it, the earliest call I'd ever had - 1:45 a.m. I never slept the night before because of the anticipation of that next day. That first morning we all dragged ourselves to the bus and off we went to location, immediately heading for our tent and to work. We set up and had our coffee and got to work. Our thousand extras were all ready by the time Production was ready to shoot.

We stood on the set watching the five hundred wagons, eight hundred horses and a thousand extras line up for the first shot. Rudy Ugland, our head wrangler had given a speech and explained to all the extras and everyone involved about safety. In no uncertain terms, he told them to forget going out and trying to become a "star". If they did, they could cause injury to themselves and others. Our first aid man was very thorough and he had done a study of possible injuries, even figuring that someone could possibly be killed in the scene. He was prepared for anything with a helicopter standing by to transfer any injured to the hospital.

The first scene took forever to set up and then suddenly they were ready. We held our collective breath as the horn blew and off they went. It was an exciting moment, horses galloping, wagons flying, people running, whooping and yelling with the larger-covered wagons slowly coming behind. I prayed that everyone would be safe, but one extra decided to be a star and did get hurt, but not badly. The only other injury was to a horse, which was sad. I felt as though I was right there when the real race had taken place in Oklahoma a hundred years before. We were reliving history that day, and I understood the Reinactor's fascination and enthusiasm,

The first day of the race, we worked seventeen and a half hours. We continued for five more days filming the huge scenes and later we picked up stunts with a smaller crew. My extra help, with the exception of Shirley, went back home.

Then in no time at all, we were back to our basic crew that had begun the film. Our last big scene, which was minute compared to the great race, took place in a chicken-plucking factory where Nicole had to go to work. It was a terrible place and we all had sweat pouring off us in that heat. The women's faces were all red and their hair was bound up with rags. I sprayed them with cool water whenever it was possible. Lynne actually told me she was very pleased with my work on this scene.

It was almost the end of the location in Montana and I was beginning to pack up my things to send back to Los Angeles. Most of the crew was packing to go on to Ireland. Dublin would become Boston of the 1880's and Dingle, on the west coast of Ireland would become the birthplace of the character Tom Cruise played in the beginning of the film. I had not even thought of going to Ireland and I was so happy Barbara was going to get the chance to go.

The last weekend the company threw a huge party, inviting all the crew, and all the locals that had worked on the

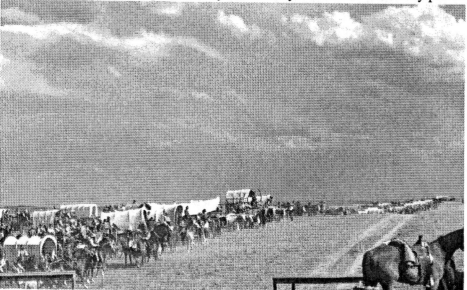

On Location of *Far & Away*

film. The charter for Ireland was due to leave the next Friday. Pat, Barbara and I arrived at the party early. We walked in, helped ourselves to hors d'oeuvres and walked up to the bar to get ourselves a drink. Barbara ended up with a drink in each hand, but she never had a chance to take a sip, when suddenly she tripped and fell on a tiny stair on the way to our table. She landed on her right shoulder.

We helped her up, but she was in a lot of pain and it only got worse. We realized she needed to go to the hospital. The diagnosis wasn't good. She was all set to go to Ireland in a few days and now she had injured her shoulder. All along, she had been saying she couldn't believe she was going to Ireland. I had told her not to say that. Lynn gave Barbara a few days to see if she might heal quickly, but she couldn't even lift her arm. Finally the doctor said there was no way she would be able to do anyone's hair. Lynn was not happy. I felt so sorry for Barbara. What a disappointment.

After the doctor pronounced the verdict and Barbara knew she wouldn't be able to go, I told Lynn that I had my passport and I'd be willing to help out if she needed me. She said, "I don't think that will be necessary." I kept on packing, addressing and sending my things back to Los Angeles.

Suddenly Lynne decided that she wanted me to go to Ireland after all. I reminded her that I didn't have a work permit, but she said we could get around that. I agreed to go to Ireland and that night I hurried home to re-pack. I had so much to do and so little time to get it done. Lynn remarked, "Sugar, you don't seem to be excited about going to Ireland." I explained that I needed to stay calm and focused if I was going to be ready in time. I did manage to get everything done and as I boarded the plane to Ireland, I was finally able to relax.

I missed my mother's eightieth birthday party in Los Angeles. My mother had suffered a stroke three years before. She had worked until she was nearly seventy-seven. She had never been a truly happy person, but she had been brave and coped with her life and what it had offered, in the best way she knew. Since her stroke, she seemed to be closer to God, more forgiving. She looked quite beautiful in the photo I received from my sisters. Her hair was very white and her eyes a bright blue.

I was on my way to Ireland with the rest of the crew, on the chartered plane, but I had no work permit. It had taken the others three months to get one legally. Our unit manager suggested I should say I was just along for the ride, if asked about it, when I went through immigration. It reminded me of the time on *Who'll Stop the Rain* when the unit manager told me to hide in the closet of the freighter if we were boarded by the Coast Guard, because we were overloaded.

It was a very long eleven-hour flight and we snoozed all scrunched up in our seats. I awoke as we began our descent into the Dublin Airport. Looking out of the window, I could see the countryside with its hedgerows. It reminded me of a giant patchwork quilt. It was lovely. The Irish were friendly folks and I passed through customs without a hitch. We boarded a bus for Dublin where we were checked into the first-rate Westbury Hotel, right downtown. My room was pretty with flowered bedspreads and chairs, the large bathroom complete with a deep bathtub, which by now you know is one of my favorite things.

I unpacked, set up the little coffee pot and grinder that I carried everywhere. I laid out a pretty cloth on a table where I placed Adi Da Samraj's picture. Next I went in search of flowers for my room and was I surprised when I found the weather very warm.

Grafton Street was teeming with people when I stepped out the door of the hotel. A Hare Krishna group came dancing and singing down the sidewalk, beating drums and playing finger cymbals. There were girls in saris, young people sitting on the sidewalks with half-shaved, tattooed heads. Shops displayed signs warning, "Watch out for Pickpockets".

I bought a brightly colored bunch of flowers and found my way back to the hotel. I could hear sea gulls screaming through my open window and it was warm and muggy. Below my window were two pubs. I wondered just how noisy would they be at night. It didn't matter at that moment because I was so exhausted that after a hot bath I fell into bed and was in dreamland in a moment.

Because of our seven-hour time difference, we had a day to rest before going back to work. I just relaxed. That night I ordered a cucumber sandwich and a draft Guinness Stout, brewed right there in Dublin. From that night on I enjoyed a pint while I took my bath in the evenings.

Our first day of work took us to a huge estate in Kilruddery. I'd read about these wonderful places, but had never seen one. It was impressive. Martin, our driver for the duration, drove us there in his VW bus. He was a big, jolly, kind man who loved his beer and his pub.

The weather was damp and foggy, giving an almost mystical feeling which enhanced the marvelous setting. Set away from the main house was the production area. We had a huge makeup trailer for the stars and a smaller one for the extras. I introduced myself to Ann, the Irish head hairdresser who was taking Barbara's place beside Lynne. She appeared friendly enough, but later I discovered that wasn't the case at all.

It was early and the extras weren't there yet, so we went to breakfast. I'd never seen anything like this elegant set up. Astro-turf had been laid on the wet lawn so our shoes wouldn't get wet. The tent was "brilliant" as the British say - huge, puffy, inflated, pink and white. Inside there was every kind of breakfast food you could imagine: hot cereal, coffee, tea, rolls, toast, butter, honey, jam, fruit, juice and more. Just outside the tent, in a small trailer, was a grill where we could order anything such as eggs, bacon, ham, sausages, potatoes, kippers, pancakes or waffles. It was as classy a setup as I'd ever seen.

Breakfast finished, with full bellies, we began dressing the ladies' hair. That day's scene took place inside the elegant home and the costumes and hairdos' were fancy. I warned Ann that Lynne preferred the hairdos to be rather flat than full and that she tended to yell when she wasn't pleased. It was to no avail. Ann didn't like having an "American" tell her what to do, so she didn't listen. And just like I'd warned her, Lynn yelled. Oh well, I tried.

After we finished with all the ladies, I went to check out the set before I left for the warehouse. The crew was preparing for the first shot. The house was perfect, with hounds and the owners dressed in tweeds, just like one would expect. It must have been hundreds of years old.

Our warehouse in Dublin was located beside the River Liffy. It was similar to our Montana setup. It housed the wardrobe, the tailors, makeup and hair plus a lunchroom. Our American cook Mary prepared the most sumptuous vegetarian lunches and there was always the Irish Tea and soda bread with jam available all day long.

My two co-workers were terrific girls, both of them great characters. Martina was a high-spirited tiny redhead. Driscoll had long black Rastafarian extensions and wore them tied up on top of her head with a scarf, which gave the illusion that she was wearing a black palm tree. Our head makeup woman from Ireland was Toni. She, like Ann, appeared to be so nice and friendly. She reminded me of an opossum. She was short and round and her voice purred. Later I discovered she was sort of a Godfather/Mother (Mafia style) who had great power over many of the Irish people in our company. People feared her because she could make or break their careers. I wondered how this worked, but never found out. Sometimes she and Ann teamed up to make it miserable for all of us including the Irish girls. I didn't get it.

Each morning I called a taxi to take me to the warehouse. I charged it to the company. Soon the dispatcher knew my voice and would say "Is this Sugar?" I began to feel he was an old friend. Martina and Driscoll and I set up our haircutting stations and the extras began to arrive. Just as they had done in Montana, they came to us dressed in costumes so we could design their hair.

In Dublin there was an area called Temple Bar that doubled as Boston 1890. The streets were cobblestones and the buildings ancient. Our production designer had built the whorehouse to fit right in with all the rest of the buildings. I could hardly distinguish it from the real ones. By the time the props had been dressed around the area, it looked and felt just like the 1890's.

The crew moved to Temple Bar and we had a makeup set up in a building down there. In the mornings I'd oversee the extras for Lynne, so there would be continuity between what we had filmed in Montana and what we were filming in Dublin. Ann resented my help. She didn't care how the hair looked, she just wanted it done her way - an attitude I found difficult to understand. I was relieved when I finished each morning and was able to return to the warehouse and my friends and those great lunches.

It was unusually hot for Dublin and the hotel had no air-conditioning. To make matters worse I had difficulty sleeping, thanks to the noise from the two pubs outside my window. If I wanted to be cool at night I needed to have my windows open, but then there was too much noise. I soon bought a fan and kept the windows closed.

The shooting company worked at night and we did the fitting during the days. It was like we had two separate film companies. We never saw each other. One evening the company threw a party for everyone, but it didn't start until eleven o'clock. I took a nap and went for a little while, but was ready to leave by the time the rest of the crew arrived. Eventually we, the day crew threw our own party and it was far more fun.

Unfortunately, I wasn't very happy in Dublin. After the jet lag wore off, I got an ear virus. I also missed my family. Often I felt like the unwanted stepchild. Production wanted me to hurry and finish and go home, so they could cut costs. I was working as fast as I could. I wasn't the only unhappy person. Nobody liked the way we were all treated in the warehouse. Toni and Ann's bitchiness took its toll. All of us felt we were being treated like servants. I finally gave up on our American crew. I felt far more connected with my new Irish friends anyway. At least we had fun together. They had the ability to laugh at themselves. They lived for the moment or the day and weren't impressed by wealth at all. I liked that.

The final straw came one night when they were filming the burning of the estate. An extra had come to us with a weird haircut, long on top and short all around the bottom. I tried to make it look presentable and it looked just all right. Besides he played the part of a terrorist and was wearing a burlap bag over his head in the scene. I wasn't worried about it. He never took the bag off his head.

Early the next morning, Lynn called yelling loudly. "How could you give such a terrible haircut?" She told me not to do any more haircuts, just to oversee the others cutting hair. I couldn't believe it; in fact, I truly had no idea what she was talking about and asked her to send a photo of the extra. Later I found out that Ann and Toni had brought this man to her attention to show her what awful work I did. I sensed they made it look as bad as they could on their own. Anyway by this time I was in tears. Everyone in the warehouse was furious with Lynne. They knew how hard I had worked. I pleaded with Lynne to see clearly how devious Toni and Ann were and how they always tried to stir up trouble to make themselves look better. Lynne was the head of the Hair Department and I told her she shouldn't be intimidated by them.

Later Lynne seemed to come to her senses and called back to apologize. By now I understood she was insecure and sometimes became hysterical and tended to take it out on me. Understanding it didn't make me like it any better. I knew I'd done a great job. On the plus side, I figured I'd given more than a thousand haircuts that summer and earned almost $40,000 which was why I took the job, after all.

The day of our big set arrived. We had been preparing for it for a month. The Guinness Brewery was supposed to be Ellis Island where Immigration was located at the time, in America. It looked very much like the real thing. Once again, just like our big race, we reported to work at 1:00 a.m. The extras piled in and kept coming for hours. It was never ending. When we finished, I walked out into the street and it looked fabulous. There were horses and buggies, little pushcarts, crowds of people everywhere. In this scene Nicole and Tom have arrived in America and immediately are robbed by a swindler. As I stood observing the scene, I was proud and knew it had been worth all the work I had done. My department had run smoothly and I was pleased with my work despite the painful aspects.

That morning, for the first time, Lynne congratulated and thanked me. Then she said, "Sugar, why don't you just take a vacation and see some of Ireland before you leave. These ladies are never going to be nice to you. You've finished what you came to do and I am grateful." She was right too. I hadn't seen much of anything, so I gave her a hug and kiss and said good-by. I rushed to the hotel to pack and by 10:00 a.m. was on the train to Galway, heading west. My trip was perfect. I saw the green fields with sheep grazing, the beauty of the true Ireland.

Upon my arrival in Galway, I walked to the tourist bureau and booked myself into a B&B outside of town and found a taxi to take me there. As the drive took me past Galway Bay and out of town, the countryside became more picturesque as we drove on. The B&B was in a modern house, but my room was cozy.

Although weary from my early morning, I decided to take a short walk down the dirt road toward the bay that was glistening in the afternoon light. I was met and greeted by an old man leading his cows down the road past a thatched-roof cottage. After an early dinner, I crawled under the down comforter and went to sleep, even though it wasn't yet dark. I was exhausted, relieved and very happy. I left for Dingle the next morning, well rested.

Once in Dingle, I walked up a hill and checked into the quaint Brenner Hotel where our crew would also stay when they arrived. Natalie, our location girl, called and we planned to meet the next day so she could show me around the area. I walked around Dingle that afternoon, investigating the beautiful gardens and back roads. I found a bookstore where they had a bar and enjoyed my lunch among the books. The next morning Natalie picked me up and we drove up the coast. She asked if I'd mind stopping by her cottage. "Of course not." I replied. What a sweet white cottage, surrounded by fuchsia bushes with a walled herb garden. The rooms inside were small and cozy. I could picture myself there on a vacation some day.

Across from Natalie's cottage was an orange caravan and she introduced me to the two men and a woman who lived there. The men were fishermen. They served us coffee in handmade cups along with homemade bread and honey. As we talked, I observed the men. They were very attractive in a boyish way and very charming. The woman seemed much harder. Many of the Irish women seemed to take on masculine qualities that their lovely mates lacked.

After a delightful visit, we took off for the set. Off the shore I could see mystical islands in the distance. Natalie described how many poets and writers had lived on those islands centuries before. I loved the mystery and history that were so much a part of Ireland and I enjoyed myself completely. I felt like a totally different person than I had been in Dublin.

The first set we came to was the cottage overlooking the ocean. It would be burned down at the beginning of the film. I slipped off my sandals and walked barefoot down the hill, toward it. I wanted to get a better look and see how a thatched roof was actually made. I pictured my ancestors living in a place like this generations earlier. Next we went to see the little poverty stricken village set where Tom's character had grown up. They were just putting the finishing touches on it, but it looked as if it had been there for more than a hundred years. As we drove through the countryside, I could see the results of the glaciers and Roman rock walls. It was fascinating.

We had breakfast the next morning and before I knew it, I was waiting for the 5:35 p.m. train back to Dublin. When I arrived in Dublin, I went straight to the hotel and to my room. The next day I want by the studio to settle everything and said good-by to my friends in the office. I didn't go to the set. I wanted to retain my happy memories of the last three days and forget the conflict.

The next day I flew home. In the end, I was happy I had gone to Ireland. I found a love for the Irish people, learned something about my heritage and had enjoyed working with my crew in the warehouse. My only regret was that Barbara hadn't been able to be there too.

Chapter 72

STAY TUNED
Vancouver, Canada; Tucson, Arizona

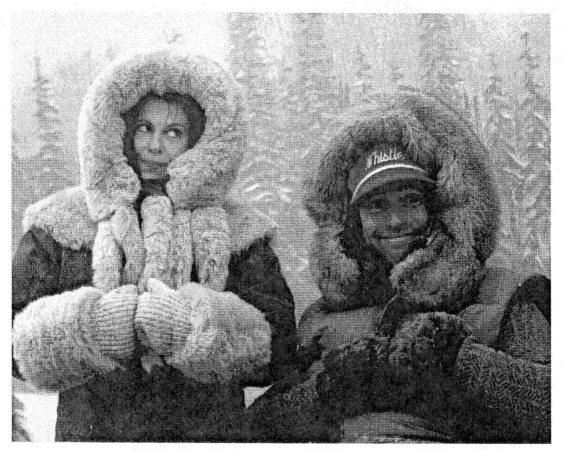

Pam Dawber and John Ritter, *Stay Tuned*

By the time I arrived home from Ireland, I'd had enough of location. It felt so good to be home with my family. My bookstore had grown. My inner life had become full and rich. I noticed that I no longer reacted to everything that happened. I was beginning to pause and observe and then make a choice on how to respond to a situation or not respond at all. I realized that all my high and low adventures could come and go and I was still free to enjoy whatever came up.

Our taxes were being audited. I went to see my accountant, Millie. She explained how much work she would need to do and I casually remarked, "At $80.00 an hour for you, I'd better get right back to work." As soon as those words were out of my mouth, I got a call from Peter Hyams' company, which was shooting in Vancouver, Canada. He was directing a film called *Stay Tuned*. It was a silly film about a couple that get sucked up into a television dish and spend time in TV Hell trying to escape. It starred Pam Dawber, John Ritter, and Jeffrey Jones. Lee Harmon, my old friend was going to do the makeup.

Thinking back to my summer prayer, I realized that once again my wishes had been granted. "I'd love to come," was my answer. There was a plus factor. Pat was working on *An American Heart* in nearby Seattle. I could visit him on the weekends seeing as we only worked a five-day week in Canada.

I fell in love with Vancouver. It became one of my all time favorite cities. As the plane came in for a landing, I could see mountains, oceans, trees, and it was lovely. My home was the luxurious Meridian Hotel. It was in the downtown area that consisted of wonderful shops and restaurants. When I checked in, I expected to be shown to a normal hotel room. Instead, to my delight, when the door opened, I found that it was a large apartment. It was a perfect place to live for a few months. It was in the hotel complex and I had all the amenities, like maid and room service. It was a lovely apartment, the furniture rich and traditional in lovely colors. There was a fully equipped kitchen and a balcony where I could watch the sunset over the ocean. I couldn't have asked for more.

As soon as I was unpacked, the driver took me to pick up a rental car provided by the company. I was concerned about driving myself in a strange city, so always gave myself extra time to get lost each morning.

Our studio was called the Bridge Studio. It was a strange name, but it was where they had made bridges in the past. A part of the Golden Gate Bridge in San Francisco had been constructed there. A couple of the stages had strange shapes, because they had accommodated bridge parts. Peter greeted me with a hug, happy to see me again. I was given a script to study and eventually Lee arrived from Oregon.

We decided to get reacquainted over lunch, down by the ocean. I hadn't seen him for a few years. He had finally convinced his wife to move from Arizona to Corvallis Oregon. During college, he'd been a basketball star at the college and always been looked up to since then. He was a big fish in a little pond. He'd driven his large motor home to Vancouver to live in so he could save the per diem they paid him for his room. It wasn't as comfortable as my place, but he was able save a lot of money.

We ordered lunch and I had a beer. Lee was surprised at me. He assumed I'd order a glass of wine and wondered when I'd become so common. He talked about how he loved golf so much that he had a golf cart complete with curtains that was rain proof. He could golf in any weather. I didn't understand how golf could be all that encompassing, but it appeared to be his main interest.

Wanting to be fully prepared for anything, I'd brought all my wigs with me. We were going to shoot a scene from the French Revolution and I knew I would use them. I hired a perfect assistant, Kandace Loewen. She was young and lovely, smart and capable. Lee hired Sandy, a great makeup artist. Sandy developed a crush on Lee. He reminded her of her father, with his gray beard and teddy bear body. I liked Sandy, but I think she was a little jealous of my friendship with Lee and never warmed up to me.

Pam Dawber was fabulous. I'd met her when she was filming *An American Geisha* in Kyoto, Japan. She remembered Pat, and said she sort of remembered me. It

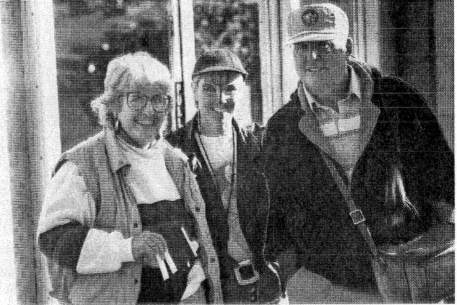

Sugar on the set of *Stay Tuned* with Kandace and Lee

wasn't really important. I liked her immediately. She became one of my favorite people. Pam was genuine, intelligent, and well traveled, and her lovely, thick brown hair was great to work with. We found we had many things in common.

John Ritter was likable, and would do anything not to offend. He was funny and sweet, but I sensed there was a lot going on inside him that had never been expressed. He would zone out and fall asleep while I was fixing his hair. He loved to have a shoulder rub and was grateful for that if I had time. I found his assistant Chad to be spiritually inclined and we became friends.

This film was a real challenge, the kind of challenge I loved. There were scenes from many different time periods because our stars were going from TV film to TV film in this TV Hell. John's character was a major couch potato and he sells his soul to the devil, played by Jeffrey Jones. When the TV dish sucks him up, his wife Pam has to rescue him.

We set up our makeup and hair trailer and I put a photo of Adi Da Samraj up on my mirror so I could always see Him and introduce Him to others. I kept some of his books to offer people who might be interested in His Teaching, in the trailer. My life had changed in such a positive way; I wanted to share it with everyone who might be interested. They would ask about Him and then sort of zone out after a little bit. They appeared to be satisfied with their lives and weren't ready to question or look for answers. I didn't push, but I longed to be able to find people who wanted a spiritual life and were willing to get into a discussion. Pam was the only one interested. I gave her some of my books to take home.

My first weekend, I took off for Seattle, heading to the waterfront and Pat's delightful little waterfront condo. I arrived early and was there before he got home. We walked to the nearby market and had dinner. The next day he showed me around Seattle. The weather was perfect.

The next weekend I was able to go to Seattle again. This time I visited the set. They were shooting at a lovely house on an island. The director, Martin Bell, had worked with Pat on a commercial earlier that year and Pat had expressed a desire to do a film in Seattle. Martin obliged him. Martin's wife, Mary Ellen Mark, was the still photographer, famous in her own right. Jeff Bridges and Edward Furlong played father and son. Jeff was attractive, nice and charming. I saw some of my friends from Los Angeles who were working on the crew and had fun visiting.

My favorite place in all of Seattle was the huge bookstore in Pioneer Square. I'd never seen anything like it. There was a coffee shop right inside it. My second favorite thing was a Starbuck's coffee house. They were just coming into their own. I loved their fresh ground coffee and espresso.

We began filming at the tract house where John Ritter and the family lived. It was where the devil, in the guise of a TV repairman, shows up. Jeffrey made a wonderful devil.

I had lots of preparation to do. We had many extras to get ready for the big scenes. We had a 1940's nightclub, a wrestling event, a French Revolution, a quiz show, scenes from the far north and the Wild West. I hired many Canadian hairstylists to help me. We set up our Hair Department on one of the stages. It was so much fun. In the mornings, I'd fix Pam's hair and then go to help with the extras. The Canadians were thrilled that I would work with them. Their experience with most Americans who came to work in Canada was not good. They said they felt looked down upon and most Americans kept to themselves and even never invited the Canadians into their trailer to visit. They never offered to help out on the big calls. They described the Americans as looking and treating them like they were like peasants or something of the sort. I could appreciate their complaints, because of my recent experience in Ireland. But still, I didn't understand it.

I loved the Canadian crew. They reminded me of what it had been like when I first started out working in the movie business. They were sweet, kind people, ready to assist each another, not out do, or do in, each other. It was refreshing. Our unit manager, from the USA, was an old friend of mine, Arnie Schmidt. I'd worked with him on *Who'll Stop the Rain*. He was a good person and especially kind. His Canadian counterpart was Michael McDonald.

The company had been generous with me and my salary matched Lee's salary. I was paid $3000 a week, and case rental. They couldn't pay into my medical plan, but I was compensated for that. I was very happy with my deal. Lee commented in his pessimistic way. "It's so good, how can it last?" I wasn't worried. I had a truly abundant year's earning, over a $100,000 with three months off. Amazing!

Our 1940 nightclub looked absolutely fabulous. There was a fight and we dressed our boyish stunt girl all up in satin, high heels and a snazzy hairdo. She looked so cute, but was quite uncomfortable. She'd never worn high heels in her life.

I needed some special wigs for our actors and there was nobody in Canada to supply them. I called Mathew Mungle, who I worked with on *The Doctor,* and he gave me the name of a wig maker, who made them quickly. They were beautiful wigs. Lee had to order total facemasks for doubles for a sword fight in the castle for John and Jeffrey. I needed two wigs for John during the French Revolution. He had to have one for the time period. I used a long blond wig Madeleine Kahn had worn in *High Anxiety* for the part of the female. John looked quite attractive in those long blond curls, if a bit large of face.

When the facemasks arrived they didn't look like John or Jeffrey. They had such serious expressions. Nobody had given a thought to the fact that when someone has their face cast in plaster; it is not a pleasant procedure. The facial expressions of the masks reflected that.

In the beginning, Lee and I would bicker, like we always had done, just for fun. Kandace and Sandy said we were like an old married couple. Lee would say, "Well, I've known her for thirty years, but I can't divorce her." He'd talk about all the women who had loved him in the past - Barbra Streisand, Faye Dunaway and more. All stories I'd heard before, but I didn't hold up any fingers like he had done to me in Chicago, years before. These young women couldn't imagine us two old timers in our heyday. They didn't realize that even though we'd changed a lot on the outside, inside our young spirits remained alive. They laughed at us all the time. Lee would tell me how I reminded him of his mother. At first I thought that was nice, but later I found out that when he was growing up, she had done everything for him, including his homework. She even helped him win a basketball scholarship. I later began to realize underneath it all, he might have resented her.

The French Revolution was superb. My hairstylists outdid themselves. The extras looked glorious. They had taken my wigs, built them up, powdered them and it amazed me. Peter came up to me and said, "Hot Stuff, Sugar." I started to give the hairstylists the credit when Peter stopped me. "Stop," he said. "Sugar, take the credit. If it hadn't been good, you would have had to take responsibility for that too. So accept the praise." It was a good lesson to learn.

Pam and I became very good friends. We had a great time communicating and talking about life in general while I did her hair. She had traveled all over the world and lived a full life for which she was grateful. Now she was married to Mark Harmon and had one darling son and was pregnant with her second child. She was having troubles keeping the baby and had to go for shots, but later had a healthy son. They were buying and refurbishing a new home at the same time. I loved her describing *Mork and Mindy* and her experiences with Robin Williams and Jonathan Winter. What insanity that must have been. She had such respect for Robin's talent.

John Ritter was always kind, but disconnected, off on a cloud. I felt sorry for him and one day offered to give him some of Adi Da's writings, thinking it might be helpful. He gracefully changed the subject after I mentioned it, as though he hadn't heard me. I guess he didn't want to say that he didn't want it. I would have understood.

One night while filming a scene, I found myself walking the streets of downtown Vancouver at 3:00 a.m. I began to think to myself. When I was younger, I could never have imagined myself at fifty-seven doing things like this. I was amazed.

Peter Hyams, our director, loved to talk about the making of movies. He said he hoped nobody ever realized how much he loved directing because they could probably get him for free, if they only knew. He preferred making a million. He loved Nick, our key grip, who was a passionate man. Peter began to describe the great beauty of a passionate person. "That's what attracts us to them," he said. "Passionate people are willing to expose themselves, take chances, and put themselves on the line. They put their essential selves into living their lives as children do." I agreed with Peter. He was passionate himself and that was why I loved working with him.

As work progressed Lee became more sarcastic and even mean at times, always putting me down. I'd been through this before in Chicago, so I tried to keep from reacting. One day on the set, Peter asked, "Why do you let him get away with that?" I thought for a moment and announced, "Well if he wants to make an ass out of himself, that's his problem." The crew all laughed and Lee didn't like that. Still, he didn't stop. One afternoon while I was listening to John Ritter talk about something, Lee walked up to John and butted right into our conversation. "Oh, how is it she isn't talking for a change, just listening?' Seeing as he was so rude, I decided to be evil and replied. "I am listening because he has something interesting to say."

Xochi came to visit and we toured that weekend. John, the double for John in the sword fight, called me one weekend and asked if I'd like to go to Victoria Island. It was already one o'clock on a Sunday afternoon. I said sure, I was curious. We caught the 3:00 p.m. ferry to Victoria. It was a beautiful ride; we passed by many small islands. We took a short drive through the town and it began to pour. Not wanting to walk around in the rain, we came back on the 6:00 p.m. ferry, but at least I got to see the island.

My favorite crewmember was Joel Whist, who worked in special effects. He told me about his father who had been in the Norwegian underground during the Second World War. He described his parents' home on Salt Sea Island, which his mother had designed. She had put sculptures of their faces on the ceiling of the rooms on the top floor. I hoped to see it one day. Joel had fallen in love with Thailand and told me he wanted to open up a snack bar on the beach. A few years later I went there and fully understood why he loved it so much.

The wardrobe women were such fun. Debbie Douglas, one of them told me that if I ever worked on a film with Mel Gibson, I should drop a water balloon on him for her. She had worked with him and he had thrown them at her. Mel was going to film in Maine the next summer and there was a possibility I could have worked with him.

Lee no longer enjoyed my company. I realize now that I had changed over the years and grown. He had remained the same. He still wore the facade of the "ex-jock" and told the same stories over and over. The guys all liked him because he was an athlete, but it was wearing thin. His twin brother, who he didn't get along with, had cancer. I kept after him telling him to make up and deal with it before his brother died. Being my most Pollyanna self, I brought him books and tapes to help. Sometimes Lee's mind appeared to be elsewhere. He tried to keep his work as simple as possible so he could return to his Oregon home early. Often I wondered why he had even taken this job. Now he was boring with the same old sarcasm each day. I realized it was his defense, but I was tired of being the butt of his jokes. Foolishly I continued to cope, instead of letting him know how I felt.

Pat finished in Seattle and flew off to Atlanta to work for a few weeks on *Free Jack*. When he finished, he flew back to Seattle, picked up his car and drove to Vancouver to stay with me. He loved the city. The parks were perfect for walking. He stayed for Thanksgiving and although the Canadians celebrate on a different day, our caterer cooked a traditional Thanksgiving dinner for us with turkey and all the trimmings.

The company threw a party at a lovely restaurant for Christmas and I decided to go all out with my look. There was a huge East Indian section in Vancouver. I found a beauty shop that did henna art on my hands and I bought a Punjab outfit to wear. It was fun to be with the crew away from work. Ralph Gerling, the camera operator was always so gruff at work and I often wondered if he even liked me. That evening, Ralph and his wife, Pat and I sat together and we got to know each other and I realized his gruffness was all just a cover up.

I flew home for Christmas. It had been dark and rainy in Vancouver and New Hampshire's brightness with the snow and sunshine was just what I needed. I spent the holidays with the family and did my Christmas shopping in Conway. My dollars went much farther at home than in Canada. I liked bringing money home to my town.

Following Christmas vacation we left for Whistler, a ski resort north of Vancouver. It was a huge ski complex and resort. What a set up. All the hotels were located at the foot of the mountains and the skiers never had to get in a vehicle to get to the slopes, shops or restaurants. We stayed at yet another lovely hotel. This was where we shot the scene that was the far north in which Pam and John were being pursued by wolves.

Our wolf trainer was an old friend of Clint Rowe. Clint had become my friend on *Turner & Hooch*. I had great fun listening to stories about their early adventures. The wolves were very interesting. I'd never been close to one before. With their yellow eyes, long back legs and nervous energy it was easy to see they were not dogs at all. They were very well trained and did their work without a hitch.

During the time we were at Whistler, things came to a head in my relationship with Lee. Lee, Sandy and Kandace hung around together in the evenings. They never once invited me to go with them. Normally I liked to go to bed early, but I felt left out this time. One day, while we were shooting on a set inside a hanger, I began talking with Arnie Schmidt. Lee walked up and made a sarcastic comment and then began talking about the next week's work. Lee wanted enough time off to drive his motor home back to Oregon before we went to Tucson. We still had shooting to do before we left for Tucson. I didn't want time off and it made me angry that he hadn't consulted me; he just made arrangements to suit himself. At that moment, I realized that I'd had it with him. I looked straight at Lee and gave him the finger. I'd never done that in my life to anybody. I had to be quiet because they were shooting. Next I held up all ten fingers. I truly meant what I felt, ten times over. I was furious. I burst into tears and ran off the set. I didn't want to ruin the scene.

A few minutes later, Lee followed me to the trailer. He came in, saying, "That wasn't a very nice thing to do to me." I couldn't believe him. I began to pour my hurt feelings out, letting him know how I felt when he ridiculed me in front of everyone every time I opened my mouth. The whole crew had commented on it. I had tried to cope, but that had been my mistake. He then confessed that I made him feel inferior because I read so much. (Maybe he didn't really love his mother so much.) I understood that he had been defensive, but I no longer was going to stand by with a smile on my face and take his harassment. I was fed up. He needed to take the responsibility for his own pain. I finally understood that. Lee was right. I had changed. It wasn't easy and yet, I knew it was time I began to be honest.

The crew was glad I'd finally stood up for myself. I know Arnie was happy I'd blown up because he told me he wondered why I'd taken the abuse for so long. I wondered myself. The next morning Lee tried to talk to me and I told him I wasn't ready; I was still too upset and didn't want to break into tears. I never talked to him until I saw him in Arizona a couple of weeks later.

I had hoped to be able to take Kandace with me to Arizona and she wanted to go. They said they couldn't take many Canadians so I bid her a tearful farewell. She had been a big support and help to me. I sadly took leave of all my Canadian friends, hoping I'd return one day soon. We flew to Tucson on Jan 23. The pale sunlight felt so good. It wasn't really warm, but felt perfect after all the rain in Vancouver. Our motel was seedy. I'd stayed there years before, but now time had taken its toll. It was far past its heyday.

We had been apart for a couple of weeks and Lee was pleasant. When he called to ask if I wanted a ride to Old

Tucson the next morning I accepted his offer. We were friendly on the ride out there. It was all going great until Pam came in. "Have you two made up?" she teased. "Yes," I answered. And then she looked straight at Lee and remarked, "You really were hard on her, you know." That was it. Lee remained cool to me for the rest of the shoot. I never heard from him for ten years. Finally, I called him and he apologized. I cried I was so happy.

Old Tucson was often used as a movie set. Whenever I was there I always wondered if this was the kind of town where my father had hung out when he was a sheriff back in 1890.

There were general stores, restaurants, saddle makers, and stunt men giving hourly performances.

In the film, we had a shootout between John and Jeffrey and later we tied Pam to the train tracks while a train hurtled toward her. All of a sudden it was all over, finished and we wrapped. Later that spring, I got a surprise call from the production office of *Stay Tuned*. They had cut the film and now they were going to do three weeks of retakes to try to add more humor. Delighted to return to Canada, I got right to work preparing for it.

What they planned to film were many vignettes, spoofing the most popular television shows of the season. I was baffled at first because I seldom watched television. I had to do lots of research to find out what my actors were supposed to look like. I went to the Wig Department at Warners where I got lots of help from John Norin and Lee Crawford.

All at once a whirlwind took over my life. On my arrival in Vancouver, it was a complete madhouse at the studio and I was totally psyched. One after another, we filmed vignettes of *Star Trek, Three's Company* and *Seinfield*. We filmed a rap video starring Salt-N-Pepa, a crash car dummy vignette and more.

Lee wasn't available to do the makeup, which was fine with me. I told production that Sandy was perfectly capable of taking Lee's place, so they happily hired her. Candice wasn't available so I hired another hairstylist, who was a real character and talented. I missed Candice and her calm demeanor, my new partner tended to be hysterical at times. It was crazy enough on this retake without it being crazy in our trailer.

The Burmans from Hollywood were hired to do the special makeup and masks. It was fun to work with the female part of the Burman team. They also had to rush everything together and they did a fine job.

Sandy's first makeup job was to paint red lips on a cow. She was so funny, carefully painting those big bow lips on the calm cow. I laughed to myself, remarking "I don't think Lee would have done nearly as good a job as you did." She smiled, pleased with herself.

John Ritter looked great as the Captain on *Star Trek* Jeffrey was a Klingon and he looked menacing. There was a *Three's Company* skit in which John had a nightmare about that show coming back to life and happening all over again to him. *Wayne's World* had Garth and Wayne sitting on the couch talking. I was proud of myself for learning about all these funny folks so quickly.

They had planned to shoot the rock video at a live location, but changed plans when they found it was far too noisy. They had to come up with something on stage and quick. For three days things poured into the long stage, day and night. I peeked in and there were parallels going up three stories and huge pipes, lots of funky things. It was the "reel" hell. The pipes had fires inside of them and there was lots of smoke and noise. Then it was ready - a real miracle. The creation of that set was a true example of people working together toward an end.

Salt-N-Pepa were the star performers and they were great. Jeffrey, the devil was dressed as Vanilla Ice. (He had just been discredited in real life.) John Ritter was dressed as Prince (or whatever his name was at the time) in a banana yellow outfit with a turban headpiece. It was so hilarious watching them dance up one parallel and down another - a chase with Salt-N-Pepa singing all the way through. The music thumped loud and we tapped our feet along with the music, getting caught up in the scene.

The video took three days to film and again we were finished. It had been so exhilarating and had taken me back to the good old days when movie making was really a joint effort. It was the last time I ever experienced that. I wanted to continue working in Canada as often as I could. I didn't realize at the time that this was a kind of finale gift for my movie career. It had topped everything I'd done in years and I had enjoyed myself to the fullest.

I went home to Snowville and worked in my garden, wondering if another film might be on the horizon. But nothing appeared and I realized how lucky I had been to work as much as I had that last year. It had been very slow in Hollywood. It was the middle of the recession in New England also.

The bookstore was costing us more than $2,000 a month for Bette's salary. While I was working, we could afford to pay her. I couldn't manage it otherwise. Without any work in sight, I had to tell Bette that I would be taking over the store. I didn't have a choice at that point. The business was growing, but there wasn't much profit, even on the good days. It was a specialty store and appealed to a small number of people. I don't know why I was so hesitant to tell her. It was my store after all. Still, I felt as if I was making her give up her child.

I began running the store in September. At first, I had a great time. It was so much fun ordering lots of neat things for Christmas. I was on my own for the first time. Bette had done a great job, but she had her style and I had mine. In retrospect, maybe I should have stuck to hers, she was far more frugal. In any case, the Christmas season in the store was fabulous. We brought in more money that December than we had in nearly the whole preceding year. It was exciting and festive. As I closed the store that Christmas Eve and Pat and I took off for Boston to spend Christmas with Tanya and her family, the snow began to fall gently. I had left the Christmas lights on inside the store and it looked beautiful.

The store grew in size and eventually we ended up taking over the whole house. It was a place of calmness and peace, with wonderful smells from the candles and incense. People stopped in just to unwind. I had a couch and chairs in the living room and a pot of tea was always on. At the front counter I met nearly everyone who came through the door. Eventually I began to feel like a counselor - free of charge. Teenagers came by every afternoon and I was happy to have them, because my shop exposed them to new ideas and ways of seeing the world. I hoped it would help them to stay away from drugs or booze. It would be better to be high on meditation.

Pat had been in Minneapolis all winter working on *Grumpy Old Men*. I hadn't been able to leave the store to go visit him on location. I missed him. I felt tied down. When that film ended in the spring, he headed straight to Jupiter, Florida to work on a Movie of the Week with Burt Reynolds. He asked me to come down to be with him. Laurie was living at home again and she agreed to watch the store for me while I was gone.

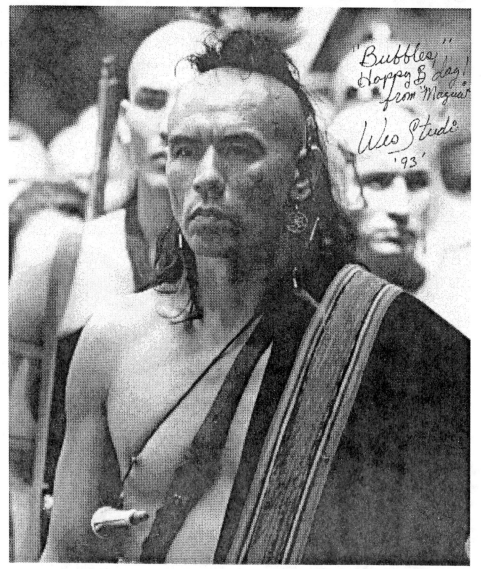

Wes Studi, *Geronimo*

It was May and the weather was still pleasant in Jupiter, not too hot. In fact it felt wonderful to be in the warm climate. Spring in New Hampshire came slowly that year and I appreciated the warm vacation. Pat had a lovely, roomy condo near the beach and it was beautiful there. I spent three weeks relaxing, drinking in the sun and then headed home to meet my newest grandson Connor who was born just hours before I arrived in Boston. I had promised to stay in Boston for a few days and help Tanya after she came home with the baby. They sent her home after just one day which I thought was heartless and much too soon. I loved being there, able to take care of Tyler then two and Brittany nine.

When I got home from Boston there was a call from Moab, Utah. They wanted me to go work on *Geronimo* for a week. Laurie said, "Go, I'll stay here at the store for you." So off I went. Xochi was working on the show as a second, second assistant. Walter Hill was the director. There were large calls with lots of Indians and they needed extra help.

Getting to Moab was a crazy experience. There were many plane changes, but finally I arrived. A driver and a couple of other new crewmembers that arrived at the same time from

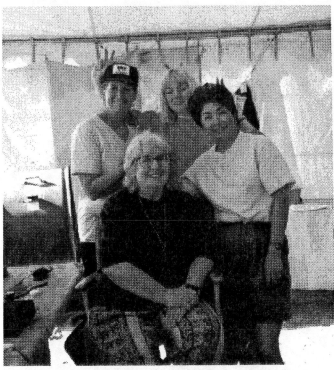

Sugar and hair stylist friends on the set of
Geronimo

various locations met me. We were all very hungry and stopped to have a tasty Mexican dinner something I couldn't find in New England.

Peter Tothpal, Arnold Swarzenagger's hairstylist was our boss and Gary Liddiard, who I hadn't seen since *Havana* was the head makeup man. My good hairdresser friends, Chris Lee, Cheryl Ross and Charlene Johnson were already there. We spent hours catching up on our lives.

Makeup was done in a big tent. First the extras went to the Wardrobe, next to Makeup and last to Hair. We took a bus to the set, which was sometimes up a mountain. It was hot and I was getting up early, spending long days out in the heat. Strangely enough, I began to realize that I hadn't felt so good in a year.

Moab was even prettier and more spectacular than I remembered. It had changed since I'd been there on *Blue*. There were many great little shops now and a brewpub and great restaurants. But best of all were the mountains and the sunsets that were spectacular in shades of orange, red and gold.

On June 17 we celebrated two birthdays, mine and Jason Patric's. They had a cake for each of us and Wes Duty, who played Geronimo gave me a happy birthday photo that read "To Bubbles" (Pat's newest nick name for me.) The caterers, Frank and Michelle of For Stars, staged a spectacular scene too. Frank and friends parachuted down from the sky in brightly colored parachutes as part of the celebration.

I worked that week and returned home. A week later they called me to come back to work for two more weeks. By then Bette had come back to work at the store. She was thrilled. I had realized that I didn't want to be there all the time. I was happy to have my freedom back.

At the end of the location in Moab, I had come to the conclusion that retail just wasn't for me. I was much happier out among people, on location. Being in the store, trying to solve people's problems, listening to them, drained me and I didn't know how to prevent it. Bette was far better than I at cutting people off who drained her energy. I didn't like having a regular schedule and routine. It didn't agree with me.

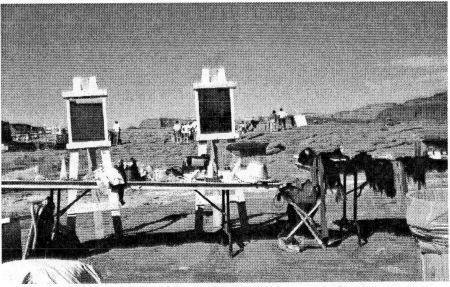

Hairdressers' arrangements on the set of *Geronimo*

While I'd been in Utah, Michael McDonald, the Canadian unit manager on *Stay Tuned* called to check my availability for a film that was starting in Toronto. I didn't give it a thought. I longed to work in Canada again. I realized I didn't belong in the bookshop and I took this as a sign that I go ahead and take the job. No questions asked. Dumb move, in hindsight I realized that I should have thought more about it and made some inquiries, but I said "Yes."

Chapter 73
TRIAL BY JURY

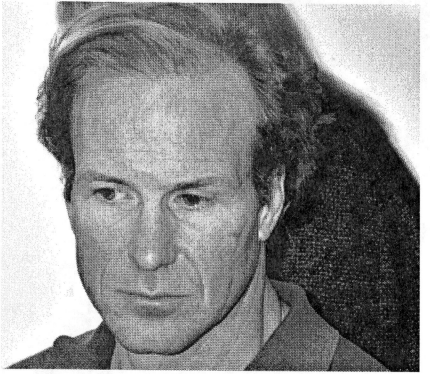

William Hurt, Trial by Jury

I did it again. I accepted a job without looking into the circumstances. Hard to believe I could repeat my mistake. Obviously I hadn't learned from my experience on *Havana*. All I could think about were the great memories I had of when I worked in Vancouver. I had longed to go back to work in Canada, any time I could.

Michael McDonald was truthful with me about *Trial by Jury*. He'd tried for the "big guns" like Kathy Blondell or Susie Germaine to do the female star's hair. Joanne Whaley Kilmer, at the time still married to Val Kilmer, had a reputation for being difficult. I realized by now I was considered second string, but that didn't bother me. I was so excited that I didn't hear what Michael said about how difficult Joanne could be.

I would also do William Hurt's hair, which was a nice surprise. Although we'd been friends for a long time, I'd never done his hair. Our other actors were Armand Assante, Gabriel Byrne, Kathleen Quinlin and Margaret Whitton. Our director was a lovely, genuine person who had also written the script, Heywood Gould. Our cameraman was straight from television's Northern Exposure, Frederick Elmes.

Michael described Joanne's part in the film. Joanne ran an antique clothing store and the clothes designer had suggested she have hairstyles from the Forties. The wigs had been ordered even before I came into the picture. I had no say about that. Joanne insisted on wigs, for some reason she was under the impression that she could never use her own hair and therefore always demanded wigs.

Armed with that information, I collected my research I'd collected for *The Other Side of Midnight* to take with me. It was the correct time period.

I have to say that the Canadians have class. Once again I was given a nice apartment, although not as classy as the Meridian in Vancouver. I also had my own car. My only problem was my apartment was right across the street from the giant underground shopping centers. Temptation was always staring me in the eye.

I was taken to the production office where I was delighted to see old friends, Michael MacDonald and Mandy the production secretary from *Stay Tuned*. To my delight I discovered an old friend would be the first assistant, Albert Shapiro. When I met Heywood Gould, our director, I took an immediate liking to him.

There was a stage below the office and our makeup room was right off that. It was large, roomy and bright. I was introduced to the two Canadian women, Jennifer the hairstylist and Ann, the makeup artist. Along with them was Katherine James, an American makeup artist, recently returned from New Zealand where she had done Holly Hunter's makeup for *The Piano*.

Joanne Whaley Kilmer walked through the door and I felt an air of electricity. She brought Natalie Wood to my mind in some ways. She was petite, cute and charming as could be. We discussed hairstyles and I showed her the photos I had considered. She appeared to like the Forty's styles. The next day the wig designer from New York delivered the wigs and gave her a fitting. The wigs looked quite nice and appeared to fit well.

William Hurt was next to arrive. He amused me. What a perfect politician. He walked into the makeup room and spied me. He winked and then went straight toward Joanne and greeted her first. That was smart; he knew the pecking order and wanted to start out on the right foot with her. Then a few minutes later, he came over and gave me a hug. I understood.

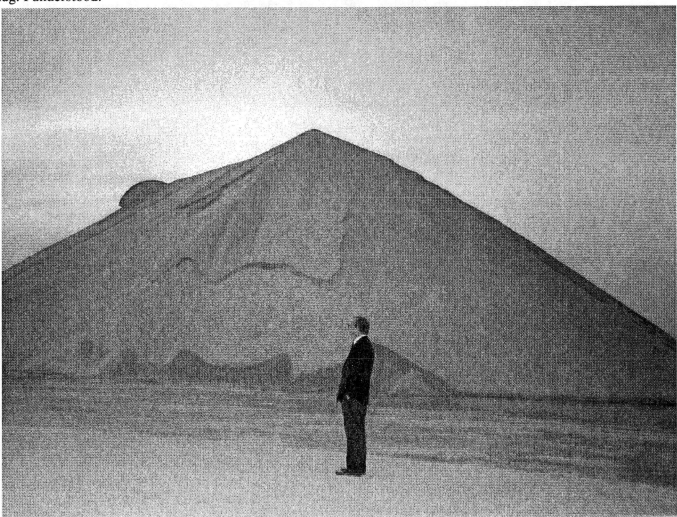

William Hurt, *Trial by Jury*

Katherine began doing Bill's makeup for the test. He was supposed to be a more rugged character than usual. Katherine wanted to lose his regular "wasp" look. She suggested curling his smooth hair and proceeded to take out her curling iron and curl. I was surprised at this, because that was my job. Nicely, but firmly, I told her I was there to do the hair, but would be happy to take her suggestions.

Joanne's wig overpowered her small face and I worked to make it look like less hair. The producers hated the way it looked, so I cut more hair out. By this time it looked more natural, but then Joanne had her own ideas and began to pull it farther back on her head, than it was made to go. It never really looked good after that. To make matters worse, the cameraman seemed to have forgotten he was no longer doing *Northern Exposure* and failed to light Joanne so that she looked good, instead he lit for atmosphere and Joanne didn't look pretty at all.

Joanne might have had some similarity to Natalie, but her features were not so sweet and the camera didn't love her like it did Natalie. The producers were not happy with our work and Katherine was worried, because there was little she could do with the makeup, if the cameraman wasn't willing to light it right. I tried to explain to the producers that the tests were what they were called "tests" so that we could see what needed to be changed. The sad part was, nobody wanted to cross the cameraman, so we all suffered.

I was having a difficult time. Katherine was always putting her hands in Joanne's hair and Mary our designer got into the act too. Normally the Makeup and Hair support each another. I felt Katherine was working against me. I was uncomfortable. I wanted to try using Joanne's own hair, thinking it would surely look better than the wigs, but Joanne wouldn't even give me a chance to try.

One Saturday, Joanne finished early and I took her wig off, I left it on the block. I had to get back to the set to watch Bill's hair so I planned to dress it later. That night, when I came back to Makeup, the wig had disappeared and on the wig block was a note from Joanne, saying she had taken the wig home with her. She wanted to work with it. I didn't even call her, I was so angry. It was wrong of her to do that.

Bill and I got along very well. He was straight with his needs. He instructed me never to speak to him while he was working, or while I was dressing his hair, unless he spoke to me first. I followed his directions, because on *The Doctor* I had seen him blow up when someone wrecked his concentration. I liked his new "do". I used a small curling iron and his hair looked curly and made him look more rugged.

The other actors were fantastic people. Armand Assante had matured from the young man I met on *Little Darlings* He'd been through many life changes and was a terrific human being. I loved talking with him about life in general. Gabriel Byrne was a sweet, genuine person. He often brought his children to the set and I could feel his love for them. The only mystery was how he had ever ended up with such a tough woman as Ellen Barkin. Kathleen Quinlin was beautiful in person and so nice. Unfortunately, Fred the cameraman seemed intent on making her look dreadful with his red lighting. Margaret Whitton arrived later and was lots of fun. She had worked with Mel Gibson, the previous summer, and told me her horror stories about the hairdresser in Maine. She wished that they had hired me when I had called because the hairdresser on that film knew nothing about wigs. She had to do her own.

It was fortunate that all those other people were there because Bill was definitely no fun. Not that he was supposed to fill my life with laughter, it was just that he seemed so angry all the time and I couldn't escape that. One day he lectured the director in front of the whole crew, humiliating him. That wasn't done, it should have happened in private. I figured he had taken this film to pay his alimony, not because he really wanted to do it. It's a shame for an actor to have to do that.

My relationship with Joanne was getting more and more uncomfortable. I could see her whispering to Katherine, who kept fiddling with her hair. I was confused. At one point we had been worried that Katherine might get fired because of how Joanne's makeup looked. Now it appeared that I was on the hot spot. I was upset. Each morning before work, I'd meditate and ask for guidance, but it didn't seem to help. Finally one morning I put my head down on the floor in surrender and asked Adi Da Samraj to show me what to do. My prayers were soon answered.

When Joanne came in that morning, I bit the bullet and asked, "Are you angry with me?" She answered "Yes. I'm furious with you. I don't think you even care about my hair." At first I was confused, because I certainly did care, but then I realized that Katherine had been trying to undermine me for some reason. In the beginning I had asked Joanne to be honest with me if she didn't like something. She never did that. So even though it was uncomfortable, I was happy everything had come to a head. I had been at my wit's end.

I called Albert Shapiro, our first assistant, and explained what had happened. He had intuited that something like this might take place. He knew Joanne hated the way she looked in the film, and he felt I was being made the scapegoat. But there was nothing he could do to prevent it. Whatever the reason, it was too tense and I wanted to be out of there as quickly as possible. I told Michael that I would do Bill's hair until they could find a replacement for me. We were working at a university that day and so I just walked away and found a place to sit by myself and I broke down into tears. I was unhappy and confused, but at the same time relieved.

It was strange, in many ways, because Joanne was still very friendly with me. She appeared to like me as a friend, but not as a hairstylist. It was uncomfortable for me though, because Bill and Joanne sat side by side in the makeup trailer while I curled Bill's hair and Katherine did Joanne's makeup. Jennifer, the Canadian hairstylist, began to do Joanne's hair until the new hairstylist arrived.

The day before the new hairdresser was to arrive, I told Bill I'd show the new hairdresser just how I did his hair and leave the little iron I used on him. "Why?" he asked. "Because I am leaving." "You can't go now." He began to get agitated. I had wondered why he hadn't asked me to stay earlier, but realized that he thought I wanted to go and didn't want to keep me there against my will. I had a hunch that Michael McDonald had convinced him I wanted to leave. After all, his budget didn't allow for two hairstylists from the USA. Bill got on the phone to his agent and then handed me the phone and told me to explain the situation to his agent.

Unfortunately, Joanne was still having her hair done down below in the trailer and while I was explaining what had happened she heard every word. I had only told the truth, but it wasn't pretty. The Canadian women were angry with me for saying what I said and I felt like an outcast for a while. They were so polite and would never have told the truth if it would hurt or insult a person. I hadn't meant to upset Joanne, but I guess the truth hurt and to be truthful I really didn't care anymore.

A few moments later Michael McDonald rushed into the trailer and called me aside. "Sugar, can you stay and do Bill's hair?" I told him that I guessed I could do that. From then on, I only had to do Bill's hair and come in while he worked. I'd been demoted, but upgraded. Not bad, $3000 a week to do one person's hair and he didn't work every day. The best-paying job I ever had in fact.

When the new hairstylist arrived there was no room in the makeup trailer for me, not even enough chairs. Bill said, "Never mind, you can come and stay in my trailer." He was very sweet to me. From then on I kept a chair outside his trailer and waited for him. I went inside if it was cold, but it was more pleasant to sit outside.

Nobody really enjoyed that film. It was tough, too much tension, right from the very beginning. Morgan Creek the producing company had shaved two million dollars off the budget at the last minute. It didn't give Heywood Gould, our director, the freedom he needed. Actually I don't think Heywood was equipped to deal with Bill Hurt either. I'll bet he went back to writing his books after he finished that film.

I used shopping to distract myself for the first time. The underground, right near my apartment, was full of wonderful places and so cool during that hot summer. I'd shop and return home with bags of stylish clothes from Le Chateau and many other great stores. My charge account balances grew, but it kept me sane. I longed to go home.

Pat came to visit right at the time I began to do only Bill's hair. It was remarkable the change that came over Bill when he was around Pat. They laughed and talked about old times when they had been drinking together. Sometimes I wondered to myself if it had been better for Bill when he drank. He was so intense now. Michael MacDonald asked if Pat could stay. It made life much easier for us all to have him there. Bill's mood had improved so much.

I would have been out of there, but I didn't want to let Bill down. I had about three more weeks left to go, but they crept by so slowly, it seemed much longer. At last Bill was finished and I was free to go. It was such a relief.

I told everyone good-by and Jennifer, the Canadian hairstylist, gave me a big hug saying I had taught her a lot by enduring everything so graciously. A couple of years later a crewmember called our house looking for Pat and we discussed that production. He told me that he had never been on such a miserable film, before or since then. It wasn't only me who felt that way. I had gotten one more push to quit the business and it was time to pay attention.

Chapter 74

AFTERWARD

I left Toronto emotionally exhausted. I never wanted to do another film. I sensed that my experiences had finally alerted me to the future of the movie business and I didn't want to have anything to do with it.

For years I'd tried to get out of the business. I'd gone to the farm in 1970, to the inn in 1977 and to my bookstore in 1990. Yet I kept letting myself get lured back. Was it the money? Possibly. But a part of me kept remembering how much fun I'd had at times and optimist that I was, I kept hoping the next film might be different. The definition of insanity is doing the same thing over and over again hoping things will change. Perhaps I was insane. It was time to acknowledge the old days were gone forever.

I'd always wanted to write, to be a writer, to have a career as a writer. My cabinets were full of the piles of things I'd written over the years. I just hadn't taken myself seriously. I realize now I had to come up against a brick wall before I'd allow myself to do what I knew in my heart was the right thing. I don't know why it took me so long to say no to Hollywood.

That fall I had been getting calls from my sister Fortune, who lived in San Diego. She had moved my mother in with her, now that she was unable to live on her own any longer. It was difficult; Fortune wasn't used to living with anyone, let alone a difficult mother. She wanted me to come out and give her a break for a few weeks.

The day after Christmas, I got a desperate call for help from Fortune. She was exhausted – no longer able to take care of our mother on her own. Not knowing what to do, I talked with Laurie, my oldest daughter who had just moved to the San Diego area for a new job. She was managing Pick Up Stix, a fast food Chinese restaurant. Fortunately there was a small apartment available in her complex and she offered to watch over my mother if she wanted to rent it. My mother had always been independent and very much wanted her own place. Laurie could keep a close eye on her and my sister wouldn't have all the responsibility. Fortune was hurt and furious with me for making those arrangements. I didn't understand. I figured that I was relieving her of her problems. I did what I thought was best. Since then I have warned people who ask for my help, to let them know, I help in the way I see best and it may not be just what they planned on.

As things turned out, I didn't have much time to worry about it. I moved my mother into the little apartment and got her settled. She was very happy. The next day, I went to La Costa Spa and treated myself to a massage. That afternoon I began to feel ill. Thinking it was my gall bladder I treated myself with herbs. Early Monday morning, Laurie insisted on taking me to the emergency room at the hospital. I didn't argue. By the time we go to the hospital, I was so weak I could hardly walk. They took me into the emergency room at Scripps and after the x-rays were done they realized that it was very serious. My appendix had already ruptured. They rushed me into surgery.

While I was on the gurney, waiting to be wheeled into surgery, I heard loud rock music playing, shades of *The Doctor*. I remember asking the nurse if they could turn off the music. As sick as I was, I had to chuckle. The next thing I remembered, I was waking up after the operation, free of pain.

How lucky I was to be so close to Scripps Hospital. If I'd been home alone, I might not have gotten to the hospital in time. After surgery, I was so weak and exhausted that I didn't want to see anyone. I had almost died and had a lot of recovering to do. Pat called me from New Hampshire, shocked by what had happened. I could hardly talk to him.

At first they gave me morphine for the pain, but then they switched to Demerol, which made me sick to my stomach and didn't agree with me. I felt sicker and sicker.

Four days after the operation, I was so low that for the first time in my life, I didn't care if I lived or died. In fact, I would have been happy to die. I didn't want to leave my family, but I was so sick that I didn't think I could hang on.

In Adi Da Samraj's Teaching, there is no fear of death. He had pointed out that most of us spend all our lives trying to avoid death. He is the Dawn Horse. I had read that when death was approaching all I needed to do was take the Horse's tail and hold onto it. He would take me through the tunnel to the light. As I lay there, I remembered that Teaching. His picture was on the table by my bedside. In surrender I looked at Him and asked if He could intertwine my fingers in the horse's tail. I was too weak to do it myself. I dropped off to sleep in total surrender.

January 11, 1994, I awoke, still alive. When I looked over at His picture, it seemed as though He was smiling at me, letting me know that I wasn't getting out of there so easily. I knew I would recover.

From then on, my life became different. I understood I had been given a gift and I needed to pay attention. In retrospect, I can see that this experience was the final push to get me to quit the movie business and get on with what my real life was about.

I stayed in the hospital for ten days, thankful, totally awake and clear. While I was there the big Los Angeles earthquake awakened us and shook our room in a rolling fashion. I had escaped it, but still experienced it in a way. That was enough for me.

I stayed with Laurie during my recovery. She and Patrick took excellent care of me and I ate lots of great Chinese food. It was nice to be with them. I spent time with my mother. In the beginning my mother was able to walk faster than I was able to walk. She and I talked about many things we'd never discussed before. She knew that her will needed to be straightened out and that her taxes were behind, so we worked on those things. We talked about her funeral arrangements. She was adamant that she wanted to be cremated. "Sprinkle me somewhere and I don't want to pay for a grave site." She said she wasn't afraid to die which made me feel good. She had always been so private that this time was a gift for me. After that she became more and more vague.

I returned to New Hampshire in the middle of March, still very weak, but much better. Pat was still in Los Angeles working on *Dirty Rotten Shame*. He was able to make it home for a couple of weeks in April between shows.

The antibiotics had taken a great toll on my body and for a long time I had no energy. I spent lots of time sleeping and resting and was almost afraid to go out at night. I was beginning to write and I kept my word processor beside the bed, so I couldn't avoid seeing it and each day I wrote.

Writing was a lonely job and I decided to become a realtor, hoping I could combine the two, balancing my life by being a realtor part time. I also wanted to earn some money. To my great surprise I passed the test on the first try. I was a realtor for two years when the recession was in full swing. I didn't sell much, but had fun anyway. Though at first I thought I could combine my writing and real estate, I was wrong. The computer at the office spoiled me. My word processor, at home, was no longer adequate. My writing was ignored. I was very busy, not making money, just busy. In my defense, it was the bottom of the recession and nothing was selling.

Although I had no desire to work in films again, I didn't want to burn any bridges so I wanted to keep my union dues current, just in case I should ever need it. That meant that every two years I had to work for five days to be re-certified. My two years were nearly up. (Working in Canada hadn't counted.) I heard that Adi Da Samraj, who normally lived in Fiji, might be coming to California. He had a form of inherited Glaucoma and needed an operation on both eyes.

One day I got a call from the Mountain of Attention. I was asked if I still had any contact with film stars. This was going to be the first time in years that people would have the opportunity to sit with Adi Da Samraj. I couldn't think of anyone, but I asked if I could come out for the advocate's conference that was being held in October. I wanted more than anything to see Beloved Adi Da Samraj. I always wanted to share His Teaching with everyone.

Looking back, I wished that I'd come to Adi Da's Teachings, long before I actually did at the age of fifty-six. When I worked with Natalie Wood, Elizabeth Montgomery and Inger Stevens, I gave them my love and support, but I'd never actually had a Teaching like His to share or offer them. Now it was too late for those friends, but I yearned to bring this awareness to others. In my life I had always shared everything wonderful that happened to me with those who would listen.

I flew to California and Pat rented a lavender Cadillac and drove me up north to Clearlake to the Mountain of Attention Sanctuary. There was no guarantee that I would see Adi Da Samraj, but I prayed I would be able to.

Miracles do happen. Although Adi Da Samraj's eyes had been operated upon and the light was not good for His eyes and made it difficult for Him, He agreed to sit with us.

Dennis Quaid had become aware of Adi Da Samraj. He took the opportunity to come and sit with Him that same day. It amused me to see Dennis, all decked out in white, surrounded by his entourage. Nervously, he glanced about, as I walked up to him and said "Hello." We had met at *The Presidio* when I was doing Meg Ryan's hair on *The Presidio*. She was now his wife. I asked him to tell her hello for Sugar and then walked away, seeing how uneasy and guarded he was.

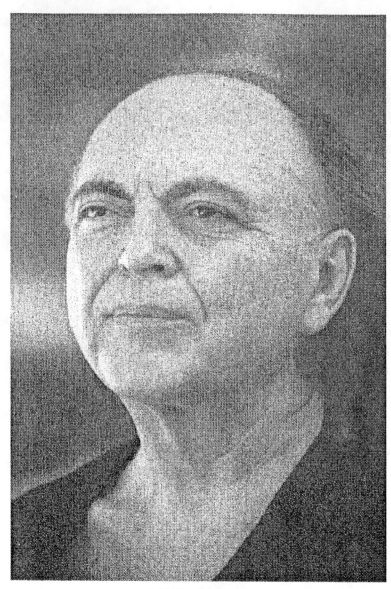

Adi Da Samraj

During that afternoon, we were notified we would be able to sit in Darshan (where you sit with Adi Da Samraj, in silence and breathe in all the love that He is). The moment I began to walk toward the sanctuary, my tears began to fall. I wasn't sure why I was crying. I had wanted to see Him, be in His presence for so long. Now I could feel the tears well up and my heart began to break open. I could feel His love penetrating me, long before He arrived.

The Conch shell sounded and slowly Adi Da Samraj was driven up in a golf cart. One of the Adidama (the women who serve Him) took his arm as He walked slowly to the chair that had been prepared for Him. The sun was very bright and He was wearing dark glasses to protect His eyes. He walked carefully to His seat in front of us.

All my life, I'd pictured God looking like an old man, with long white hair, a beard, loving and passive. I'd been wrong. At that moment, with my first glimpse of Adi Da Samraj, I knew God was not tall. He was round. His hair was dark and flowing and this moment, He was dressed in orange. It was a revelation. The love flowed from Him penetrating directly into my heart. I was truly heartbroken.

They say He changes your life; mine was changed in a moment. They say He works with your karma. Whatever He does, I knew my life was changed the moment I knelt down before Him, offering my gift, uttering only, "I love You."

Later that evening, I noticed that Dennis Quaid appeared to be more relaxed, not so paranoid. I had no idea how he was affected, but he hadn't done the preparation most of us had done. I am sure he must have felt all the love surrounding Him that I felt that day.

Back in Los Angeles, still walking on a cloud, I went to work with my friend Shirley Dolle on *Deep Space Nine* at Paramount, my old haunt. The whole studio was totally occupied by *Star Trek* and it's off shoot productions.

My old friend Cherie Huffman and I worked on the extras. We laughed with each other about our adventures in the movie business, wondering what we were doing there, sitting in caves with all these strange creatures wandering about. We were just putting in time.

But I found out that there was a reason I was there. One morning our call was 4:00 a.m. at the Japanese Gardens, near Sepulveda. It was dark and foggy that morning and I could hardly see where I was going. I was nervous. Cherie had told me that she drove wearing a man's hat and had a gun between the car seats. I didn't want to be that fearful. I missed the turn off in the fog and had to retrace my steps. Finally I found the parking lot. There, I was met by a driver, who took me to the makeup trailer. We set up for our extras and then went for breakfast. In the meantime the sun rose and the beautiful Japanese gardens were revealed.

There are no mistakes and I realized that, when Robert Foxworth, Elizabeth Montgomery's husband, walked into the trailer that morning. Lizzie had died of cancer earlier that year at the age of sixty-two. What a tragedy. Bob and I had known each other since he met Lizzie on *Mrs. Sundance*, more than twenty-four years before. His eyes opened wide. "Sugar" he said and walked over. He took me in his arms and hugged me for a long, long time. We stood back and looked at each other and hugged again. We talked, trying to catch up on so many years. We talked about Lizzie's house. His friends had advised him to sell. "No, I love that house," I advised. "It's a perfect place." He agreed. We talked until it was time for him to go to work.

Later that day, I was taking a break and I walked past his dressing room. He was sitting on the steps. We resumed our conversation on a deeper, more personal level. I asked him how he was doing. "Okay," he began to tell me about Lizzie's last days. "She never wanted to get old." "Well, she didn't, did she?" I replied.

He went on to tell me how difficult her dying had been because she wouldn't let anyone talk about it. She wouldn't discuss it with her children, her doctor, not even Bob. One night, longing to release her from her pain, willing her to let go, he told her she could go home. Angrily, she told him never to say anything like that again. He was at a loss and so very sad. He said she looked like a little bird by the time she died.

Oh, my delicate friends. I was saddened that she'd been in that frame of mind, so full of denial. She never gave her family the chance for closure. It made me want to cry all over again.

Chapter 75

EXPECT THE UNEXPECTED

I went home from my last stint in the movie business thinking that I was done at last, unless something really amazing happened. It did.

May rolled around and Adi Da was on His way to Cape Cod. It was a miracle; He had never been to the Boston area before. I was so excited, I could hardly wait. After feeling His love permeate my heart, I couldn't wait to be with Him again. I took time off from my work as a realtor and beat it down to Boston, where I was told I could go to Cape Cod on retreat.

Beloved Adi Da Samraj was staying in a wonderful estate on a little island one of the devotees had provided for Him. All my life, working in films I'd been near and worked with famous people, but this was different. It was a powerful experience and a privilege to serve the Guru.

Adi Da Samraj gave Darshan at the house and I was able to attend. He sat with us in the middle of the night. We'd sit there quietly and suddenly He would appear. I could feel my heart breaking open once again. He sat down, arranged His clothes and closed His eyes. I began to breathe with Him, losing all thoughts, just being with Him, drinking in His love.

The first night I left the house about three o'clock and went home to sleep. The next day I got a call from Godfrey, a devotee who kept things organized at the house. In his very elegant English way, he said he'd heard I worked as a hairdresser on films and Beloved's family needed some advice about their hair. Could I possibly come to the house and advise them? I had brought a few hair cutting things, just in case a fellow devotee needed a haircut, but I had no idea I'd be asked to do the family's hair.

I was told I would meet with the Adidama Sukha Dham after Darshan. I became nervous. Seeing as I was not a night person, I hoped I wouldn't be too sleepy to think straight. During Darshan that second night, my mind didn't rest, my ego was too busy worrying about doing things right. I needn't have worried. When I met Adidama Sukha Dham, she radiated love. She was one of the loveliest women I'd ever met. She was in the ultimate stages of life, yet totally in the moment. She gave me a hug and then we talked. Her hair was long and very fine, and it lay flat on her head. Most of the time she lived on the island in Fiji and she had stuck with her hairstyle for many years. Now she had matured and needed a change. Adi Da, who is ever caring, wanted her to go to a salon, have a perm and enjoy the experience. She'd never been to one. But both Yuki, the traveling hairstylist and I felt it would be a mistake to entrust her hair to a stranger who'd never even met her. She took our advice and Yuki gave her the perm. She looked beautiful.

Later I met the others, including Adidama Jangama Hriddaya and Beloved's daughter Namleela. Namleela is an accomplished pianist and at sixteen had graduated from high school and was ready for college. Namleela asked if I could trim her hair and happily I did. I felt so privileged to be in such intimate circumstances with Adi Da's family. When you give the Guru a gift, it is actually a gift for you.

Earlier that year Pat had called, lamenting "We're never together. You're there and I'm here. When is it going to change?" I heard him, but didn't know what to do about it. However, on my return from Cape Cod, it was clear to me what needed to be done. I had to quit my realtor's job. I quit at the end of June. I knew at the moment I left Cape Cod that it was time to declare myself a writer. It was what I'd wanted to do for such a long time.

My sudden decision shocked Pat. His complaint had been heard, now we could be together all the time. We had been apart for so many years. When I finally decided, I realized that he wasn't quite prepared for my availability. Pat finished *Star Trek: First Contact* and came home for the summer on the Fourth of July. It was a busy summer, full of fun. Pat pointed out that even though I'd been so afraid of retirement, I seemed to be enjoying myself.

John Leonetti was asked to direct *Mortal Kombat: Annihilation*. John wanted his brother, Matt Leonetti, to be cameraman and Pat to be the gaffer. At first it was going to be filmed in Los Angeles and Pat wasn't really interested. Suddenly things changed.

The movie business was busier than it had ever been and there was no available stage space in Los Angeles. As a result, they decided to shoot the film overseas, beginning in London, then Israel, Jordan and finally Thailand. All of a sudden I decided to join Pat. In fact I wanted to go so badly, I promised Pat I would finish my book. I bought a laptop computer to take with me on the trip. Pat's take was that I was a fair-weather friend. I wouldn't come visit him in Los Angeles, but I was off in a moment on a trip like this. I guess he was right. But then you can write nearly anywhere.

Pat took the film and left for a whirlwind trip around the world on September 20. They flew to Thailand, Jordan, Israel and finally to London where I joined him on October 16, 1996.

I finally had to admit that I was addicted to the excitement the movie world provided. I loved movies, but I no longer wanted to work on them as a hairdresser. I did love to travel. Maybe I was too old to want to work the long hours even if the business hadn't changed. Or was I wiser?

In England, we found an apartment in Watford near Leavesdon Studio where they were shooting. The first scenes were filmed in Wales and I spent a week in Llanidloes, a wonderful place by the sea. It was stormy, wild and cold upon our arrival and it made me realize how much Wales had influenced the personalities of Richard Burton and Dylan Thomas.

We spent six weeks in England and the thought that I'd like to live there disappeared in the cold and damp, as my bones began to ache. In December I left for home to prepare for Christmas and Pat flew to Jordan.

Pat had told me that Thailand would be too hot for me, but everyone I knew who had been there, loved it. While arranging for my retirement, I had spoken with Jon Laurence about my trip. He convinced me to go. "Don't miss it! I've been there seventeen times." He proceeded to tell me the wonders of it.

My retirement pay was minimal. I had made a mistake when I went to the farm and also to the inn. I had taken it out, not expecting to come back into the business. It had not been a good move. I ended up with $149 a month. Not much

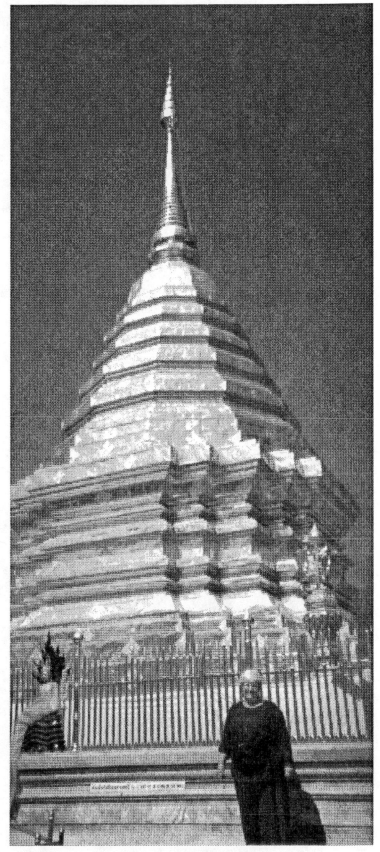

Sugar in Thailand

after forty years in the business.

I was happy as could be in Thailand. It was perfect weather in January, February and March. In all my travels I had never met such sweet, kind, patient people. I left Thailand in tears not wanting to leave the people I had grown to love. Maybe I'd been Anna who taught there in another life. Before I had gone to Thailand, I was becoming content to stay at home and slow down. After that trip I was ready to return at any time. In fact my next book is going to be based in Thailand. I'll have to go back for research.

Chapter 76

AN ORDINARY WOMAN'S LIFE GONE RIGHT

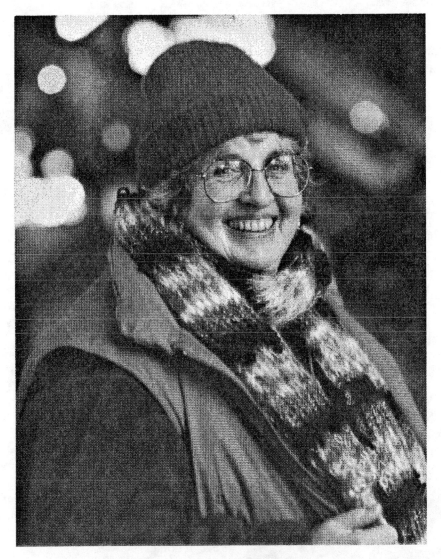

Ginger "Sugar" Blymyer

Just like in the movies, there are sequels and remakes. There are still actors and actresses I want to know. Many actors give me great pleasure. Often their acting is exquisite and so subtle that I must see them a few times before I'm able to discover how complete and complex their talent truly is. Jonathan Pryce, beginning with *Brazil*, was wonderful. In *Carrington* he was fabulous and as Peron in *Evita* he made me fall in love with him. The excellence of his acting inspires me to give my all whenever I am trying to create. Aidan Quinn is very special. He subtly sneaked his way into my heart in *Avalon*. Those blue eyes are amazing. He has continued to delight me whenever he appears. I admire Johnny

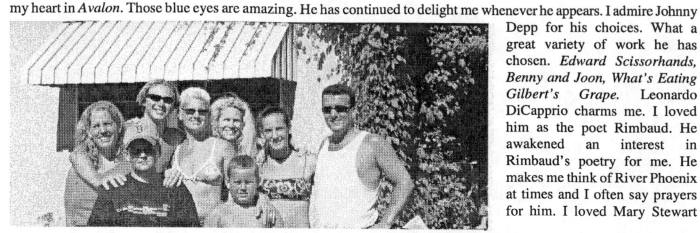

Sugar's family, all grown up

Depp for his choices. What a great variety of work he has chosen. *Edward Scissorhands, Benny and Joon, What's Eating Gilbert's Grape.* Leonardo DiCapprio charms me. I loved him as the poet Rimbaud. He awakened an interest in Rimbaud's poetry for me. He makes me think of River Phoenix at times and I often say prayers for him. I loved Mary Stewart Masterson, in *Fried Green Tomatoes*. It is interesting that many of these people have worked together. I am proud to have been a part of the business in which these people work.

Undoubtedly, in the future I will fall in love with other actors who are also remarkable. I like to believe that there will always be someone to inspire and charm me no matter how long I live.

True, the movie business has changed. It used to be a family and there was respect by and for all parties. The producers respected the crew and their abilities and the crew respected the producers, because they created projects for them to work on. The people who begin their careers at the present time won't know the difference. I almost feel sorry for them. In looking back, I realize how fortunate I was. I was given a magical opportunity. It seems to have disappeared now.

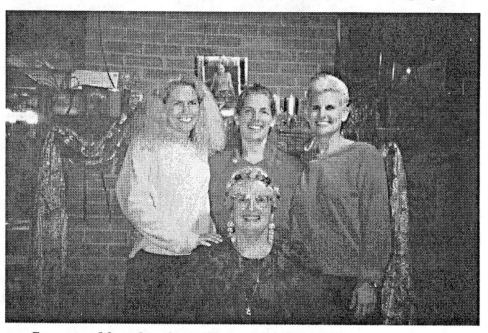

Sugar and her daughters (from left) Xochi, Tanya and Laurie

It is my hope that everyone will bring back the respect in all areas of the industry.

Because of my work in the movie world, I have seen more in my life than most people ever see or experience in ten lives. Traveling the world over has given me an education I could never have found in any school. My experience has taught me to live in the moment and to enjoy life as it comes.

Pat, my husband, helped me edit the book for content. He says I seldom have an unexpressed thought and in that he is absolutely right. I want to share my experiences with you, and inspire you to a life of passion and learning and excitement. Pat also commented after finishing the book that I came off as a rather loose woman at times. That tickled me, I always thought of myself as a free spirit. But perhaps I

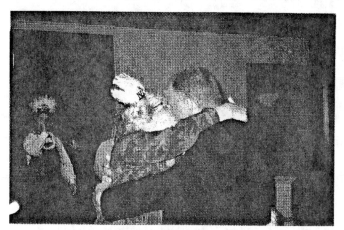

Sugar and her husband. Pat

was ahead of my time. Whatever I have done in my life seemed the right thing at the time and I have no regrets. Living this life in my own way has made me a happy woman, still ready to learn and looking forward to more life of adventure wherever that takes me. I thank Pat for his support through the years. It has taken me nearly fifteen years to get this finished. I feel that now is the right time to bring out the book though life has added many extra Chapters to it.

I feel so happy to have found my Spiritual Teacher Adi Da Samraj. My life has changed and no longer do I search for happiness, yet my life continues to be more wonderful and happy every day.

My advice to anyone who wants to be in the "biz" is to go for it. If you don't find it to be for you, at least you tried. And to those who find it as wonderful as I have so much of the time, I wish you a wonderful life of film. And when you look back, may you also be AN ORDINARY PERSON, WHOSE LIFE HAS GONE RIGHT.

I want to give thanks to my writers group in Snowville who have encouraged me to keep going all these years. Also thanks to the many people who have given input, done some editing and listened to me. Of course I give thanks to all the people who experienced my adventures along with me during the many years of my movie work. There is so much more that happened, but enough is enough.

If you have questions please write me at *ginger@hairdressertothestars.com* or take a look at my Web site at www.hairdressertothestars.com. It will keep you apprised of any upcoming adventures.

Become interested in the Teaching of Adi Da Samraj, you can find a wonderful Web site on the Internet at www.adidam.org.

Photo Credits

A very special thank you to Dianne Wells who provided many of the photos in this book from her collection and for sharing her personal experiences with Natalie. Her contributions helped to make the book possible.

The Baby Jane Collection
Pages 3, 40, 45, 66, 84, 89, 90 and 140

Peter Sorel
Page 136

Gwen Nagel
Page 173, Painting of Snowvillage Inn

Bill Ray
Cover Photo

INDEX

A

A Book of Numbers · 125
A Case of Rape · 133
A Time to Run · 125
A. C. Lyles · 90
Adam Arkin · 280, 281, 282
Adam at Six a.m. · 113
Adi Da Samraj · 3, 273, 278, 282, 287, 291, 296, 304, 307, 308, 310, 315
Adidama Jangama Hriddaya · 310
Adidama Sukha Dham · 310
Aidan Quinn · 313
Al Pacino · 165
Alan Pakula · 63, 66
Alan Rudolph · 234
Alan Watts · 160
Albert De Salvo · 94
Albert Shapiro · 303, 304
Alfred Hitchcock · 33, 195
Alien · 225
All Fall Down · 27, 28
All the Right Moves · 228, 230, 289
Alma Johnson · 145
Aloha Bobby and Rose · 152
Altered States · 225
American Ballet · 178
Amidou · 168
An American Geisha · 239, 295
An American Heart · 295
An American in Paris · 18
Andre Previn · 63
Andy Griffith · 231
Andy McLagen · 35
Angela Lansbury · 27
Ann Bancroft · 178
Another 48 Hours · 268
Anthony Quinn · 108, 109, 110
Apocalypse Now · 165
Apples Way · 136
Armand Assante · 302, 304
Arnie Schmidt · 193, 296, 298
Arnold Schwarzenegger · 264
Arthur Freed · 14, 17
Arthur Hiller · 209
Arthur Lowe, Jr. · 82
Arthur Miller · 82
Audrey Hepburn · 47
Audrey Rose · 179
Ava Gardner · 18
Avalon · 314
Awakening Land · 196, 202, 207, 212

B

Baby Maker · 113, 114, 115
Bachelor Father · 36
Barbara Hershey · 114
Barbara Lampson · 268, 285
Barbara Leonetti · 125, 272
Barbara Lorenz · 161
Barbara Walters · 261
Barbra Streisand · 106, 189, 297
Barefoot in the Park · 85, 270
Barry Fitzgerald · 36
Beatrice Arthur · 85, 152
Beau Bridges · 99
Ben Hecht · 99
Ben Nye, Jr. · 161, 169
Beneath the Planet of the Apes · 98
Benji · 167, 212
Benny and Joon · 314
Bernadette Peters · 228
Bernie Pollack · 161, 270
Beta Batka · 216, 217
Bette Snow · 268
Bewitched · 133, 206
Bill Fraker · 80, 126, 129, 131, 138, 150, 152, 155
Bill Hurt · *See* William Hurt
Bill Tompkins · 26
Bill Turner · 216, 217
Bill Tuttle · 17, 19, 80
Billy Burton · 87
Billy Crystal · 241
Billy Graham · 125
Black Sunday · 157, 163, 169, 173
Blake Edwards · 49, 50
Blue · 88, 89, 90, 133, 249, 301
Bob & Carol & Ted & Alice · 106
Bob Clatworthy · 63
Bob Dawn · 163, 164, 169, 170, 171, 173
Bob Foxworth · 133, 140, 204, 206
Bob Jiras · 41, 42, 54, 56
Bob Mulligan · 42, 63, 64, 67
Bob Norin · 213, 231
Bobbie Morse · 152
Boris Segal · 202
Brad Wilder · 258
Brandon De Wilde · 27
Brazil · 313
Breaking Away · 225
Brenda Vaccaro · 119
Brian Keith · 100, 102, 209
Brigadoon · 14, 16
Bronson Gate · 36
Brothers Grimm · 23
Bruce Barrenger · 187

Bruce Dern · 163, 164, 165
Bruno Cremer · 168
Buddy Holly Story · 234
Burgess Meredith · 26, 276
Burt Reynolds · 89, 216, 300

C

Camelot · 90, 111
Captain from Castile · 82
Carla Hadly · 99
Carlos Thompson · 16
Carol Schwartz · 275
Carrington · 313
Cary Grant · 162
Charlene Johnson · 301
Charles Bludhorn · 88
Charles Boyer · 85
Charles Bronson · 70, 74, 158
Charles Jarrot · 179, 185
Charles Manson · 157
Charlie Lang · 63
Charlie Schram · 18, 19
Charlton Heston · 98
Cherie Huffman · 308
Cheryl Ross · 289, 301
Children of a Lesser God · 226, 281
Chopper I · 135
Chris Lee · 301
Christine Lahti · 280, 281
Christopher Plummer · 63, 66
Christopher Walken · 223
Chuck Hayward · 36, 59, 289
Chuck Roberson · 31, 35
Chuck Rocher · 113, 114, 121
Clark Gable · 15, 17
Clark Paylow · 112, 123
Cleopatra · 56
Clint Althouse · 184, 185
Clint Eastwood · 26, 267
Clint Rowe · 265, 298
Cloris Leachman · 152, 195
Cocktail · 228
Cold Turkey · 112
Colin Wilcox · 114
Colombia Studios · 106
Commando · 238
Conrad Hall · 137, 161
Conrad Hilton · 63
Courtney
    Natalie Wood's Daughter · 154, 219
Craig T. Nelson · 228, 264
Crowning Glory · 19
Curly Linden · 28
Cyd Charisse · 18

D

Dan Haggerty · 121
Danny Mann · 109
Danny Streipecke · 264, 266
Dave Salvin · 156
David Carradine · 114
David Jansen · 69
David Lang · 222
David Niven Jr. · 58, 64
David Niven, Jr. · 56
David Quaid · 213
David Salvin · 155
Day of the Dolphin · 126, 127, 134, 142, 269
Day of the Locust · 133, 135, 136, 137, 161
Dean Jones · 49
Dean Tavalaris · 63
Death Becomes Her · 273
Debbie Douglas · 297
Debbie Reynolds · 15, 18, 29
Deborah Kerr · 22
Deep Space Nine · 308
Deep Throat · 131
Del Ree Todd · 144
Delia Shep · 275
Dennis Quaid · 261, 307, 308
Dick Bush · 155, 175, 176
Dick Hart · 141, 142, 231
Dick Kline · 97, 99, 107, 111, 112, 141, 144, 145, 192
Dick Shawn · 80
Dick Van Dyke · 112
Dinah Shore Show · 152
Dino Conte · 258
Dino De Laurentis · 145
Dionne Warwick · 152
Dirty Rotten Shame · 307
Disney · 35, 49, 264, 265, 266, 280, 281, 282
Dog Soldiers · *See* Who'll Stop the Rain
Don Cash, Sr. · 29
Don Feld · 50, 58
Don Gallagher · 23
Don Merritt · 140, 163
Don Schoenfield · 26
Donna McDonough · 25
Dore Schary · 14
Doris Day · 46
Dorothy White Byrne · 21, 92, 128
Down and Out in Beverly Hills · 266
Dr. Zhivago · 166
Dream of Kings · 107, 108, 111, 113
Dudley Moore · 156, 165, 192
Dustin Hoffman · 161, 165
Dyan Cannon · 106

E

E.T. · 228
Earl Rath · 141
Ed Feldman · 281
Ed Ternes · 234
Eddie Butterworth · 41, 74, 80, 128, 136, 206
Edie Hubner · 18
Edith Head · 46, 64, 66, 70
Edmund Gwenn · 11
Edmund Purdom · 15
Edward Furlong · 296
Edward Scissorhands · 314
Elizabeth Ashley · 38, 138
Elizabeth McGovern · 263, 264
Elizabeth Montgomery · 133, 140, 148, 150, 196, 202, 219, 222, 307, 308
Elizabeth Perkins · 280, 281
Elizabeth Taylor · 15, 18
Ellen Barkin · 263, 264, 304
Ellen Burstyn · 39
Elliot Gould · 106, 107
Elvis · 15, 38
Ernest Borgnine · 211
Esther Williams · 18
Ethel Merman · 152
Eva Marie Saint · 27, 28
Evita · 282, 313
Extreme Prejudice · 253
Eyewitness · 225

F

Facts of Life · 211
Fade In · 89
Family Matters · 266
Far and Away · 284, 285, 286
Fat Chance · 139, 143, 147
Faye Dunaway · 189, 297
Fiddler on the Roof · 223
Flush · 178
For Lovers Only · 231
For Those Who Think Young · 39
Forrest Whitaker · 263
Fox Studios · 23, 87, 98, 113, 123, 135, 181
Francis Ford Coppola · 63
Frank Bauer · 208
Frank McCoy · 85
Frank Perez · 275
Frank Perry · 138
Frank Raymond · 125
Frank Yablans · 186, 188, 190
Fred Brost · 184
Fred Konacamp · 185
Fred MacMurray · 34
Frederick Elmes · 302
Free Jack · 298
Fried Green Tomatoes · 314

Fritz Weaver · 163
Frontier Circus · 33
Fun in Acapulco · 38

G

Gabriel Byrne · 302, 304
Gaily, Gaily · 99, 103, 104, 105, 109, 111, 289
Gary Busey · 121, 122, 206, 219
Gary Liddiard · 269, 301
Gary Morris · 89
Gene Kearney · 144
Gene Kelly · 18, 19, 36
Gene Reynolds · 34
Gene Sax · 85
George Axelrod · 69
George C. Scott · 127, 128
George Hamilton · 28
George Justin · 170
George Kennedy · 211
George Peppard · 38
Georgy Girl · 89
Geronimo · 300, 301
Godfather II · 152
Godfrey Cambridge · 80
Going Home · 119
Going My Way · 36
Going South · 196
Gone With the Wind · 109
Gordon Bau · 51
Grace Kelly · 22, 33, 132
Grasslands · 121, 131
Gregory Hines · 241, 244
Greta Garbo · 14, 18, 50, 189
Greystroke · 6
Grizzly Adams · 121
Grumpy Old Men · 300
Gulf & Western · 88
Gunn · 80

H

Hal Holbrook · 204
Hal Lierly · 148, 153
Hal Polar · 160
Hal Wallis · 85
Hamlet · 161
Handbook to Higher Consciousness by Ken Keyes · 153
Hank · 68, 144
Harry Ray · 50, 56, 58
Harry Stradling, Sr. · 80, 82
Havana · 268, 271, 272, 285, 301, 302
Hayley Mills · 69
Helen Gruzik · 58, 232
Helen Gurly Brown · 44
Helen Rose · 15, 22

Hello, Dolly · 98
Helter Skelter · 157, 159, 161, 242
Henry Fonda · 44, 46, 97
Henry Hathaway · 29
Henry Mancini · 60
Henry Winkler · 265
Hex · 121, 131
High Anxiety · 195, 196, 197, 296
Hillary Thompson · 121
Holly Hunter · 303
Holy Jumping Off Place · 278
Honey I Blew Up the Kids · 282
Hooch · 264, 265, 266, 267
Hope Lang · 222
How the West Was Won · 26, 28, 30, 35, 158
Howard Koch, Jr. · 76, 161, 179, 188, 213
Howard Koch, Sr. · 39, 179

I

Ian Bannon · 80
Inger Stevens · 107, 108, 109, 307
Inside Daisy Clover · 63, 219, 270
Invasion of the Earth · 155
Irene Papas · 108, 109
Irene Sharaff · 179, 181, 188
Irwin Allen · 219

J

Jack Bernstein · 178, 181
Jack Fear · 68
Jack Freeman · 28
Jack Gorton · 98
Jack Jones · 144
Jack Lemmon · 50, 51, 54, 56, 59
Jack Nicholson · 196
Jack Stone · 19, 102, 228
Jack Warden · 257, 260
Jack Young · 17
Jackie Gleason · 48
Jackie Kennedy · 47, 101
Jacqueline Bisset · 112, 170, 172
James Bridges · 114
James Colburn · 80
James Darren · 39
James Dean · 16, 20, 277
James Drury · 15, 17, 33
James Mason · 144, 146, 147, 149
Jan Brandow · 206
Jan Michael Vincent · 119
Jane Fonda · 85, 159, 160
Jane Ross · 232
Jane Seymour · 204
Janet Leigh · 38
Janie Gorton · 86
Jean Burt Reilly · 51

Jean Harlow · 18
Jeff Bridges · 138, 296
Jeffrey Jones · 294, 296
Jerry Gatlin · 36, 289
Jerry Lewis · 38, 134
Jerry O'Dell · 144
Jim Bridges · 114
Jim Brown · 112
Jimmy Smitts · 241
Jimmy Wong Howe · 70, 74, 75, 83
Joanna Pettit · 89
Joanne Whaley Kilmer · 302, 303
Joe Camp · 212
Joe Pantoliano · 241
Joe Pasternak · 14
Joe Sargent · 155
Joel Whist · 297
John Agar · 156
John Avildsen · 275
John Beck · 178, 179, 186, 187
John Derek · 33
John F. Kennedy · 47
John Forsythe · 36
John Frankenheimer · 28, 157, 163, 166
John Houseman · 14, 70
John Ritter · 294, 295, 296, 297, 299
John Schlesinger · 137, 161, 163
John Seale · 281
John Stephens · 142
John Wayne · 31, 35, 51
John Zuckerman · 256
Johnny Baron · 243
Johnny Depp · 314
Johnny Handsome · 263, 264
Johnny Jenson · 114
Johnny Truee · 19, 22
Jonathan Pryce · 313
Jonathan Winter · 297
Jonathon Gries · 242, 244
Judy Garland · 17, 107
Jupiter's Darling · 18

K

Kandace Loewen · 295
Karate Kid · 275
Karel Reisz · 192
Karen Black · 136
Karl Malden · 27, 89, 209
Katalin Elek · 275
Katherine Bard · 63
Katherine Helmond · 231
Katherine James · 303
Kathleen Quinlin · 302, 304
Kathy Blondell · 99, 142, 302
Kay Pownall · 189, 213, 219
Keenan Wynn · 50, 51
Keester Sweeney · 19
Keith Carradine · 121, 122
Kellie Martin · 255
Ken Hollywood · 14, 17
Kenneth of New York · 100

Kenny Chase · 136, 157
Kenny Norton · 144, 146, 148, 149, 204
King of Monaco · 132
Kiss of the Spider Woman · 226
Kris Kristofferson · 232, 233
Kristy McNichol · 216

L

Ladislav Blatnik · 64
Lana Turner · 11
Larry DeWaay · 289
Larry Tucker · 106
Lauren Bacall · 44, 46
Laurie
  Sugar's Daughter · 23, 25, 34, 74, 85, 113, 116, 117, 119, 121, 122, 129, 143, 148, 150, 154, 155, 167, 168, 170, 178, 180, 188, 190, 202, 214, 215, 219, 227, 230, 231, 232, 236, 238, 253, 254, 262, 277, 283, 285, 300, 306, 307
Lea Thompson · 228
Lee Harmon · 178, 184, 239, 241, 294
Lee Marvin · 18
Lee Stanfield · 19
Lena Olin · 268
Leo Guerrin · 121
Leo Letito · 101
Leon Uris · 82
Leonard Engleman · 281
Leonardo DiCapprio · 314
Leslie Ann Warren · 232, 234
Leslie Caron · 18
Linda Christian · 82
Linda Trainoff · 195
Linda Trichter-Metcalf · 254
Lisa Whelchel · 211, 212
Little Darlings · 214, 215, 304
Lizzie Borden · 148, 150, 151, 152
Lola Albright · 23
Lord Love a Duck · 68, 69
Lorraine Roberson · 25, 34
Lost in Space · 92
Louis Calhern · 19, 22
Louis Salon de Coiffure · 23
Love Song · 132
Love With a Proper Stranger · 41, 44, 64
Lyle Azador · 211
Lyn Quiyou · 285
Lyndel Kail · 99, 133

M

Madeleine Kahn · 296
Maharishi · 249, 250
Maharishi Mahesh Yoga · 39
Mame · 85

Mandingo · 143, 145, 146, 148, 150, 151, 154, 204, 228
Mandy Patinkin · 280, 282
Marathon Man · 161, 162, 163, 178
Mare Winningham · 264
Margaret Whitton · 302, 304
Marge Champion · 91
Marie France Pizier · 178, 179, 180, 181, 184, 185, 186, 187, 189, 190, 191
Marilyn Monroe · 18, 136
Marinello Beauty College · 21
Marjorie Main · 116
Mark Harmon · 257, 258, 261, 297
Marlee Matlin · 226
Marlon Brando · 18, 25, 32
Mart Crowley · 222
Marthe Keller · 157, 163
Martin Bell · 296
Martin Sheen · 114
Marty Feldman · 156
Marty Jurow · 56
Mary Badham · 70, 71
Mary Keats · 27, 195
Mary Stewart Masterson · 314
Mathew Mungle · 281, 296
Matt Dillon · 216
Matt Leonetti · 153, 254, 272, 311
Maude · 152
Maureen O'Hara · 35
Maureen Stapleton · 135
Max Factor · 63
Maya Angelou · 153
McLintock! · 35, 36, 289
Meg Ryan · 257, 258, 307
Mel Brooks · 153, 155, 195, 196
Mel Gibson · 297, 304
Melina Mercouri · 100, 184
Memory of Eva Ryker · 218, 222
Meteor · 206, 208, 209, 210, 258, 266
MGM · 4, 6, 9, 10, 11, 12, 13, 14, 18, 21, 23, 25, 27, 32, 33, 37, 41, 49, 80, 83, 86, 89, 102, 189, 193, 208, 209, 241
Michael Caine · 139, 142
Michael Chapman · 228
Michael Douglas · 113
Michael McDonald · 296, 301, 302, 305
Michael Moriarty · 192
Michael Todd · 18
Michele Hugo · 203
Michelle Lee · 152
Mickey Gilbert · 87
Mickey McCardle · 60
Mickey Rooney · 17
Mickey Rourke · 263, 264
Mike Glick · 275, 281, 282
Mike Mochella · 205
Mike Moder · 235
Mike Nichols · 66, 127, 128
Mikhail Baryshnikov · 178
Mildred Natwick · 85
Milt Krasner · 43
Miracle on 34th Street · 7, 11
Mission Impossible · 49

Mitzi Gaynor · 15
Models Inc. · 223
Moose · 135, 136
Morgan Freeman · 263
Mork and Mindy · 297
Mortal Combat Annihilation · 271
Mrs. Sundance · 131, 133, 308
Mutiny on the Bounty · 25, 32, 34
My Fair Lady · 47, 275
My Three Sons · 34

N

Namleela · 310
Nancy Sinatra · 39
Naomi Cavin · 99
Natalie Wood · 7, 9, 11, 41, 42, 43, 44, 45, 46, 48, 49, 50, 51, 52, 54, 56, 57, 58, 59, 60, 63, 64, 66, 67, 68, 69, 70, 71, 73, 74, 75, 76, 80, 82, 83, 94, 102, 105, 106, 107, 125, 128, 132, 133, 139, 140, 141, 142, 143, 154, 158, 161, 206, 208, 209, 210, 213, 214, 218, 219, 220, 221, 222, 223, 224, 242, 270, 277, 293, 303, 304, 307
Natasha
    Natalie Wood's Daughter · 125, 132, 154, 219, 223, 224
Nellie Manley · 7, 36, 37
Nick Nolte · 170, 172, 173, 174, 192, 193, 253
Nicole Kidman · 285, 288
Nikki Clapp · 183
No Secrets · 254
Norma Crane · 80, 223
Norman Jewison · 100, 101
Norman Steinberg · 156
Northern Exposure · 302, 304
Notre Dame Cathedral · 58

O

Oklahoma · 10, 14, 35, 286, 288, 290
Orson Welles · 155
Out of Africa · 6

P

Palladium · 22
Pam Dawber · 239, 294, 295
Pamela Tiffin · 39
Paramount · 7, 36, 38, 39, 43, 44, 47, 48, 49, 69, 70, 75, 85, 88, 89, 90, 91, 145, 148, 153, 157, 161, 166, 179, 260, 274, 308

Pat Blymyer
    Sugar's Grandson · 231, 238, 253, 254, 307
    Sugar's Husband · 94, 95, 96, 97, 98, 99, 100, 101, 102, 103, 104, 105, 106, 107, 108, 109, 110, 111, 112, 113, 114, 116, 117, 118, 119, 120, 121, 122, 123, 124, 125, 126, 127, 128, 129, 130, 131, 132, 133, 135, 138, 139, 141, 142, 143, 144, 145, 147, 148, 150, 151, 152, 153, 154, 155, 156, 157, 158, 161, 164, 165, 167, 168, 169, 170, 171, 172, 173, 174, 175, 176, 178, 180, 183, 186, 188, 189, 190, 191, 192, 193, 194, 196, 197, 198, 199, 200, 201, 203, 204, 206, 209, 210, 211, 212, 213, 214, 215, 216, 217, 218, 219, 225, 226, 227, 228, 230, 231, 232, 233, 234, 235, 236, 238, 239, 244, 245, 246, 247, 252, 253, 254, 257, 261, 262, 263, 265, 267, 268, 269, 271, 279, 280, 281, 282, 283, 285, 287, 289, 290, 295, 296, 298, 300, 301, 305, 306, 307, 310, 311, 314, 315
Pat McNalley · 49
Paul Baxley · 32
Paul Brennigan · 26
Paul Lohman · 209, 266
Paul Mazursky · 106
Paul Monte · 276
Paul Newman · 18
Peeper · 139, 143, 156, 241
Peggy Pemperton · 141
Penelope · 80, 84, 222
Pennies from Heaven · 228
Percy Kilbride · 116
Perry King · 144, 145, 146
Peter Falk · 50, 51
Peter Gunn · 23, 175
Peter Hurkos · 32
Peter Hyams · 139, 241, 242, 257, 258, 261, 294, 297
Peter Sorel · 161
Peter Tothpal · 264, 301
Peter Yates · 172, 225
Planet of the Apes · 98
Playhouse 90 · 6, 28
Please Standby · 154
Poltergeist · 227, 228, 230
Pretty Baby · 203
Punchline · 265

R

Raf Vallone · 182
Ralph Gerling · 298
Rancho Deluxe · 138
Randa Haines · 281
Rawhide · 26, 276
Ray Stark · 70, 73, 75
Raymond St. Jacques · 125

Red Heat · 257, 262
Reggie VelJohnson · 264
Revue · 33, 36
Rex Harrison · 47, 275
Ricardo Montalban · 89
Rich Man, Poor Man · 172
Richard Fleisher · 94, 144
Richard Gregson · 105, 125, 132
Richard Thorpe · 38
Richard Ward · 146
Rita Wilson · 266
River Phoenix · 255, 314
Robert Blake · 70
Robert Culp · 106
Robert Evans · 162
Robert Foxworth · 133, 150, 219, 308
Robert Mitchum · 11, 119
Robert Mulligan · 41
Robert Redford · 63, 70, 71, 85, 98, 139, 268, 269, 286
Robert Russell Bennet · 17
Robert Ryan · 131
Robert Shaw · 163, 165, 169, 172
Robert Wagner · 125, 132, 133, 161
Robert Walker, Jr. · 121, 122
Robert Watts · 182
Robin Clark · 196
Robin Knight · 281
Robin Williams · 297
Rock Hudson · 18, 21, 168
Rockateer · 282
Rocky V · 274, 276, 278, 280, 281
Rod Taylor · 33
Rod Wilson · 285
Roddy McDowell · 63, 68, 222
Rodger Spottiswoode · 265, 266
Roe vs. Wade · 267
Roger Moore · 15
Roger Vadim · 85
Rolf Miller · 133, 136
Ron Howard · 285, 286, 288
Ron Maxwell · 216
Ron Schwary · 268
Ronald Neame · 209
Ross Mahl · 144
Roy Scheider · 168
Rudy Ugland · 290
Running Scared · 239, 240, 261, 286
Rusty Tamblin · 17
Ruth Gordon · 63, 68, 69
Ruth Montgomery · 136

S

Sage Stallone · 275, 276
Sally Kellerman · 97
Sally Kirkland · 89, 119
Salt-N-Pepa · 299
Sam Waterston · 138
Sand Pebbles · 217
Scott Glen · 121, 122
Sean Connery · 209, 210, 257, 258

Seconds · 168
Seinfield · 299
Selznick Studios · 109
Seven Arts · 70, 74
Seven Brides for Seven Brothers · 17
Severn Darden · 80
Sex and the Single Girl · 44, 47
Sharon Tate · 157, 158
Sheb Wooley · 26
Sheila O'Connell · 253
Shel Schrager · 192
Shelly Winters · 36, 38
Sherry Wilson · 28, 39, 155
Shirley Dolle · 274, 280, 289, 308
Shirley MacLaine · 52, 178
Sid Caesar · 156
Sidney Sheldon · 187
Sigourney Weaver · 225
Silver Streak · 186
Sir Laurence Olivier · 161, 178, 223
Snow Village Lodge · *See* Snowvillage Inn
Snowville Inn · 200, 211, 212, 261
Soldier in the Rain · 48, 69, 267
Somebody Up There Likes Me · 18
Something of Value · 18, 21
Songwriter · 232, 233, 237, 258
Sorcerer · 155, 157, 164, 167, 168, 169, 176, 196, 269
Splendor in the Grass · 7
Stacy Keach · 145
Stan Smith · 19, 29
Star Trek · 299, 308, 310
Star Wars · 6, 196
Stay Tuned · 294, 299, 301, 303
Steve Abrums · 258
Steve McQueen · 7, 42, 43, 48, 217
Steve Rash · 234
Steven Bauer · 242, 244
Steven Railsback · 157
Steven Spielberg · 228
Susan Sarandon · 178, 179, 187, 203
Susan Schwary · 268
Susie Germaine · 50, 56, 302
Suzanne George · 144
Suzanne Plechette · 49, 113
Sydney Guilleroff · 18, 19, 44, 80, 101, 161, 188
Sydney Pollack · 70, 73, 92, 268, 269, 270
Sylvester Stallone · 275, 276, 277
Sylvio Narizzano · 89

7

Talia Shire · 275
Taming of the Shrew · 35
Tanya
  Sugar's Daughter · 24, 25, 34, 97, 113, 116, 118, 122, 139, 143, 145, 146, 147, 167, 176, 177, 188, 189, 190, 213, 214, 220, 238, 239, 254,

267, 268, 279, 300
Tap · 241
Tatum O'Neil · 216
Teahouse of the August Moon · 18
Tennessee Ernie Ford · 152
Tennessee Williams · 70
Terrance Stamp · 89, 90
Terry Lewis · 185, 187, 188
Terry Miles · 196
That's Entertainment · 145
The Abyss · 266
The Affair · 131, 132
The Birds · 32, 33, 34, 36
The Boston Strangler · 92, 94, 97, 144
The Cher Show · 152, 195
The Deep · 169, 170, 171, 172, 173
The Doctor · 280, 284, 296, 304, 306
The Double McGuffin · 211, 216
The Egyptian · 15
The Farmer's Daughter · 107
The Fugitive · 69
The Grasshopper · 111, 112, 172
The Great Race · 49, 50, 51, 52, 60, 219
The Harrod Experiment · 124
The Janitor Doesn't Dance · *See* Eyewitness
The Jumping Off Place · 278, 279
The Killer Inside Me · 145
The Mission · 6
The Monkees · 97
The Munsters · 36
The Naked City · 49
The Other Side of Midnight · 178, 179, 181, 190, 196, 241, 303
The Piano · 303
The President's Analyst · 80
The Presidio · 257, 260, 263, 281, 307
The Prodigal, a Biblical Story · 18
The Soul of Nigger Charlie · 126
The Sound of Music · 56
The Sting · 139
The Swan · 22
The Sweetheart Tree · 60
The Three Caballeros · 35
The Ugly Dachshund · 49
The Virginian · 15, 33
The Wages of Fear · 168
The Yellow Rolls Royce · 52
This Property is Condemned · 7, 70, 79, 158, 161, 268, 270
Three's Company · 299
Tina Raines · 121
Tippi Hendren · 33
To Kill a Mocking Bird · 70
Toby Simon · 254
Tom Cruise · 227, 228, 260, 285, 288, 289, 290
Tom Ellingwood · 216
Tom Gries · 157, 158, 242
Tom Hanks · 264, 265, 266
Tommy Miller · 155
Tommy Morrison · 275, 276
Tommy Tuttle · 205
Tony Curtis · 38, 44, 46, 50, 51, 54, 56, 57, 59, 92, 97

T., Tall Jones · 211
Transcendental Meditation · 135, 253, 273
Trial By Jury · 302
Trish Vandeveer · 127
Tuesday Weld · 48, 68, 192
Turner & Hooch · 264, 298
Turning Point · 178
Twilight Zone · 23
Tyrone Power · 82

U

Universal Studios · 33
Ursula Andress · 38

V

Val Kilmer · 302
Van Johnson · 38
Vanilla Ice · 299
Verne Caruso · 213
Vertigo · 195
Victor Hammer · 277
Vincent Buglosi · 159

Visions · 152, 153
Vivian Macateer · 23, 203, 289

W

Wally Westmore · 37, 39
Walter Hill · 245, 263, 300
Walter Pigeon · 15, 17
Warner Brothers · 24, 47, 49, 50, 51, 59, 68, 90, 157, 219
Warren Beatty · 7, 27, 28, 42, 165
Wayne Maunder · 87
Wayne's World · 299
Weird Science · 238
Wes Duty · 301
What's Eating Gilbert's Grape · 314
When Things Were Rotten · 153, 154, 155, 165
Whitey Snyder · 50, 56, 92
Who'll Stop the Rain · 172, 192, 195, 291, 296
Who's Afraid of Virginia Wolf · 66
William Freidkin · 155, 169, 175
William Hurt · 225, 280, 281, 302, 303, 305
Willie Nelson · 6, 232, 233, 234
Wives and Lovers · 36, 38
Won Ton Ton · 156

X

Xochi
    Sugar's Daughter · 32, 34, 35, 113, 116, 117, 118, 122, 123, 139, 143, 145, 147, 167, 176, 177, 178, 189, 190, 213, 214, 223, 224, 226, 232, 241, 244, 254, 257, 264, 297, 300

Y

You're Going to Hear From Me · 63
Yul Brynner · 183
Yvonne De Carlo · 36

Z

Ziggy · 174, 179, 192